Fundamental Themes in Clinical Supervision

Edited by

Dr John R. Cutcliffe
Professor Tony Butterworth
and Brigid Proctor

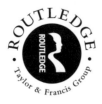

London and New York

NLaIB   GSTK   (CESJJK)

First published 2001
by Routledge
11 New Fetter Lane, London EC4P 4EE

Simultaneously published in the USA and Canada
by Routledge
29 West 25th Street, New York, NY 10001

Routledge is an imprint of the Taylor & Francis Group

© 2001 John R. Cutcliffe, Tony Butterworth and Brigid Proctor

Typeset in Sabon by The Midlands Book Typesetting Company,
Loughborough
Printed and bound in Great Britain by University Press, Cambridge

British Library Cataloguing in Publication Data
A catalogue record for this book is available from the British Library

Library of Congress Cataloging-in-Publication Data
Fundamental themes in clinical supervision / edited by John R. Cutcliffe,
Tony Butterworth, and Brigid Proctor; foreword by Sarah Mullally.
    p.   cm.
   Includes bibliographical references and index.
   ISBN 0-415-22886-7 – ISBN 0-415-22887-5 (pbk.)
   1. Nurses – Supervision of. I. Cutcliffe, John R., 1966- II.
Butterworth, Tony. III. Proctor, Brigid.

  RT86.45 .F86 2001
  362.1′73′0683–dc21

                          00-045951

ISBN 0-415-22887-5 (pbk)
     0-415-22886-7 (hbk)

ok into

6

17

08

9

Fundamental Themes in Clinical Supervision

Clinical supervision has been available to nurses for over a decade. This book, edited by leading practitioners in the field, looks at how clinical supervision has developed during this period and what the issues are for the future, including:

- education and training in clinical supervision;
- the introduction of clinical supervision into policy and practice;
- the practice of clinical supervision within the different nurse specialists;
- current research activity;
- international perspectives and experiences.

The book is firmly grounded in clinical practice and all the contributors write from real experience. They include clinicians, educationalists, researchers and policy makers from the UK, Finland, America and Australia.

Containing the latest research evidence, *Fundamental themes in clinical supervision* demonstrates the potential of this form of training to support staff and improve client care – an essential tool for nurses and other health professionals.

John Cutcliffe is a Senior Lecturer at the school of Health Sciences, University of Ulster. **Tony Butterworth** is a Pro-Vice Chancellor, University of Manchester. **Brigid Proctor** is a counselling supervisor and trainer and a supervision consultant.

E5JJK

Contents

Figures

Tables

Editors

Dr John R. Cutcliffe RMN, RGN, BSc(Hons) Nrsg, PhD
Senior Lecturer in Mental Health Nursing and Practice Development
Co-ordinator, University of Ulster and RCN Institute, Oxford

John's interest in clinical supervision began during his mental health nurse training in 1987, where he was fortunate enough to receive supervision throughout his training. Since then, whatever the speciality of his practice, he has received clinical supervision. He has provided supervision to various grades of nurses since 1990 and continues to do so, in addition to providing supervision to many students on various courses.

He also runs a clinical supervision training course, which is currently being attended by practice nurses, mental health nurses, health visitors, general nurses, occupational therapists, physiotherapists, speech therapists, and chiropodists, and offers several teaching sessions within the university.

His writing and research activity on supervision is extensive and he has ten publications, focusing on supervision, in professional and peer reviewed nursing journals. He has several ongoing evaluatory research studies into the benefit of receiving supervision, the latest focusing on practice nurses' experiences of clinical supervision. He is a member of the editorial boards for five nursing journals.

Professor Tony Butterworth CBE, FRCN, FRC (Psych), FAMS, PhD, MSc, RGN, RMN, RNT, FRSA
Pro-Vice-Chancellor of the University of Manchester

Tony Butterworth is a qualified mental and general nurse. He is the Queens Nursing Institute Professor of Community Nursing and a Pro-Vice Chancellor of the University of Manchester. He is also Director of a World Health Organisation Collaborating Centre for Primary Health Care Nursing Education and Research and presently the Secretary-General of the Global Network of the World Health Collaborating Centres for Nursing and Midwifery.

Tony has a practice and teaching background in community mental health nursing and he has published research into schizophrenia, community nursing and HIV disease and clinical supervision.

He has served as a panel member in the United Kingdom Research

Selectivity Exercise and has a wide experience in the dissemination and development of research.

His work in mental health nursing has been complemented by sustained research into clinical supervision of practitioners and the evaluation of clinical supervision and its effectiveness on practice and patients.

He was elected to be the first Chairman of the Council of Deans and Heads of United Kingdom Faculties for Nursing, Midwifery and Health Visiting in April 1997.

Tony was made a Commander of the British Empire (CBE) in the Queen's New Year's Honours list in 1996 for services to nursing and awarded a Fellowship of the Royal College of Nursing (FRCN) in the same year.

He is one of only two founding fellows of the United Kingdom Academy of Medical Sciences who are nurses and the only nurse to have been made an honorary fellow of the Royal College of Psychiatrists.

He is the author of three text books and numerous academic papers and is an Editorial Board member of four scientific journals.

Brigid Proctor BA(Oxon), DipSocSci(Edin), CertApplSocStud(LSE)
Fellow and Accredited Supervisor, BAC

In her fourth stage of retirement, Brigid has previously been Director of South West London Counselling Course Centre. She has since had a small private counselling practice, and a large individual and group supervision and supervision training practice. Brigid presently does occasional one-off consultancy and trainings. She is co-author with Francesca Inskipp of supervision learning materials, including those referenced in her chapter, and author of *Group Supervision: a guide to create practice* (Sage, London 2000).

Contributors

Jenny Bennett RGN, Lead Professional for Community Hospital Nursing.

Bob Gardener RMN, RGN, MA, CPN Cert, IHSM (postgrad cert), Lead Professional for Mental Health Nursing.

Fiona James RGN, HV, BN, MSc, Lead Professional Health Visiting and Community Health Care Service. These three authors are all based at North Derbyshire Community NHS Trust. As a team they have facilitated the implementation of clinical supervision in their disciplines. Part of their work has been to develop a five-year multi-disciplinary strategy for the implementation of CS across the organisation. They have designed, organised and facilitated CS awareness training for supervisors and supervisees for various disciplines. At present they all receive CS and are supervisors for individuals and groups in the Trust.

Paul Cassedy RMN, Cert Ed, RNT, Dip Humanistic Psychology, MA Counselling Practice, Mental Health Lecturer, The University of Nottingham. Paul is a teacher to the Clinical Supervision course in the School of Nursing. As a counsellor, he receives both individual and group supervision. He also provides supervision for health care staff who have a counselling role, and new supervisors within an adult nurse setting.

Mick Coleman RMN, RGN, FETC, DipN, CertEd, MSc, Programme Manager, Mental Health Studies, University of Wales, Swansea. Mick has been involved in clinical supervision for many years, as a supervisor and supervisee in mental health settings. His recent area of interest is the development of clinical supervision and allied interpersonal skills amongst health care workers.

James Dooher RMN, MA, FHE Cert, Dip HCR, Senior Lecturer, De Montfort University. Jim is actively involved in the practice of clinical supervision through his clinical work. He promotes its further development in both educational and practice settings. He is currently undertaking further research in this area.

Mike Epling RMN, FETC, Cert Ed (HE/FE) RNT, Dip Ed Counselling, M Ed, Mental Health Lecturer, University of Nottingham. Mike is a teacher to the clinical supervision course in the School of Nursing. He is involved in providing supervision to staff within health care settings and counselling settings, as well as providing supervision to groups of supervisors.

John Fowler MA, BA, DipN, Cert Ed, RGN, RMN, RNCT, RNT, Principal Lecturer, De Montfort University. John is the programme leader for the Post Registration BSc (Hons) Health Care practice programme. He has a particular interest in clinical supervision, has published several articles on the subject, and is currently completing a PhD which focuses on the implementation and evaluation of clinical supervision.

Annette Gilmore RGN, BSc, MSc, European Haemoglobulinopathy Registry Co-ordinator, Central Middlesex Hospital. Annette was commissioned in 1998 by the UKCC to review the UK evaluative literature relating to clinical supervision for nurses and health visitors.

Peter Goward RMN, RNT, MSc, Head of Department, Mental Health and Learning Disability, University of Sheffield. Peter is involved in student and peer clinical supervision within undergraduate and postgraduate health-focused programmes. He is also involved in providing supervision for senior trust managers and clinicians within mental health settings.

Denise Hadfield RGN, RMN, MSc, Dip (Coun), Teaching Fellow/Clinical Supervision Consultant, University of Manchester. Denise has provided clinical supervision to a variety of disciplines over the last 15 years. She was the site co-ordinator for the evaluation project and co-ordinator for the implementation of clinical supervision of Stockport Hospitals Trust. She also currently provides advice regarding implementation and training in clinical supervision for NHS trusts within the UK.

Kristiina Hykräs LicNSe, MNSc, RN, Researcher, Department of Nursing Science, University of Tampere. Kristina has recently completed various research projects which focused on several aspects of clinical supervision, and she has several publications arising from this work. She is currently undertaking a PhD which has clinical supervision as the focus.

Joe Kellett RMN, RGN, DN (Lond), STD, RNT, BEd (Hons), MSc (Ed Man), PgCert (PSI), Senior Lecturer, University of Sheffield. Joe currently provides group supervision to students on the PostGrad (Pre-Registration Diploma in Mental Health Nursing studies. He also provides ongoing clinical supervision to mental health nursing staff at local trusts.

Billy Kelly BA, MSc, M.Res, RGN, RMN, RNT, RCNT
Ann Long PhD, RGN, RMN, HV, DipN, RNT, RHVT, BSc(Hons)
Hugh McKenna RMN, RGN, BSc(Hons), DipN(Lond), DPhil, AdDipEd, RNT, FFN, RCSI, Head of School of Health Sciences, University of Ulster. Billy, Ann and Hugh have been interested in clinical supervision for many years, have published widely on the subject and have spoken about clinical supervision at several conferences. Hugh has a particular interest in the use of reflection within clinical supervision.

Mike Nolan BEd, MA, MSc, PhD, RGN, RMN, Professor of Gerontological Nursing, University of Sheffield. Mike has worked with older people and their carers for the last 18 years. In addition to interests in the support of frail older people and their carers, Mike is exploring factors promoting job satisfaction and morale, especially for staff in continuing care settings.

Marita Paunonen PhS, Med, RN, Dean and Professor, Department of Nursing Science, University of Tampere. Marita completed her PhD, which focused on clinical supervision, in 1989. Since then she has made a significant contribution to this substantive area by developing supervisor education for healthcare professionals in Finland. Her current work is concerned with developing the SUED supervision model.

Mick Rafferty RGN, RMN, MN, PGCE (FE), Cassel Hosp. Cert in Psychosocial Nursing, Programme Manager, Clinical Developments, School of Health Sciences, University of Wales, Swansea. Mick is involved in a range of practice developments and educational courses about clinical supervision. He is currently working on a PhD which charts the developing social meaning of clinical supervision practice and education in West Wales.

Linda R. Rounds PhD, RN, FNP, Associate Professor, School of Nursing, University of Texas, Galveston. Linda has been involved in the education of nurse practitioners for 15 years. Much of this has involved the clinical supervision of students. She also serves as the external examiner to the MSc in Clinical Supervision at the University of Manchester.

Sue Smit RMN, BSc(Hons), Senior Clinical Nurse, Independent Sector Care Home, West Yorkshire. Sue has undertaken previous research into the area of support and clinical supervision, specifically for mental health nurses working in the private sector.

Paul Smith RGN, RMN, Dip (NS), Dip (UTR), Psychiatric Charge Nurse, Barnsley Community and Priority NHS Trust. Paul has received and provided clinical supervision for the large majority of his nursing career. He is currently developing clinical supervision structures for his team.

Liz Williamson RGN, BSc(Hons) Senior Nurse, Surgery (previously Senior Nurse, Research and Development), Nottingham City Hospital NHS Trust, **Gale Harvey** RGN, BSc(Hons), Clinical Leader, Burns Unit (previously, Clinical Supervision Project Co-ordinator). Together, Gale and Liz were responsible for leading, planning and implementing clinical supervision for the Trust. This included a comprehensive in-house training programme, which was devised and delivered by them.

Julie Winstanley PhD, MSc BSc CStat, Senior Research Fellow/Statistician, University of Manchester. Julie was a member of the research team, with Butterworth *et al* (1997) which conducted the 23-site clinical supervision evaluation study. She is the co-author of several papers and has since published a single-authored text for *Nursing Times* books entitled *Evaluation of the Efficacy of Clinical Supervision*.

John Wren RMN, RGN, BA (Hons), Cert Ed, PGCE, Lecturer in Mental Health Nursing, University of Sheffield. Provides clinical supervision to students on the PostGrad Pre-Registration Diploma in Mental Health Nursing studies. He has worked as part of a professional development team to provide a supervision framework for a local Trust.

Tania Yegdich MN, RPN, Clinical Nurse Consultant (Education), Royal Brisbane Hospital. Tania has advocated the introduction of clinical supervision since the early 1990s. She has developed clinically based courses and seminars which incorporate clinical supervision as part of the learning process. She provides clinical supervision to nurses in a variety of areas within her region. She has participated in her own supervision over the last 17 years and has published several articles. Her PhD studies focus on the use of clinical supervision to develop nurses' capacity to 'know the patient'.

Acknowledgements

To all of our supervisors and supervisees we have engaged with over the years; we thank you.
And for Louise, thanks for the support.

Foreword

The importance of clinical supervision for nurses, midwives and health visitors has long been recognised. *'Making a difference. Strengthening the nursing, midwifery and health visiting contribution to health and health care'* (Department of Health, 1999) sets a clear direction for the future of professional development activities such as clinical supervision, integrating them into the clinical governance programmes of every NHS organisation. So I am delighted to see this new book on clinical supervision which provides such a wide and practical perspective on this important topic.

The authors' international perspectives are matched with the experience of implementing clinical supervision in NHS Trusts, and the vital underpinning themes of education and research provide a firm foundation for practice. I am delighted to see so many nurses who have themselves implemented and experienced clinical supervision contributing chapters to this book, alongside teachers and academics well known for their contribution to research and development in this field.

There have never been so many new challenges and opportunities available to nurses, midwives and health visitors, nor a greater emphasis on individual clinicians taking responsibility for their personal professional development. Clinical supervision is key to this process, and I share these authors' enthusiasm and commitment to it.

Sarah Mullally
Chief Nursing Officer
Department of Health
London 2000

1 Introduction

Fundamental themes in clinical supervision: national and international perspectives of education, policy, research and practice

John R. Cutcliffe, Tony Butterworth and Brigid Proctor

Why another clinical supervision book?

Examination of the relevant healthcare literature will show that there is a growing number of books that focus on clinical supervision. Indeed, each of the editors has contributed significantly to this growing body of literature, having written a number of academic and professional papers, in addition to books on clinical supervision. So the reader could be forgiven for asking; why another book?

Our experience (and many of the findings in the research studies detailed in this book) suggest that when people have had some experience of clinical supervision, they appreciate it, understand it, become aware of its application and worth, and want it. Consequently, rather than a book that is based on theoretical perspectives, this book is comprised of a collection of chapters from authors who are involved in practice relating to supervision. Each of them has experienced supervision and it has left a lasting impression. Those chapters on education have been written by authors who provide training (and receive supervision) themselves. Furthermore, those that discuss attempts to introduce/implement it have experience of these very endeavours: each of the research chapters is written by authors who have carried out the research. Given the variety in the nature of the chapters, some have a more academic sense or flavour than others.

In addition to this, an examination of the relevant empirical literature highlighted certain gaps in the knowledge of the substantive area of clinical supervision. The editors noted gaps in the particular areas of:

- literature that examines and brings together national and international perspectives of clinical supervision;
- literature that encapsulates the current research endeavours in clinical supervision, highlights current key research questions and summarises the current findings;

- literature that provides experiential evidence from the various specialities/ disciplines of nursing that illustrates the process, value and application of supervision in their clinical practice.

The structure of the book

The book was designed in order to address the question: given that clinical supervision has been available to nurses for over a decade, where are we now with regard to the education/training in supervision, the introduction/policy of supervision, and the practice/research of supervision from both a national and international perspective? Hence the book has the following structure:

Part 1 of the text is concerned with current education and training for clinical supervision. Consequently, chapter 2 focuses on the background of clinical supervision in Northern Ireland and provides an overview of the education developments in clinical supervision courses. Chapter 3 examines the 'how and the why' of Brigid Proctor's supervision alliance model, and looks at some of the open learning methods of training in clinical supervision. Chapter 4 concentrates on training practitioners to become competent supervisees rather than supervisors, and suggests a possible structure for such training. Chapter 5 features the development and delivery of a diploma level clinical supervision training course at the University of Nottingham. Chapter 6 concludes this section by describing the development and delivery of a diploma level clinical supervision module at the University of Swansea.

Part II of the text is concerned with the introduction or implementation of clinical supervision into practice. Therefore, chapter 7 outlines how a group of lead professionals facilitated the widespread implementation and development of clinical supervision within a NHS Community Trust. Chapter 8 reports on the experiences of a former clinical supervision co-ordinator and her attempts to implement clinical supervision within a medium sized NHS Trust. Chapter 9 provides a summary of the literature review of clinical supervision, commissioned by the UKCC, and reiterates the UKCC's current position on clinical supervision. Chapter 10 concludes this section by focusing on attempts to introduce clinical supervision within a large NHS acute Trust.

Part III of the text is concerned with the actual practice of clinical supervision within the different nurse specialisms or disciplines, and with the current research activity into clinical supervision within Britain. Consequently, Chapter 11 leads with a focus on the experiences of a Community Mental Health nurse. Chapter 12 looks at supervision for nurses in the private sector and working within gerontological nursing. Chapter 13 considers clinical supervision for nurse educationalists and sets this practice within the context of a postgraduate mental health nursing course. Chapter 14 explores the practice of cross discipline group supervision, in this instance examining the experiences of Registered General Nurses who were new to the role of clinical supervisor. Chapter 15 focuses on the methods that are being developed to evaluate clinical supervision and highlights the latest attempts to evaluate supervision using the Manchester University Clinical Supervision scale. Chapter 16 considers the argument and evidence for using case studies to provide the qualitative data needed to evaluate supervision. Three case studies are provided in addition to a critique of the use of case studies. Chapter 17 concludes this section by reporting on the findings from a qualitative study that used multi-disciplinary groups to evaluate the experience of receiving clinical supervision.

Part IV of the text is concerned with presenting the international perspective on, and experiences of, clinical supervision. Therefore, Chapter 18 focuses on the Australian perspectives of clinical supervision. Chapter 19 provides a Scandinavian perspective in that it highlights the development of clinical supervision training and practice in Finland. Chapter 20 concludes this section by providing the North American perspectives of supervision. The book concludes by considering: where do we go from here? Consequently, Chapter 21 draws attention to the links between clinical supervision and clinical governance, points out that new ways of working (e.g. NHS direct) demand new models of clinical supervision and considers the future of clinical supervision.

Wherever findings and thinking are considered of fundamental importance to the ideology and practice of clinical supervision, these key statements have been emphasised in bold type.

The editors' position on clinical supervision

We would suggest that there is no one single correct way to carry out supervision. Any activity is based on certain implicit or explicit assumptions. Rather than give yet another definition of clinical supervision, we want to spell out some of those assumptions, of what we think it is or is not in our considered opinion. The contributors to this book are all talking about the kind of supervision that fits within these parameters. In no particular order of priority, the editors posit that these parameters indicate clinical supervision is necessarily:

- supportive;
- safe, because of clear, negotiated agreements by all parties with regard to the extent and limits of confidentiality;
- centred on developing best practice for service users;
- brave, because practitioners are encouraged to talk about the realities of their practice;
- a chance to talk about difficult areas of work in an environment where the person attempts to understand;
- an opportunity to ventilate emotion without comeback;
- the opportunity to deal with material and issues that practitioners may have been carrying for many years (the chance to talk about issues which cannot easily be talked about elsewhere and which may have been previously unexplored);

- not to be confused with or amalgamated with managerial supervision;
- not to be confused with or amalgamated with personal therapy/counselling;
- regular;
- protected time;
- offered equally to all practitioners;
- involve a committed relationship (from both parties);
- separate and distinct from preceptorship or mentorship;
- a facilitative relationship;
- challenging;
- an invitation to be self-monitoring and self-accountable;
- at times hard work and at others enjoyable;
- involves learning to be reflective and becoming a reflective practitioner;
- an activity that continues throughout one's working life.

We would argue that, ultimately, clinical supervision has to be concerned with benefiting service users. The truth of the matter is that we are all potential clients or users of health care. Additionally, each of us has, in some way, paid for such care and it is entirely understandable that when we are to be recipients of health care, we would all want the best care possible for ourselves and our significant others. We posit that this 'best care possible' can only be delivered by the front line staff, who are competent enough and healthy enough. We believe that engaging in clinical supervision has the potential to encourage precisely that. It can help keep practitioners competent and healthy enough to provide this best care possible. Unless clinical supervision ultimately does have an influence on the care provided, it ceases to be what it was designed to be and becomes something of a rather narcissistic, self-absorbed activity for staff.

There is an increasing requirement for staff who are engaged in helping relationships within health care to be accountable for their actions. However, the mechanisms for encouraging, nurturing and monitoring this accountability are vague. At the same time there is an ongoing requirement for such individuals to re-register as competent practitioners. Inextricably linked with one's eligibility for re-registration is the need to demonstrate a commitment to continuous and ongoing professional development and, at the same time, a degree of individual accountability. In order to operate as a autonomous practitioner, one first needs to be accountable to oneself and then accountable to another. It is the belief of the editors (and the authors in this book) that clinical supervision provides one mechanism whereby these processes can be achieved.

What should you gain from this book?

Having identified that this book offers the reader something different from other books on clinical supervision, the reader ought to gain something different from reading it. So what should the reader be able to gain as a result of reading this book? Perhaps you should first ask yourself: what do I want to know about supervision?

Then, if you are interested in becoming a supervisor (or supervisee), you should turn to the 'Education' section and there you will discover what type of training/education is available, what options you can pursue and at what academic level.

If you are interested in implementing supervision in practice, you should examine the 'Introduction' section and can then see some options of the ways this can be brought about, and identify some of the hurdles to the introduction of supervision.

If you are interested in the practice of supervision, you should look to the 'Practice' section and become aware of what practice is occurring, how practitioners are experiencing supervision and how it might be of benefit to them.

If you are interested in research, then you should examine the 'Research' section and can then determine what are the next logical questions to be asked in supervision, where the current knowledge base is and where future research should be focused.

It is the editors' opinion that this book identifies the real benefits of receiving supervision and this evidence has been obtained from 'real' experiences. The evidence has been provided by practitioners who share the difficulties, constraints and dilemmas that many hard pressed and busy health care practitioners experience. The writing does not come from a collection of academics, who live in a world far from the realities of clinical practice. As a result, the editors view this book as a 'carrot' book, rather than another 'stick' book. It provides readers with some hope, something to encourage them, rather than adding to the already stifling load of 'shoulds and oughts' that practitioners bear. It demonstrates, as a result of the international chapters, how different countries interpret clinical supervision within their national context. It is interesting and illuminating to see different perspectives and such perspectives might make British practitioners think about supervision in a different way. It shows that in the substantive area of clinical supervision, Britain is influential, we have something to teach other countries and something we can learn from other countries. Finally, it sets clinical supervision in context within nursing, and reflects that whilst supervision may have been available for ten years, its potential to support staff, to help them become more individually accountable, and to improve client care has not yet been fully realised.

To borrow an expression that arises from contemporary parlance: we have come far, but there is still a long way to go.

Part I

2 Clinical supervision

Personal and professional development or the nursing novelty of the 1990s?

Billy Kelly, Ann Long and Hugh McKenna

Editorial

This chapter includes an exploration of the background to the development of clinical supervision in nursing, and reviews the body of scholarly work that has been written on clinical supervision. It then offers the Northern Ireland perspective on the practice and training of, and research into, supervision, paying particular attention to the degree module course in clinical supervision provided by the University of Ulster. Lastly, the chapter includes research findings which indicate how valuable practitioners in Northern Ireland find clinical supervision.

We believe that this chapter highlights a key issue, and that is the problems that can occur when clinical supervision is not maintained as a distinct and separate practice to managerial supervision. It is interesting to note that this is a theme (and research finding) which recurs throughout the book. Both practices are legitimate and valuable, however, the overlap of boundaries leads to confusion regarding power issues in supervision. Concerns regarding confidentiality may inappropriately emphasise the normative aspects of supervision, and focus on the needs of the organisation rather than the individual. Therefore, we would suggest that the practices of clinical and managerial supervision remain separate yet complementary to one another.

Introduction

Since the early 1990s clinical supervision has been debated by nurse academics and practitioners, and they have argued for its adoption throughout the United Kingdom (Bishop, 1998a; Crowe and Wilkes, 1998). Simms (1993) reported a growing awareness of, and commitment to, the value of supervision and the supervisory relationship. However, she also referred to the dearth of published research on the subject. While serious consideration has been given to the theoretical aspects and relevance to practice of clinical supervision, (Butterworth and Faugier, 1992; Faugier and Butterworth, 1994; Kohner, 1994), according to Faugier (1996), prior to 1996, little of any substance had been published on the topic in the nursing literature.

Hill (1989), in a review of the literature on supervision in the caring professions, indicated surprise that supervision had not gained greater ground in nursing. Since then, interest has been stimulated by the activities of other professions, where parallels in practice have been demonstrated (Bond and Holland, 1998). These professions include psychotherapy, social work and midwifery (where there is a form of statutory supervision). In addition, community workers are dependent increasingly on forms of supervision directly related to child protection. According to White (1990), mental health nursing adopted clinical supervision based on its close relationship with the therapies and counselling.

However, given the need to tailor supervision to the specific requirements of nursing, caution was urged when adopting approaches to supervision favoured by other disciplines. Faugier (1992) warns against embracing approaches where the therapeutic interventions involved in the supervisory interaction may be inappropriate. Moreover, midwifery and child protection models of supervision are highly managerial in character and may not be an appropriate template for nursing. This is especially so given the emphasis on personal and professional development as important components of clinical supervision.

This chapter is designed to explore the background to the development of clinical supervision in nursing. It begins with a critical examination of evidence presented in the literature with particular reference to the issue of definition and models of clinical supervision. Given the focal point of the book, it continues by emphasising the available research literature on clinical supervision, particularly within the context of mental health nursing. The chapter concludes with a synopsis of a research project that was recently carried out in Northern Ireland (Kelly *et al.*, 2000).

Background and context

The conceptualisation and subsequent implementation of clinical supervision have taken place alongside the reorganisation and revitalisation of nursing's education system. Having moved away from a task to a process-oriented approach to the delivery of nursing care, the nursing profession committed itself to an expanded and extended role for its members. The introduction of the Code of Professional Conduct (UKCC, 1984) emphasised the importance of professional accountability. Since then, government policy on the management of the health service has been influential in changing the focus of nursing practice and education, and the nurse's role has altered to include practices that were once the remit of junior doctors (UKCC, 1992).

Within a period of radical education reforms, prominence was given to concepts such as mentorship, preceptorship and clinical supervision (Butterworth and Faugier, 1992; DoH, 1993). These concepts aimed to stimulate and forge new relationships amongst registered nurses and learners, and among and between registered nurses. However, with their introduction came confusion regarding their definition and the differentiation of their applicability to practice (Fowler, 1996a).

The traditional view of nursing and the paternalistic relationship with the medical profession began to be eroded (in theory anyway). In its place came a more dynamic interpretation of the nurse's role with a focus upon independent practice, with concomitant autonomy and high standards of care. The paradigm shift brought with it increased responsibility (Butterworth and Faugier, 1992).

A number of health and social care failures also contributed to the debate on the need for clinical supervision. The Allitt affair concentrated attention on the issue of safe and accountable practice in nursing (Clothier Report, DoH, 1994). Following this, two distinct types of supervision became the subject of much debate, namely managerial supervision and facilitative clinical supervision (DoH, 1993).

Managerial supervision is concerned with controlling standards and a clear distinction must be made between this approach and a personal/professional development style of clinical supervision. This could not be more dramatically illustrated than in the Shipman case involving the multiple murders of patients by a GP. This tragedy must raise fundamental questions concerning the need for clinical supervision for all health care practitioners. **The incorporation of clinical supervision within management strategy forms the basis of one of the significant debates on its implementation in nursing.** Supervision related to competency and efficiency is essentially managerially orientated. This approach, with its emphasis on resources, market orientation and quality of care assessment, is at odds with a professional developmental approach. Detailed discussion of this bi-polar issue and the resulting tension it creates may be gauged from the growing literature on the issue (Burrow, 1995; Nicklin, 1997; Darley, 1995; Fowler, 1996a,b; Wolsey and Leach, 1997; Cutcliffe and Proctor, 1998; Bond and Holland, 1998; Jones, 1998a; Lowry, 1998).

Clearly a number of important and interrelated issues influenced the introduction of clinical supervision. The 'push' factors have been summarised by Bond and Holland (1998) as:

- broad organisational changes;
- policy directives;
- concerns about accountability;
- quality initiatives for improving standards of care;
- concepts of empowerment and partnership becoming integrated into nursing philosophy;
- educational drives towards reflective practice;
- concern about practitioner health and the prevention of burn-out;
- increased value placed on therapeutic intervention and concomitant requirements for self-awareness.

The UKCC set out its initial position on clinical supervision in 1995 and the following year published definitive guidance for the nursing and health visiting professions (UKCC, 1996). The report defines broadly the purpose of clinical supervision. It also verified its worthiness in the interests of maintaining and improving standards of care in an often uncertain and rapidly changing health and social care environment. Clinical supervision was marketed as the channel through which nurses could explore, sustain and develop their personal development and professional practice. Its overall aim was to improve standards of care and, in an ideal NHS, promote the health of the nation.

Definitions of clinical supervision

As far back as 1986, Platt-Koch defined the goals of clinical supervision as: expanding the therapist's knowledge base; assisting in developing clinical proficiency; and developing the practitioner's professional autonomy. Since then, theorists have expressed concern about prescribing tight definitions that induce rigidity of thinking and practice (Cutcliffe and Proctor, 1998). While Bond and Holland (1998) claim that there are as many written definitions of clinical supervision as there are books and papers on the subject, there is no widely accepted definition. Indeed, Butterworth and Faugier (1992) cautioned about the difficulty of defining clinical supervision when the field of knowledge is in such an early period of growth.

Butterworth and Faugier (1992) describe clinical supervision as an enabling process, providing opportunities for personal and professional growth. They emphasise that it involves not penalties but opportunities for development. Two years later, the same authors claimed that clinical supervision is an exchange between practising professionals about their practice that enables the development of professional skills (Faugier and Butterworth, 1994). More recently, clinical supervision has been defined as a designated interaction between two or more practitioners to ensure quality patient services within a safe/supportive environment, enabling a continuum of reflective and critical analysis of care (Bishop, 1998a).

Bond and Holland (1998) put forward an important analysis of clinical supervision. Examination of their work demonstrates that their contribution to the debate is all encompassing and valuable both for its clarity and its contribution to an inherent understanding of the skills and processes involved in clinical supervision. Scrutiny and synthesis of their writings reveal that they have defined clinical supervision as:

- regular protected time for facilitated, in-depth reflection on professional practice;
- an interaction that is facilitated by one or more experienced colleagues who have expertise in facilitation;
- facilitation of time and venue for the provision of frequent, ongoing sessions led by the supervisee's agenda;
- an enabling process that permits supervisees to achieve, sustain and develop creatively a high quality of practice through means of focused support and development;
- a reflective process that permits the supervisees to explore and examine

the part they play in the complexities of the events within the therapeutic relationship as well as the quality of their practices;

- a life-long learning experience that should continue throughout the practitioners' careers, whether they remain in clinical practice, or move into management, research or education;
- a unique characteristic of the nursing profession, as it focuses on clinical practice.

Bishop (1998a) supports the view that the terminology used in defining clinical supervision must focus on clinical practice and attempt to describe a mechanism to support the development of the 'best possible' standards of care. While that would seem to hold true for the range of definitions available, there must be a danger that such a degree of flexibility will serve to dilute the essence of clinical supervision and to confuse further the wider profession, other professions and the public. In particular, the degree to which some definitions may endorse a managerial context has been referred to as a growth block within the ongoing development of clinical supervision. Clearly there remains insufficient differentiation between managerial and clinical supervision (Burrow, 1995).

Models of clinical supervision

Given the diversity of nursing specialities there is general acceptance that models of supervision should recognise the particular needs of specific groups of nurses. This has stimulated interest in the theoretical basis of clinical supervision and differing approaches to models of supervision. Faugier (1992) developed a 'growth and support' model that emphasised the supervisor–supervisee relationship within the process. Butterworth and Faugier (1992) advanced this argument and devised a model that incorporated clinical supervision and mentorship in nursing practice.

Dealing specifically with community psychiatric nursing, Wilkin (1992) developed an 'interactive' model linking casework skills, personal feelings, managerial overview and an educative process. More recently, a facilitative, supportive model of clinical supervision designed by Chambers and Long (1995) supports the concept of developing a dynamic triangular relationship that promotes personal and professional development and higher standards of patient/client care. This model also emphasises the benefits of using helping communication skills and key caring concepts such as valuation, empathy, congruence and commitment.

Proctor (1986) described a model of clinical supervision that addresses its formative, normative and restorative functions. A decade later, Fowler (1996b) proposed a framework which merged Proctor's ideas with John Heron's six categories of intervention. This was designed to provide structure to both the purpose and the direction of supervisory interventions. Proctor's model has also been very influential within the wider nursing profession, having been selected as a template by scholars from a diversity of nursing specialities (Nicklin 1997; McGibbon, 1996; Waterworth *et al.*, 1997, Butterworth 1996; Bishop 1998b).

Bond and Holland (1998) have advanced Proctor's model, emphasising the means by which the normative function, (quality/standards/accountability), might be addressed through the medium of the restorative and formative functions. This is an important analysis, given the authors' contention that these principles provide practitioners in diverse settings with a flexible framework of clinical supervision that can benefit practitioners, their practice and ultimately clients/patients.

Synthesising the scholarship

There is no shortage of scholarly discussion on the topic of clinical supervision. In particular, clinical supervision in mental health nursing has attracted considerable interest. The Community Psychiatric Nursing Association (1989) asserted that supervision is a cornerstone of clinical practice. Following this, White (1990) endorsed the view that clinical supervision was well developed among nurses working in psychiatry. In a commentary on the position of clinical supervision in community psychiatric nursing, Wilkin (1992) argued that clinical supervision was the very lifeblood of CPN work.

A number of scholarly papers were written on clinical supervision in 1995. Oxley (1995) claimed that clinical supervision was particularly pertinent to community mental health nurses whose work often involves complex emotional interactions with clients, and who work largely on their own in the community. Oxley posed the key unanswered question concerning the diversity of opinions *à propos* of the professional/management accountability interface. Other scholars have theorised on issues relevant to the overall framework, structural and organisational arrangements within which clinical supervision might operate (Friedman and Marr, 1995). The relevance of leadership in the management of the process of clinical supervision has also been analysed (McCormack and Hopkins, 1995), as has the opportunity for personal development of both supervisors and supervisees (Chambers and Long, 1995). The relevance of supervision as a self-actualising process has been addressed by Farkas-Cameron (1995). While Morris (1995) argued in favour of the need for clinical supervision in mental health nursing, Burrow (1995) claimed that mental health nurses within a post-registration specialist model were no strangers to the notion of clinical supervision. An interesting study by Thomas and Reid (1995) argued fervently about the potential for multidisciplinary clinical supervision. However, Thomas (1995) asserted that while clinical supervision might be happening in some areas it was certainly not taking place in others. The degree to which clinical supervision has become an established reality was also questioned (Carson *et al.*, 1995). Despite these cerebral scrutinies, impassioned debates about the topic continued unabated in the nursing journals.

In 1997 there was a call for a model of clinical supervision for mental health nurses working in forensic situations (Rogers and Topping-Morris, 1997) and Mahood *et al.* (1998) provided some insight into the complexity of implementing clinical supervision in a mental health nursing development unit.

A number of writers have addressed the use of clinical supervision in areas of general and community nursing specialities. For example, these studies examined nurses' views on the effects of clinical supervision in a medical department (Begat *et al.*, 1997), in palliative care (Jones, 1997; 1998a), in practice nursing (Trotter and Nimmo, 1998) and in a community Macmillan nursing setting (Jones, 1998b).

A Northern Ireland perspective

Education and training

The School of Health Sciences at the University of Ulster has designed a degree level module on clinical supervision. The module introduces students to the history and foundation of clinical supervision and a range of theoretical models of clinical supervision are analysed. Ways in which effective supervision can promote and advance professional and personal development of nurses are highlighted. Anonymous examples from practice are provided to demonstrate how and why clinical supervision impacts positively on patient care. Supervisees are involved in examining elements of clinical practice. Furthermore, the enhancement of self-confidence and self-valuation of nurses who risk disclosing their practice in the safe environment of the supervisor-supervisee encounter are explored and debated. The practice element of the module consists of focusing on the use of appropriate communication skills and dimensions. Chambers and Long's (1995) work on congruence, empathy, valuation and commitment is used to process the communication principles and value sets that underpin the practice of clinical supervision.

Practice and protocols

In Northern Ireland implementation of clinical supervision is taking place on the same basis as in the rest of the UK. A deficit of published literature beyond local reports of projects and initiatives limits the amount of information on the practice of, and attitudes to, clinical supervision. However, high quality unpublished research has been carried out on the uptake and benefit of clinical supervision. For example, the Northern Health and Social Services Board (NHSSB, 1996) established a senior nurses' working group in an attempt to define clinical supervision (NHSSB, 1998). The working group defined clinical supervision as:

A practice focused, professional relationship to ensure high quality nursing practice and care to patients and clients and to provide support to staff in their professional role (p.2).

The NHSSB subsequently carried out a study using a structured interview as the research instrument. Key findings demonstrated that the ultimate aim of clinical supervision is to improve the welfare of the nurse and improve patient care. All three Trusts within the Board area demonstrated that they had embraced positively the concept of clinical supervision and were working towards adopting a model that best suits their local situation, needs and services. None of the Trusts is prescribing any specific model; rather each aims to discover and develop a framework that best suits its own unique situation. Findings also indicated that some level of training in clinical supervision was required, with one Trust suggesting a half-day training session for all staff and a further half-day for supervisors. All the Trusts were anxious that the implementation process should be undertaken correctly. The importance of, and difficulties relating to, monitoring clinical supervision and its effectiveness with regard to patient care were recognised.

The Down Lisburn Trust in the Eastern Health and Social Services Board (EHSSB) implemented a facilitative/supportive model of peer group clinical supervision in health visiting and district nursing. Staff members in these disciplines undertook education and training in clinical supervision and were given the opportunity to select a suitable model and to elect supervisors from within their own disciplines. Twelve months later a questionnaire survey was carried out to evaluate progress (Down Lisburn Trust, 1999). Key findings demonstrated that 93.2 per cent of the twenty-eight staff targeted found clinical supervision to be either very helpful or satisfactory in relation to the support and guidance that was provided for professional practice and 76.6 per cent of the sample group found clinical supervision to be either useful or very useful to them. Respondents were asked to comment on the usefulness of clinical supervision. Results demonstrated that clinical supervision:

- challenges practice;
- prevents isolation;
- provides opportunities to reflect, discuss, gain support, give support and affirm practice in a non-threatening environment;
- maintains confidence in their professional role;
- helps to improve and update practice 'on the ground';
- provides a safe environment to discuss practice and resolve problems;
- provides much valued and needed support from colleagues;
- permits individuals to admit that they do not know everything;
- is essential and nurturing.

The Northern Ireland Hospice and Marie Curie (Northern Ireland) have been very innovative and proactive in implementing clinical supervision. The overall aims of clinical supervision in both voluntary organisations can be synthesised as:

- safeguarding standards;
- developing expertise;

- advancing the delivery of high quality care;
- facilitating ongoing personal and professional development within a safe forum;
- nurturing a sense of empowerment in all nurses by having the opportunity, either as individuals or in groups, to reflect on aspects of their clinical practice and on what nursing/caring is;
- focusing on how nursing is distinct from other allied professions who work in the culture of health and social care.

In both organisations, clinical supervision is being cascaded to reach all members of nursing staff. Methods of evaluation are being identified and introduced to investigate the benefits to participants and improvement in nursing practice. The authors are aware that clinical supervision is being carried out in other areas in the province. Nonetheless, further research needs to be carried out to investigate the part it plays in promoting the health and wellbeing of nurses and, in pursuing excellence in the provision of nursing care.

Policies on clinical supervision within mental health nursing

Although clinical supervision has been implemented within mental health nursing in Northern Ireland, the distribution and uptake across the Health and Social Services Boards and Trusts is unclear. Board and Trust policy and procedures on clinical supervision within mental health nursing are not stan- dardised. This would be in keeping with the position adopted by UKCC (1996), which recognised the need for local flexibility. Written policies and procedures do however contain common features, which are fundamental to the process and recognise the relationship between the clinical supervision and standards of practice, development of the practitioner and professional accountability.

There is general acceptance that clinical supervision must be seen to operate in the best interests of patients and clients, that all clinical staff are involved in a clinical supervision relationship and that it should enable and empower prac- titioners.

The need for supervisory sessions to be on a regular basis is recognised and while a variety of methods are suggested within local policies, clinical super- vision on a one-to-one or group basis would appear to be the commonly adopted approaches. The process acknowledged the need for training of super- visors and, to a lesser extent, training for supervisees.

Procedures specify, sometimes in considerable detail, the nature of the clinical supervisory meeting and how the exchange should be managed and recorded. This involves a written contract between the supervisor and super- visee. The issues of confidentiality and the storage of records are addressed and in some cases this requires the supervisee to be wholly responsible for any written record.

While there is a strong emphasis on clinical supervision being practitioner led and practice focused, these principles do not always permeate the practice of clinical supervision. In some instances there is a clear recognition that clinical supervision is distinct from managerial control but there are also examples of policy and procedure that are implicitly management focused. As in other countries, the interface between managerial control and a personal/ professional development model of clinical supervision appears to have created problems in Northern Ireland. This can be evidenced through the different approaches used for dealing with situations that involve the nursing code of professional conduct or where management intervention is deemed to be required because the competence of the practitioner is questioned. The involvement of senior management is often the preferred approach to resolution as opposed to a counselling approach that places responsibility for action on the supervisee. The direct involvement of line managers acting as clinical supervisors for staff who are contractually responsible to them does little to ameliorate these problems.

Northern Ireland mental health nurses have embraced clinical supervision in the spirit of advancing standards of clinical practice and the personal/professional development of practitioners. In common with colleagues in the rest of the United Kingdom, they encounter difficulties in the implementation and practice of clinical supervision. There is, however, a recognition of the inherent value of clinical supervision in advancing mental health nursing and this will fuel the desire to ensure its availability to all mental health nurse practitioners and to overcome any identified deficits in the process.

Research on clinical supervision in Northern Ireland

Brooker and White's (1997) survey on Community Mental Health Nursing in Northern Ireland included a section on clinical supervision. The findings demonstrated that 79 per cent of those community mental health nurses (CPNs) (n=229) who were receiving clinical supervision reported positive outcomes as a result. These included additional clinical insight, increased confidence and stronger working relationships. However 13 per cent (n=15) of CPNs reported no positive outcome and of the total population of CPNs, one in five (n=33) did not receive clinical supervision (Brooker and White, 1997). Nonetheless, the identification of positive outcomes supports the findings of other UK studies (Bulmer, 1997; Butterworth, 1997, 1998; Bishop, 1998b).

Kelly *et al.* (2000) undertook a study on clinical supervision in Northern Ireland. The aim was to redress the information deficit by exploring and evaluating the current position in the province. A standardised postal questionnaire that incorporated Major's (1993) twenty-item Likert scale of attitudes towards clinical supervision was used. Prior to carrying out the study, the researchers contacted Major for permission to use her questionnaire. Data were collected from the total population of community mental health nurses (CMHNs) working within ten out of eleven HPSS Trusts in Northern Ireland. It was not possible to gain access to one of the Trusts. The sample comprised n=225 CMHNs.

To ensure content validity the questionnaire was scrutinised independently by a panel of research 'experts'. A pilot study using 18 post-registration nurses was carried out and as a result questions were modified slightly. From the pilot data, the internal consistency of the attitude component of the instrument was tested using coefficient alpha: a coefficient of 0.73 was obtained.

In the main study 153 valid questionnaires were returned, representing a response rate of 61.2 per cent. The reliability of the completed 20-item Likert scale was assessed by calculation of the coefficient alpha for the total scores in respect of the full sample. Alpha for the full sample = 0.9033 and the standardised item alpha = 0.9072. This confirmed the internal consistency of the attitude scale.

Data from the completed questionnaires were analysed using the Statistical Package for Social Scientists (SPSS: version 7.5). The key results are as follows: 66 per cent (n=101) had successfully completed a recognised, recordable community mental health nursing course, the remainder of the sample had not. Only 37.3 per cent (n=57) had received training in clinical supervision. Of those trained, 19.3 per cent (n=11) were trained in supervisory skills, while 21.1 per cent (n=12) were trained in both supervisor and supervisee skills. Eighty-one per cent of the respondents (n=124) were engaged in a clinical supervision relationship, 50.8 per cent (n=63) as supervisees only, 8.9 per cent (n=11) as supervisors only, and 40.3 per cent as both supervisors and supervisees.

It was interesting to note that management allocated the supervisors for 55.6 per cent of the supervisees and 47.6 per cent said that their line managers were their supervisors. Only 1.6 per cent indicated that their supervisor had been chosen by 'mutual agreement'. Most, 74.7 per cent (n=92), were receiving one-to-one supervision and that supervision was undertaken almost exclusively within normal working hours (98.4 per cent, n=122).

Analyses of attitudes towards clinical supervision reflect overall support for clinical supervision. This result concurs with the findings of Major (1993) who had reported favourable attitudes to clinical supervision by both managers and CPNs. However, readers should note that the present study is not a replication of Major's study; therefore it is not directly comparable.

Results of the present study indicate that there is strong agreement that all CMHNs should receive clinical supervision. This finding was reinforced further by a 100 per cent rejection of the proposition that 'experienced CMHNs do not require clinical supervision' and by endorsement of the statement that 'supervision is essential in CMH nurse education and training'. There was also agreement among respondents that supervision relieves isolation, leads to personal development and promotes greater confidence. There is firm agreement that supervisors and supervisees need appropriate training and that proactive and effective organisation and planning are important elements for successful implementation.

Findings showed majority agreement (80.4 per cent, n=153) from managers and supervisors that managers were not the best people to act as supervisors. Results also showed strong opposition to CMHNs being supervised by other disciplines.

A key finding was the high level of uncertainty expressed by those currently engaged in clinical supervision. There were uncertain responses to the following statements on clinical supervision: 'improves standards of care'; 'greater confidence results'; 'personal development'; and 'the development of new skills'. Levels of uncertainty were markedly greater among respondents who were not managers or supervisors. Those not engaged in clinical supervision recorded even higher levels of uncertainty in respect of key attitudes.

A number of important issues arose from this study and the authors believe that these have implications for research and training as well as the practice of clinical supervision. These include the training deficits in supervision skills and how this impacts on the practice of clinical supervision, (see also Cutcliffe, 1997), and the availability of skilled supervisors in the field. The effects of not being engaged in a clinical supervision relationship resulting in the loss of opportunity for personal/professional growth and development are raised. There was also the confusion as to the meaning and purpose of clinical supervision. This was particularly so with regard to supervision being viewed primarily as managerial rather than as developmental and growth enhancing. Significant uncertainty emerged among respondents as to the value of key concepts. These findings might have profound implications for nursing practice and standards of care.

Conclusion

According to the UKCC (1996) clinical supervision is designed to bring practitioners and skilled supervisors together to reflect on practice. Supervision also aims to identify solutions to problems, improve practice and increase understanding of professional issues. In particular, the UKCC emphasises that clinical supervision is not a managerial tool that encourages overt managerial responsibility or managerial supervision. In a prevailing general management environment there remain concerns that resource implications may inhibit the effectiveness of clinical supervision and managers may still need to be convinced of the long-term benefits that improvements in nursing practice and overall efficiency can produce.

Synthesis of the literature demonstrates that developments in nursing have embraced clinical supervision and that implementation, while not universal, is advancing in parts of the UK. However, significant problems and tensions remain unresolved. These relate primarily to issues concerning definition, models and systems of clinical supervision practice. There needs to be an assurance of appropriate education and training for both supervisors and of supervisees. The complexity of the bi-polar phenomenon of management/ quality control versus the personal/professional development interface is a challenging issue that may inhibit the full commitment of practitioners. Equally, any continuing uncertainty among practitioners regarding the value of clinical supervision can only result in misunderstandings regarding its purpose and in lack of commitment to the process. Even more serious, such uncertainty might have profound implications for current nursing practice, for the development of autonomous practitioners and ultimately for patient care. Because there are dangers that clinical supervision could be viewed as mere novelty it is imperative that the process is seen to contribute significantly to improvements in standards of care and to the wider provision of health care services.

Evaluation reports of clinical supervision are now emerging and first results are encouraging with a generally positive view being taken on the value of clinical supervision (Butterworth, 1997, 1998; Bulmer, 1997; Brooker and White, 1997; Bishop, 1998b; Kelly *et al.*, 2000). Research is needed to discover if improvements in nursing care and in nursing care outcomes can indeed be attributed to experiencing clinical supervision. However, it would be extremely difficult to control and isolate clinical supervision as a factor within the totality and complexities of nursing care. Hence, there are many factors within the phenomenon of clinical supervision that have not yet been seriously addressed. Very soon there will be no reasons left why these are not addressed, only excuses.

Acknowledgements

The authors would like to thank the following for the information shared on the topic of clinical supervision in NI:
Molly Kane, Assistant Director of Nursing Services, The NHSSB, NI.
Maura Devlin, Principal Nurse and Noreen Magorrian, Director of Primary Care Services, Down Lisburn Trust, EHSSB, NI.
Liz Atkinson, Director of Nursing Services and Liz Houston, Assistant Director of Nursing Services, The Northern Ireland Hospice.
Eileen Foley, Chaplain, Marie Curie Centre, NI.

References

Begat I B E Severinsson E I and Berggen I B (1997) Implementation of clinical supervision in a medical department: nurses' views of the effects. *Journal of Clinical Nursing*, 6, pp389–394.
Bishop V (1998a) (ed.) *Clinical Supervision in Practice, Some Questions, Answers and Guidelines*. London: Macmillan Press Ltd.
Bishop V (1998b) Clinical supervision: what is going on? Results of a questionnaire *NT Research*, 3, (2), pp141–149.
Bond M and Holland S (1998) The surface picture: the development and value of clinical supervision. In *Skills of Clinical Supervision for Nurses*, Ch2. Buckingham: Open University Press.
Brooker C and White E (1997) (Final Report) *The Fourth Quinquennial National Community Mental Health Nursing Census of Northern Ireland* p. 40. Sheffield: University of Sheffield and Keele University.

Bulmer C (1997) Supervision: how it works. *Nursing Times* 93, 48, pp53–54.

Burrow S (1995) Supervision: clinical development or management control. *British Journal of Nursing*, 4, 15, pp879–882.

Butterworth A and Faugier J (1992) (eds) *Clinical Supervision and Mentorship in Nursing*. London: Chapman and Hall.

Butterworth A (1996) Primary attempts at research-based evaluation of clinical supervision. *NT Research*, 1, 2, pp96–101.

Butterworth A (1997) Clinical supervision: ... or honey pot. *Nursing Times* 93, 44, pp27–29.

Butterworth A (1998) The potential of clinical supervision for nurses, midwives and health visitors. In Bishop V (ed.) *Clinical Supervision in Practice, Some Questions, Answers and Guidelines*. Ch 9. London: Macmillan Press Ltd.

Carson J Fagin L and Ritter S A (eds) (1995) *Stress and Coping in Mental Health Nursing*. London: Chapman and Hall.

Chambers M and Long A (1995) Supportive clinical supervision: A crucible for personal and professional change. *Journal of Psychiatric and Mental Health Nursing*, 2, pp311–316.

CPNA (1989) *Clinical Practice Issues for CPNs*. London: Community Psychiatric Nurses Association Publications.

Crowe F and Wilkes C (1998) Clinical supervision for specialist nurses. *Professional Nurse*, 13, 5, pp284–287.

Curtis P (1992) Supervision in clinical midwifery practice. In Butterworth A and Faugier J (eds) *Clinical Supervision and Mentorship in Nursing*. Ch 7. London: Chapman and Hall.

Cutcliffe J R (1997) Evaluating the success of clinical supervision. *British Journal of Nursing* 6, No. 13, p725.

Cutcliffe J R and Proctor B (1998) An alternative training approach to clinical supervision: 1. *British Journal of Nursing*, 7, 5, pp280–285.

Darley M (1995) Clinical supervision. *Nursing Management*, 2, (3), pp14–15.

Davies S, White E, Riley E and Twinn S (1996) How can nurse teachers be more effective in practice settings. *Nurse Education Today*, 16, (1), pp19–27.

Department of Health (1993) *A Vision for the Future*. London: National Health Service Management Executive.

Department of Health (1994) *Independent Inquiry Relating to Deaths and Injuries on the Children's Ward at Grantham and Kesteven General Hospital during the period February to April 1991* (Clothier Report) London: HMSO.

Down Lisburn Trust (1999) Audit of clinical supervision. Unpublished report. Lisburn: Down Lisburn Trust.

Farkas-Cameron M (1995) Clinical supervision in psychiatric nursing – a self-actualising process. *Journal of Psychosocial Nursing*, 33, 2, pp31–37.

Faugier J (1992) The supervisory relationship. In Butterworth T and Faugier J (eds) *Clinical Supervision and Mentorship in Nursing*. London: Chapman and Hall.

Faugier J (1996) Clinical supervision and mental health nursing. In Sandford T and Gournay K (eds) *Perspectives in Mental Health Nursing*. London: Baillière Tindall.

Faugier J and Butterworth A (1994) *Clinical Supervision. A Position Paper*. Manchester: Manchester University.

Fowler J (1996a) The organisation of clinical supervision within the nursing profession: a review of the literature. *Journal of Advanced Nursing* 23, pp471–478.

Fowler J (1996b) Clinical supervision: What do you do after saying hello? *British Journal of Nursing*, 5, (6), pp382–385.

Friedman S and Marr J (1995) A supervisory model of professional competence – a joint service/education initiative. *Nurse Education Today*, 15, (4), pp239–244.

Hill C E (1989) *Therapist Techniques and Client Outcomes*. Newbury Park, CA: Sage.

Jones A (1997) A 'bonding between strangers': a palliative model of clinical supervision. *Journal of Advanced Nursing*, 26, pp1028–1035.

Jones A (1998a) 'Out of sights' – an existential-phenomenological method of clinical supervision: the contribution to palliative care. *Journal of Advanced Nursing* 27, pp905–913.

Jones A (1998b) Clinical supervision with community Macmillan nurses: some theoretical suppositions and case work reports. *European Journal of Cancer Care* 7, pp63–69.

Kelly B Long A and McKenna H (2000) A survey of community mental health nurses' perceptions of clinical supervision in Northern Ireland. *Journal of Psychiatric and Mental Health Nursing* (In Press) .

Kohner N (1994) *Clinical Supervision in Practice*. London: King's Fund Centre.

Lowry M (1998) Clinical supervision for the development of nursing practice. *British Journal of Nursing*, 7, (9), pp553–558.

McCormick B and Hopkins E (1995) The development of clinical leadership through supported reflective practice. *Journal of Clinical Nursing*, 4, (3), pp161–168.

McGibbon G (1996) Clinical supervision for expanded practice in ENT. *Professional Nurse*, 12, 2, pp100–102.

Mahood N McFadden K Colgan L and Gadd D (1998) Clinical supervision: the Cartmel NDU experience. *Nursing Standard*, 12, (26), pp44–47.

Major S (1993) Attitudes towards supervision: a comparison of CPNs and managers. In *Community Psychiatric Nursing: A Research Perspective*, Vol. 2, Ch 12, London: Chapman and Hall.

Marrow C E Macauley D M and Crumbie A (1997) Promoting reflective practice through structured clinical supervision. *Journal of Nursing Management*, 5, (2), pp77–82.

Morris M (1995) The role of clinical supervision in mental health practice. *British Journal of Nursing*, 4, (15), pp886–888.

NHSSB (1996) Implementation of clinical supervision in the NHSSB area. Unpublished report. Belfast: Northern Health and Social Services Board.

NHSSB (1998) Update of clinical supervision in the NHSSB area. Unpublished report. Belfast: Northern Health and Social Services Board.

Nicklin P (1997) A practice-centred model of clinical supervision. *Nursing Times*, 93, (43), pp52–54.

Oxley P (1995) Clinical supervision in community psychiatric nursing. *Mental Health Nursing*, 15 (6) pp15–17.

Platt-Koch L M (1986) Clinical supervision for psychiatric nurses. *Journal of Psychosocial Nursing*, 26, (1), pp7–15.

Proctor B (1986) Supervision: a co-operative exercise in accountability. In M Marken and M Payne (eds) *Enabling and Ensuring*. Leicester: National Youth Bureau for Education in Youth and Community Work.

Ritter S Norman I J Rentoul L and Bodley D (1996) A model of clinical supervision for nurses undertaking short placements in mental health settings. *Journal of Clinical Nursing*, 5, (3), pp149–158.

Rogers P and Topping-Morris B (1997) Clinical supervision for forensic mental health nurses. *Nursing Management*, 4, (5), pp13–15.

Simms J (1993) Supervision. In Wright H and Giddey M (eds), *Mental Health Nursing: From First Principles to Professional Practice*. London: Chapman and Hall.

Thomas B (1995) Clinical supervision in mental health nursing. In Department of Health, *Clinical Supervision – Conference Proceedings*. London: Health Service Management Executive.

Thomas B and Reid J (1995) Multidisciplinary clinical supervision. *British Journal of Nursing*, 4, (15), pp883–885.

Trotter G and Ninmmo S (1998) Clinical supervision and practice nurses. *Nursing Times*, 94, (25), pp52–53.

UKCC (1984) *Code of Professional Conduct for the Nurse, Midwife and Health Visitor*. London: United Kingdom Central Council for Nursing, Midwifery and Health Visiting.

UKCC (1992) *The Scope of Professional Practice*. London: United Kingdom Central Council for Nursing, Midwifery and Health Visiting.

UKCC (1996) *Position Statement on Clinical Supervision for Nursing and Health Visiting*. London: United Kingdom Central Council for Nursing, Midwifery and Health Visiting.

Waterworth S Pillitteri L and Swift F (1997) Clinical supervision: Empowerment in practice. *Nursing Management*, 3, (9), pp14–16.

White E (1990*) Report of the Third Quinquennial National Community Psychiatric Nursing Survey*. Manchester: University of Manchester.

Wilkin P (1992) Clinical supervision in community psychiatric nursing. In Butterworth A and Faugier J (eds) *Clinical Supervision and Mentorship in Nursing*. Ch.14. London: Chapman and Hall.

Wolsey P and Leach L (1997) Clinical supervision: a hornet's nest? *Nursing Times*, 93, (44), pp24–26.

3 Training for the supervision alliance attitude, skills and intention

Brigid Proctor

Editorial

This chapter focuses on the 'supervision alliance model'. It outlines the background and antecedents to the development of the model, it describes the key components of the model and then explores the training process the author uses and makes reference to the open learning structure. Brigid's model is perhaps the most commonly used clinical supervision model within health care. The literature is replete with reference to it and explanations of it, and it should be noted that some of these do not provide an accurate representation. Consequently, there is merit in going back to the originator and having the record set straight. It is hoped that this chapter will add to the clarity and understanding of the function and purpose of the model. It is interesting to note that Brigid suggests the principal function of her model is the restorative function, that is, its supportive function. In a health care system that has witnessed the demise of traditional support systems, the importance and value of support within clinical supervision needs to be highlighted. Consequently, the editors would point out that effective supervision requires a supportive underpinning as the foundation upon which the formative and normative aspects of supervision are built.

Introduction to the supervision alliance model
Is it transferable?

When I discovered that 'the Proctor model' of supervision was quoted in the literature of clinical supervision in the Health Services, I was surprised, gratified (naturally) and then concerned. Most quoted is a framework for thinking about the sometimes conflicting tasks of supervision. That framework emerged from the practice of training and consultative supervision in counselling and related settings. The three aspects of the tasks and responsibilities of supervisor and practitioner (or supervisee) – *normative, formative,* and *restorative* – form the core of a more extended and comprehensive model. It has been developed with several colleagues over the years, but finds its fullest expression in the open learning materials developed and produced by Inskipp and Proctor (1993, 1995). We now call it the *supervision alliance model.*

I have felt concern that a model developed in a particular context might be confusing to the generality of healthcare workers. The assumptions and language of counselling and psychotherapy supervision could be inappropriate and off-putting. A mismatch of language and assumptions might hinder innovative thinking about clinical supervision for nurses as 'a welcome pause for reflection in a busy working life'. I am glad to take this opportunity to describe how and why our model has developed, and to focus on those aspects which I think could usefully transfer to other settings. In saying how we attempt to help practitioners and supervisors develop the ability to use and offer clinical supervision, I will also focus on those aspects of training which I think would be of interest to health service educators.

Antecedents

When I first started thinking seriously about supervision I was working as a trainer on a three-year, part-time counselling skills course for people who worked in a wide variety of 'helping' or 'caring' jobs. All participants offered some service to other people – clients, consumers, students, patients, whatever – who, for some of the time, were likely to be in the process of *choice or change* or to be experiencing *confusion or distress*. (Gilmore, 1973) Participants (or their managers) thought it would be helpful for them to develop a wider variety of communication and counselling skills than their previous training equipped them with.

Course members worked in education and youth work, social work, voluntary services, personnel and welfare departments. Many were health professionals – community psychiatric nurses; midwives; health visitors; specialist nurses; psychologists; occupational, speech, music and drama therapists; general practitioners, and the occasional consultant. Others worked professionally (without the title of 'professionals'), as care assistants in a variety of settings. Some participants were already 'counsellors' and many more were given that role in their organisations (at least as part of their job) as a result of doing the course.

This training context was influential when I and colleagues began to think about what we did in supervision. As we created a supervision learning forum which specifically offered an opportunity for them to become reflective practitioners, we wondered: what were our roles and responsibilities, and what were those of the course members? We were working with trainees, who were already practitioners, and whose contracted learning aims were to develop skills for being facilitative with people in 'choice, change, confusion, distress'. They were also, for the most part, working in situations where there was very little organisational or managerial understanding of this aspect of their work. They needed to be autonomous, self-monitoring, respectful, and intelligent about the nature and extent of their 'counselling skills' work.

The major effects, on our supervision model, of working in this context with this clientele were:

- Assuming that the *content* of the work being reflected on in supervision would be predominantly *interpersonal* work, with *organisational issues* coming a close second.
- That ideas and practices taken from psychotherapy and counselling were taken for granted as a starting point, the process of supervision bore resemblance to the process of counselling and supervisors looked to their own experiences of counselling and psychotherapy supervision for models.
- Practitioners were encouraged to develop considerable *self-awareness*, and awareness about *the processes of relating* with other people. Much of the course content also emphasised this.
- **Supervisors seldom had expertise in the core work and contexts of the practitioners they were working with only, usually, in the interpersonal aspects of the work (for instance, they only had lay knowledge of breast cancer, and hospitals, but had expertise in giving support and information to people in confusion or distress).**
- The *Codes of Ethics and Practice* of the British Association for Counselling – initially for Counsellors (1992) and Supervisors (1995), and adopted for some people using counselling skills – were the shared guidelines.
- Since they were unlikely to have any managerial supervision for the 'counselling skills' aspects of their work, their course supervision was *the only forum of accountability* to colleagues and 'clients'. When they finished training, any consultative supervision they continued to have served that purpose also. (If they were counsellors, ongoing supervision was a requisite; many non-counsellors chose to continue to have it as a personal and professional resource.) This normative function of being the person to whom colleagues were accountable was unfamiliar to people trained in 'acceptance' as counsellors. Emphasis was placed on taking that responsibility in an authoritative, rather than authoritarian, manner.
- Other support roles had not been thought of – so preceptor and mentor were roles which were subsumed under the auspices of supervision. Supervisors were initiators (though not 'hands on' initiators) into these particular kinds of professional practice and many also acted as informal mentors – supporting the professional progress of their supervisees, both pre- and post-qualifying.
- The work talked about in supervision was invariably not seen by the supervisor; a good deal of emphasis was placed on how to divine what was *not* being said or noticed by the supervisee in relation to her clients. This 'divining' was in line with the kinds of skills which supervisors had already developed as counsellors – 'noticing the unconscious processes'.

These influences shaped a model of consultative supervision which may be appropriate to some health workers and their clinical supervision, but which will be an inappropriate and uncomfortable fit for many. **I cannot stress enough that I believe health practitioners – and indeed each group of professionals – need to develop supervision training, models and skills which**

are immediately useful and practicable in their own context, within professionally agreed tasks and responsibilities.

A model geared to practice

I gladly come back to the theme of the absurdity of our education: its end
is not to make us good and wise but learned. And it has succeeded. It has
not taught us to seek virtue and to embrace wisdom: it has impressed upon
us their derivation and their etymology.

(Michel de Montaigne. *Essaies* From Alain de Botton *The Consolations of
Philosophy*. Hamish Hamilton 1999)

In the renaissance of classical learning, Montaigne wrote against the increasingly academic nature of education. He believed it should teach us *how to live*
– be useful in helping us to 'understand ourselves, ... confront death, quell
our wilder ambitions, appease our melancholy or our physical discomforts'.
Five hundred years later, I have the temerity to feel and think similarly. I
recognise that stake-holders in the clinical supervision enterprise need to have
access to theory and research in order to risk investing time, money and
personal resources. I also know the intimidation of the academic and professional world, where not to have *read* everything and be *doing* everything
leaves one open to discount. Professional practice which has been rooted in
practical and personal skill, and often intuitive understanding, is particularly
vulnerable to such intimidation in this time of continuous change.

Practitioners – of supervision and health care – need support and help
in 'seeking virtue and embracing wisdom' in a complex and multi-cultural
world. One way they can get this is by being offered regular space to
reflect on their moment-to-moment practice.

The picture in Figure 3.1 sketches the outline of the supervision alliance
model transposed into health care settings. The model is underpinned by
certain values and assumptions. The ones that come to mind immediately are
listed in Table 3.1 – there will be many others.

These assumptions are based on the writing and reflections of many who
have thought about and researched adult learning, reflective practice and facilitative learning environments. Most writing on clinical supervision in nursing
has a host of useful references. For me and my colleagues, they are assumptions which, having initially been borrowed, have been borne out in practice
over many years.

Contracts and agreements

The overall contract

The model illustrated by Figure 3.1 emphasises that clinical supervision always
involves more than two stakeholders. There is the paymaster – whoever that

may be – and the managers who have to manage the service within financial constraints; there is also the particular professional body to which the practitioner (and possibly the supervisor) belongs and owes professional allegiance; and the public who, in a public service, both finance the paymaster; and (to my mind, most important) are the consumers, without whom . . . .

All have a right to be respected in the process of clinical supervision. However, the central figures are, first, the recipient of the supervision – the practitioner. In the 'world out there' he or she is the channel through which the service is offered – the public face of the service and a person in his or her own right. Second, there is the supervisor who is responsible for creating a climate and a relationship in which the practitioner can reflect on his or her practice within clear boundaries of freedom and responsibility.

Those clear boundaries are first set by the contract that the employer makes with the supervisor and practitioner as to the purpose and manner of clinical supervision in a particular context. This will necessarily be bounded by guidelines or codes regarding wider professional ethics and practice.

The working agreement

Within the overall contract, we suggest that a working agreement for a particular supervision alliance is made between supervisor and practitioner. The working agreement is personal and particular. At one level, its clarification and negotiation is practical, identifying such key matters as responsibilities and roles, contextual factors, administrative arrangements, supervisor's methods of working in supervision, practitioner's developmental needs and learning goals, preferred learning styles, and supervisor and practitioner resources.

At another level, it is a shared process which gives each information about the other, verbally and intuitively. The process of clarification and negotiation begins to establish the degree of trust, safety or wariness there may be in this relationship and to shape a suitable working climate.

Some of the parameters of this agreement will be non-negotiable – set by the wider contract, circumstances of time and availability or by the particular supervisor who may choose to make them so because of his or her values and ideas of good practice (of supervision and of nursing). Others – especially issues of style and learning agenda – will be negotiable.

Some factors – time, place, overall purposes and supervisor and practitioner responsibilities – will need to be clarified before getting under way. Others may be better negotiated as the relationship becomes established. In any case the agreement written – and/or verbal – should be reviewed and appraised at stated intervals.

A working relationship

The contract and the working agreement are not seen as bureaucratic devices, but as a means of establishing sufficient safety – 'now we know where we

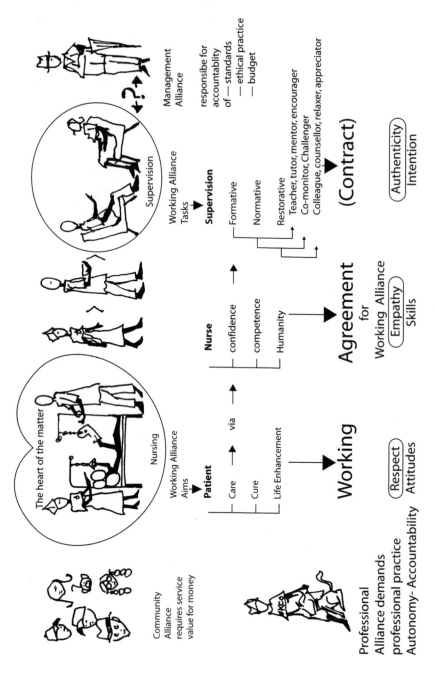

The heart of the matter

Community
Alliance
requires service
value for money

Nursing
Working Alliance
Aims

Supervision
Working Alliance
Tasks

Management
Alliance

responsibe for
accountablity
of — standards
    — ethical practice
    — budget

Patient
Care → via →
Cure
Life Enhancement

Nurse
confidence →
competence →
Humanity →

Supervision
Formative
Normative
Restorative

Teacher, tutor, mentor, encourager
Co-monitor, Challenger
Colleague, counsellor, relaxer, appreciator

Professional
Alliance demands
professional practice
Autonomy- Accountability

Working (Respect) Attitudes

Agreement for Working Alliance (Empathy) Skills

(Contract) (Authenticity) Intention

Figure 3.1 Supervision – alliance towards reflective practice

Table 3.1 Values and assumptions of the supervision alliance model

---

- It assumes that practitioners are usually keen to work well, and to be self-monitoring, if they are brought to professional maturity in a learning environment which sufficiently values, supports and challenges them.
- It values the ability to reflect on experience and practice as a major resource for life and learning.
- It presumes that reflective practice can be learned taught even but that learners require a trusting and safe environment if they are to share their experience and practice honestly with themselves or others.
- It views supervision as a co-operative enterprise between colleagues who may (or may not) be unevenly matched in work experience or age, but who share a common humanity and common professional interests, ethics and, often, ideals.

---

stand, what is in it for me and what my rights are' – and challenge – 'oh, that is what I am responsible for and what will be expected of me by this supervisor.' The overall contract signals continuing accountability to the other stake-holders in the supervision enterprise – this is both opportunity and responsibility to mature in practice and offer a better service. The working agreement signals the co-operative nature of the enterprise and the complementary roles of each party. The process, of discussing and establishing both general principles and the nitty-gritty of the alliance, is the vehicle through which an intentional and unique relationship is initiated between this particular practitioner and this particular supervisor, in this particular context.

Tasks and tension of clinical supervision

This brings us to the best known feature of the model – the complementary but sometimes contradictory tasks of clinical supervision – normative, formative and restorative. In healthcare contexts, the constituent tasks of supervision should probably be transposed.

- **Clinical supervision will be a major opportunity for professional and, hopefully, personal refreshment so the restorative task in these stressful times should, I think, be placed first. If supervision is not experienced as restorative, the other tasks will not be well done.**
- Second, the opportunity to become increasingly reflective on practice, and to learn from one's own experience and the experience of another (or 'others' in group supervision) qualifies clinical supervision as a uniquely formative process.
- Whereas in counselling contexts, supervision is the major forum of professional accountability, in most health settings there will be other places where account is rendered. Nevertheless, there will necessarily be self-monitoring elements to the work, for the practitioner. At best, clinical supervision is the safe enough setting where he or she can share and talk about practice and ethical dilemmas without jeopardising themselves.

Moreover, the supervisor cannot duck responsibility for challenging and sometimes confronting practice which causes her/him professional disquiet or concern. She/he has responsibility for making clear their own criteria of good practice, and comparing that with the practitioner's perspective. She/he may nevertheless have to decide to 'take things further' if they consider or suspect that the practitioner continues to practise unwisely or unethically. (The kind of incident which might occasion this and the procedure for addressing it would have been clearly spelled out and discussed when clarifying the overall supervision contract.) So, for both practitioner and supervisor, clinical supervision will always be a forum where normative issues are addressed and engaged with and the supervisor may, very occasionally, become a whistle blower (see Cutcliffe *et al.* 1998 a,b).

By whatever means clinical supervision is distinguished and detached from formal managerial assessment procedures, this element of monitoring will be present and both practitioner and supervisor will need to recognise the tension between the restorative and the normative tasks. In training, most supervisors and supervisees find it difficult to develop the ability to manage this tension skilfully and with integrity within a single role relationship.

Role flexibility

Each task carries attendant informal roles, which will be reciprocal for practitioner and supervisor. It can be helpful for both to recognise this, because it allows them to 'play' at relating flexibly and appropriately to the task they are engaged in at any one time.

Figure 3.1 suggests a number of complementary roles, and we have already seen that aspects of the 'preceptor–initiate' and the 'mentor–evolving practitioner' dialogue may also find a place in supervision (Morton-Cooper and Palmer, 2000).

However, the overall role responsibilities are those of supervisor and supervisee (or practitioner-in-supervision) as laid out, or negotiated, in the working agreement for the supervision. Any 'settling down' into a single set of roles (for instance, taking only restorative roles or falling regularly into a teacher–learner dyad) will not be fulfilling the working agreement.

Attitudes

So far we have looked at what clinical supervision is, and should (or could) be, according to the supervision alliance model. The next part of the model suggests what attitudes and skills are necessary, for both participants, in order to create effective working agreements and relationships, and in order to 'do' good supervision.

Attitudes are the outward expression of what we value and understand – we 'take an attitude' of approval to some things and disapproval to others. We engage in tasks with certain attitudes towards them, based on the values we consciously or unawarely espouse, and also on the understanding we have about them. If, as practitioner 'sent' to supervision, I understand clinical supervision to be an occasion for being judged and found wanting, and I value 'keeping face', I will have an attitude of wariness and possibly of appease- ment or protective aggression. If, as supervisor, I understand my role to require my being at all times more expert than the practitioner who is my supervisee, and I value performing perfectly, my attitude will demonstrate this.

A supervisor who uses this model needs to understand the underlying values of working in alliance (as opposed to hierarchically) and be prepared, at least, to test these values out in his attitude to the task. For instance, he needs to believe that 'agreements' are co-operative, and act on that. He has to assume that the practitioner he is 'supervising' has good will to her work, at least until he has clear evidence to the contrary. He has to understand that clarity of roles and responsibilities is a safeguard against oppressive supervisor (or supervisee) behaviour. He has to 'act in' to the understanding that this is a human relationship between two (or more) adult practitioners, rather than, say, a pedagogic relationship between master and pupil. A human relationship implies that either party may feel, and be, vulnerable within the relationship from time to time, so attitudes towards vulnerability need to be accepting and helpful, for the well-being of both participants and for the furtherance of the task of supervision.

The practitioner coming for supervision, in turn, has to develop certain attitudes to the task if she is to make good use of her opportunity for reflection and learning. These attitudes may be unfamiliar and 'counter- cultural'. (Hopefully this will not be the case, but especially for older practitioners, it may be more usual; and indeed more comfortable, to be reactive and compliant rather than proactive.) The title 'supervisor' has strong hierarchical connotations. A practitioner new to this kind of clinical supervi- sion may have well-founded distrust of being apparently trusted and valued as an equal contributor. The first initiation in clinical supervision will be crucial in allowing practitioners to get a feel for the potential of this unfamiliar process.

Interpersonal communication and reflective skill

These are examples of implications of the model's values for appropriate atti- tudes. But even if supervisor and supervisee identify with those values and have a similar understanding of the tasks they are engaged in, their lack of skill in communicating in this rather unusual interpersonal arena may still defeat their intentions. 'Attitudes' are what the 'receiver' sees, hears and imagines, not necessarily what the protagonist intends or imagines. So the final strand to this model is the spelling out of the micro skills which the supervisor and practitioner need to have at their disposal if they are to do 'this supervision alliance stuff' well.

Within the overall tasks, there are specific jobs which need to be done (see Table 3.2). These differ for both parties, and each needs the skills which go with his or her job. For the supervisor, there are the jobs and skills of:

- climate building, through setting up a physical environment which is welcoming, inviting information, listening without prior judgement or prejudice, checking what has been heard, sharing appropriate information, gauging the degree of appropriate formality/informality for this practitioner, licensing lightness and humour;
- clarifying and negotiating the contract and working agreement, through the key skills of clear *purpose stating* (the 'we/you must ...'s) and *preference stating* (the 'you/we may...'s) as well as listening, clarifying, and checking shared understanding;
- furthering the supervision process (This, of course, is the meat of supervision for which the clarifying and negotiating of alliance and relationship creates the culture. Skills for 'doing supervision' are what participants are expecting to be taught when they come on supervision trainings. A summary of suggested micro skills underpinning the actual supervision work is given in Table 3.2);
- *challenging* in an authoritative (as opposed to authoritarian) manner;
- *giving and receiving feedback* – both evaluative and non-evaluative;
- *acknowledging and respecting feelings* and experiences (both within the 'story' and within the supervision relationship): for instance, distress, vulnerability, confusion, anger, shame, guilt, remorse;
- *co-managing agreements* within boundaries – time management, reviews, administrative responsibilities.

For the supervisee, there are also jobs and accompanying skills to be developed. Consisting of reflective skills, as well as skill in communicating, these include:

- *preparing* for supervision, including log-keeping; identifying puzzling, interesting or upsetting experiences which could benefit from reflection; setting priorities;
- *presenting issues* in a way that makes them accessible and lively to herself and to her supervisor and is economical of time (especially in a group);
- *setting* and monitoring learning aims;
- increasingly *being open* to the supervisor's perspectives, and being able to discriminate what is useful;
- being *open to feedback*, and learning to identify if it is useful, and if necessary, to ask for no more at the moment;

- *giving feedback* to the supervisor, both spontaneously at the time when some response is helpful or confusing; and in a more considered way, at reviews.

The range and flexibility of communication asked for by this model is quite formidable when spelt out in this way. Either or both parties may already be skilled in this sort of relationship and process and everyone will have a range of transferable assets. However, in such a time-limited situation, which by its nature needs to 'feel' unhurried and to offer space for reflection, acquiring unselfconscious competence takes time, attention and openness to feedback.

Table 3.2 Supervision skills for helping practitioners reflect, learn and change

(This framework for the Helping Process is adapted from the work of Gerard Egan (1994). It is based on the systematic processes of *Exploration, Deeper Understanding, Action* – usually though not necessarily in that order. It is a useful compilation of helping skills derived from a wide range of sources which can be used flexibly. There are other frameworks e.g. the six-category intervention model (Heron, 1990) which can be used in its place within the wider model.)

Exploration

Listening empathically;
Reflecting back what has been heard about the experience being described, in its subjective and its objective aspects;
Clarifying, paraphrasing and summarising what has been heard.

Deeper Understanding

Enabling the story teller to focus in a way that makes for increased understanding
Exploring and developing the story through, for instance:
    open-ended questioning;
    awareness-raising enquiry – thinking, feeling, sensation, imagining etc.;
    deeper level empathy – testing hunches;
    making connections;
    offering alternative perspectives;
    informing;
    challenging;
    confronting.

Action

Enabling appropriate action through, for instance:
    envisaging outcomes;
    exploring options;
    cost benefit analysis;
    rehearsing;
    considering unintended consequences;
    goal setting;
    action planning.

Self-awareness

Skilful and flexible communication relies on increased self-awareness. This applies particularly for the supervisor, who has responsibility for more of the supervision jobs and necessarily takes the lead in setting the working culture. If this kind of working alliance is a new experience and the supervisor has not had the benefit of *receiving* clinical supervision of that nature, the requirement to become self-aware can be experienced as invasive. This has implications for training in the role.

The training process

Training is a slightly misleading word. The task is 'to assist practitioners to use the reflective opportunity of clinical supervision' or 'to assist the formation of clinical supervisors'. It is not 'about' supervision, but about learning 'how to do it well'. Participants usually come with the expectation that they will be *taught* 'how to do it'. But clinical supervision is a process which has no set procedures or regimen like many practical disciplines. It depends for its success on the attitudes, qualities and interpersonal skill of the participants.

The same could be said of those offering supervision 'training'. How educators assist participants to develop supervision skill, in usually very limited time, will depend on the particular skill, experience and qualities that they bring and the resources and experience that course participants bring.

The guidelines and methods offered here are those which I and my colleagues use and adapt for differing course formats and participants. Table 3.3 outlines those guidelines and methods.

The training experience

Excellent working alliances between more and less experienced workers are still relatively rare in work settings that are systematically hierarchical. This is not because workers and managers, or other senior colleagues, are inherently incapable of working co-operatively. Rather, the culture trains us in role behaviour which is appropriate to hierarchy, and can appear to punish us if we experiment with more co-operative relating. If clinical supervision is to be welcomed rather than mistrusted, these residual attitudes have to be counteracted.

I have come to believe that if people have not experienced good co-operative working relationships, they do not know what they are missing. They can be told *about* them but it is only when they experience them that the penny drops. '*Now* I understand what you are talking about.' Many people then become quite euphoric, realising that they have always known they were missing something in their lives, but not knowing what it was. Others, of course, are much more cynical, and some continue to prefer hierarchical relating.

Table 3.3 Guidelines and methods for facilitating the development of supervisors and practitioner/supervisees.

We seek to:

- Offer a *training experience* which consciously models co-operative working on tasks, values, attitudes and skills.

- Make *careful working agreements* for the course and respect them; and spend time on creating a culture of participation, safety and challenge.

- Offer opportunities for *progressive development* that is, first offer participants good clinical supervision (or audio/video taped examples) and encourage them to practise attitudes and skills for *using* supervision well; subsequently offer opportunities for developing the abilities for supervising.

- For those who necessarily start at 'supervisor' level, we still *begin* with the skills for using supervision.

- Encourage preparation through open learning materials. These include:
  simple and graphic *theoretical frameworks*;
  audio or video examples of the process and skills of supervision – acting as a 'trailer' for the subsequent course;
  simple and inviting *self-awareness* exercises which can help participants realise that they will be expected to develop self-awareness and self-management.

- Offer opportunities *to learn by experience and by doing*, so courses even one day courses – will include:
  experiential exercises, to help people know from 'inside' what the theory is 'talking about'; *attitude and skills*-modelling, and practice with feedback.

- Skills modelling allows for people to 'see for themselves' what is being talked about: practising with feedback in a safe-enough setting develops skill and self-awareness.

So I conclude that the experience of the supervision course will be the major learning medium. Carl Rogers posited '...to the extent I can create a relationship characterized on my part by a genuineness and transparency ... by a warm acceptance and prizing of the other person ... and by a sensitive ability to see his world and himself as he sees them, then (the student) will experience ... find ... become ... be more self-directing ... be more understanding ... be able to cope ...' (Rogers, 1952).

I convert these words to:

'To the extent that I can convey respect for each person in his or her social and cultural contexts; an intention for empathic understanding; a climate which is comfortable for the person – or group as a whole (warmth is not always the most appreciated attitude, initially); personal and professional authenticity; and I further add, clarity of intention: to that extent the participants will be enabled to become engaged allies in learning.'

Careful working agreements

As in supervision, safety is created by clear and open statements of set parameters and honest negotiation of what is negotiable. Overall course aims, content and any assessment methods and criteria, the extent of the staff members' responsibility and the members' responsibilities for their own learning, and the limits of staff confidentiality, can be stated ahead of time. This is the direct equivalent of the clinical supervision *contract*.

The *working agreement* is paralleled by inviting participants, in pairs or small groups, to share and then write up the kinds of ground rules they would like in order to make this a learning forum which would be both safe and risk-taking enough for them. Special needs are identified, and participants told that they will be invited to join in experiential exercises. They are also told that they can choose not to join in these and this will be honoured. They will be offered alternative 'observer' tasks, which again they have choice about taking. Time is given to set and share their own personal learning aims for the course. (They may have been asked to do this prior to the course. If time is very short, this helps but participants seem to value the chance to do it with a partner and group even if they have done it earlier.) These aims may be shared publicly on flip chart, or shared only with a partner or small group. Either way, time is allowed for re-visiting the aims along the way and at the end of the course.

As with the clinical supervision alliance, this process serves a practical purpose while it also allows the rapid building of a culture and relationship suitable for this group to work well.

Progressive development

Learning about *using* supervision is always the first step in becoming a supervisor within the supervision alliance model. We have found that informed and skilled supervisees can work well even if their supervisor is new to the role or feels less than expert. Moreover, supervisors who have experienced good supervision have already done much of the crucial learning they need in order to offer fruitful working alliances (Cutcliffe and Proctor, 1998a,b). They will be more sensitive to the vulnerability of the supervisee role and at the same time have learned to value sensitive challenge from the receiving end. They are both less intimidating and also less intimidatable.

Open learning materials

Table 3.4 shows the content of open learning materials created and produced for counsellors (Inskipp and Proctor, 1993, 1995). Part 1 is a resource for supervisees and Part 2 builds on that for supervisors. They consist of short blocks of information; self-management, self-awareness and practice exercises; and extensive audio taped illustrations and discussions. Before that, we created audiotape resources for people in helping professions in which the tapes were the main medium and were accompanied by a very brief workbook. Initially, I also made a videotape of two interviews – the first featuring the process of creating a working agreement in which supervisor and

Table 3.4 Outline of open learning materials

Part 1. Making the Most of Supervision
UNIT 1. SUPERVISION
Tasks and purposes, roles, supervisee responsibilities, contexts, arrangements
UNIT 2. YOU AS A DEVELOPING COUNSELLOR
Stage of development, theories and assumptions, as adult learner, interactive style, staying sane and competent
UNIT 3. THE WORKING ALLIANCE
Choosing a supervisor, creating a working agreement
UNIT 4. MAKING THE MOST OF THE SESSION
Self-monitoring reflections, preparing and presenting, session process and content
UNIT 5. REVIEWING
Review and evaluation, changing supervisors, where now?

Part 2. Becoming a Supervisor
UNIT 1. PREPARING FOR DEVELOPMENT: EVALUATING AS A SUPERVISOR
Where are you now as a supervisor
Who are you as a supervisor
Ways of getting started

UNIT 2. MEETING THE SUPERVISEE
The wider context
The particular context
The working alliance
The working agreement

UNIT 3. THE SUPERVISION SESSION
The management of the session
Supervising a piece of work
Guardianship of the working agreement and alliance

UNIT 4. GROUP SUPERVISION
Models of group supervision
Tasks and skills
Managing a supervision group
Case studies

UNIT 5. MONITORING, ASSESSING AND REVIEWING
Professional accountability
Evaluation and assessment
Reviewing
Self-evaluation as a supervisor

UNIT 6. 'THE BUBBLES'
Developmental stages
Working in contexts: organisations, training, volunteers
Working cross culturally and with differences
Unconscious processes and parallel process
Creativity and supervision
Use and abuse of power
Ethical and legal issues
Models of group processes
Making and keeping records
Audio-visual aids

Box 3.1: Experiential portrayal of the supervision alliance model

Having made name cards for all the characters and words in the picture (see Figure 3.1) we invite participants in turn to take a card, starting with 'the patient' (or client), and to take up a position in the centre of the room. Moving through supervisor, professional manager, Trust manager, GNC, to positions representing 'the working alliance', 'the contract', normative, formative and restorative tasks – and so on (depending on available numbers, of course) until all who choose to join in have a position. When all are in their chosen places each speaks for that role and reflects on what he or she realises when standing in that position. The exercise sounds complicated, but in practice is simple to set up.

It is invariably surprising, enlightening and humbling to hear the various insights.

practitioner explore the differences between managerial and clinical (or consultative) supervision and the second a supervision session based on that agreement. This was accompanied by a written commentary and suggested workshop formats.

There is already good material, for instance, on log keeping, which is necessary as a preparation for supervision (Morton-Cooper and Palmer, 2000) and there will be other relevant material which would be transferable.

Experiential and creative exercises

Creative exercises are those that invite participants to engage more of their senses than 'just words'. (For further information see the Group Supervision references quoted earlier.) The object is to help people have access to what they know, but do not usually 'count'. So, for instance, we often ask participants to create the supervision alliance model (as depicted in Box 3.1) as a kind of sociogram. The method is described in Box 3.2.

Box 3.3 gives a cartoon illustration of certain 'ways of being' that a supervisor needs to adopt for the different tasks and jobs she has to do within supervision. The verbal information explains the cartoons. (We now use the words 'active leadership, assertion and following' because the words 'proactive aggression, assertion and compliance' which we originally 'borrowed' from Gilmore and Fraleigh (1980) proved confusing.)

In one exercise, we ask pairs to stand up and in turn practise miming each of those ways of being in relation to their partner. In very few minutes, participants learn what they find easy and what difficult or impossible – taking a clear lead, standing their ground and holding the line, or trusting a supervisee's initiative. (Such exercises require as much time to de-role and reflect on as they do to perform.)

Box 3.2: Experiential and creative activities

Exploring resources

Mull over your network of colleagues, friends, family, supervisor, other professionals, etc., and identify and write down who or what could meet the needs listed.

1 Sharing your work in confidence.
2 Getting feedback/guidance.
3 Developing professional skills, ideas, information.
4 Letting off steam if you are angry, discouraged, fed-up.
5 Acknowledging feelings of distress, pleasure, failure, etc.
6 Feeling valued by those you count as colleagues.
7 Widening your horizons.
8 Increasing your physical, emotional or spiritual wellbeing.

Which needs do you consider well enough met at the moment?
Which of them are, or might appropriately be, met in supervision?
Which need some topping up?
How might you do this?
Which are not at all well met?
How might you meet them within your available resources?
Have you other professional needs?

(These questions can also be used in a kind of musical questions exercise to break the ice near the start of a course. Participants mill around and when the music stops, speak about one of the questions with their nearest neighbour for half a minute. Then the music starts again and at the next stop, the next question is discussed. It invariably produces quite a buzz.)

Adapted from Inskipp and Proctor (1995)

Attitude and skills practice with feedback

That exercise is an example of practising attitudes. Since one of the most difficult learnings for beginning supervisors seems to be managing formative, restorative and normative tasks within the same alliance and relationship, recognising what it takes, behaviourally and emotionally, to challenge authoritatively while remaining respectful and empathic is a first step. Developing verbal range and accuracy for communicating differing intentions follows from that. Instant feedback, about the impact on the receiver of the way chosen, or better still, on oneself when hearing or seeing video or audio recordings – is invaluable.

Participants who are learning to be supervisors need to have seen and heard a variety of supervisory interventions which illustrate specific micro-skills – either on the course or in pre-course materials. When they recognise what is

Box 3.3: Ways of being
Active Leadership, Assertion, Following

Active leadership   **Assertion**   **Following**

These cartoons illustrate three different 'ways of being' ('proactive behaviours' in a different jargon) which supervisors need to be able to call on. At points in the relationship, there will be choices – 'which is my best way of being to fulfil our present objectives?'

In **active leadership** there is a conscious and intentional will to lead, influence, take charge – in teaching, to alter the furniture in another's mind. This will be essential in initiating the working agreement and at times during the doing of the supervision work.

In **assertion** the intention is to hold firmly to rights and responsibilities – one's own and others'. The assertive supervisor will hold to agreements and boundaries despite subtle or obvious pressure from practitioner/supervisee (or, indeed, manager), but will leave initiative in the hands of the supervisee, like a dam to her stream.

Following entails trusting where the supervisee/practitioner chooses to go – trusting being possible because of the knowledge that it is possible to switch to assertion or, if necessary, leadership if agreed objectives are being lost sight of.

Adapted from Inskipp and Proctor (1995)

expected, they can go on to find ways of using those interventions in their own style and manner.

Feedback skills are some of the first that need modelling and playing with. Giving and receiving feedback and ground rules for making feedback useful – are essential for both supervisee and supervisor in the working alliance and they are also a requisite for fruitful skills learning on the course.

Doing supervision

To enable participants to develop their version of a helping process in supervision, we set up structured exercises for practising particular responses (as on most counselling skills courses). Since 'supervising' puts pressures on the supervisor to find solutions, we focus on reminding people about the skills of reflecting, paraphrasing and summarising what is being talked about, the exploration phase, before moving into focusing and action. It is this that encourages the practitioner to 'hear' what she is saying and begin to ponder and reflect.

Focusing

We have developed ways of thinking about and practising a variety of focus points to aid deeper understanding in the supervision process. These are based on the process model of Hawkins and Shohet (1989). However, I believe that a framework for focusing in settings in which practitioners are not solely, or predominantly, concerned with interpersonal issues needs to be developed. For instance, at any particular time, would it be helpful to focus on the practical aspects of a situation, on issues of responsibility, on interpersonal dilemmas, on the practitioner's feelings or thinking at the time, or on the 'buttons' which the issue had pressed for her? Or some other aspect of the situation? Without an awareness of the range of possible foci, supervisors tend to become routine in the areas they focus on or the factors or perspectives they ignore.

Having noticed the range of possible foci, it is also important to raise awareness about *how* focus is determined. Experienced counsellors, when developing as supervisors, tend to feel it is their responsibility to identify and pick a focus for the supervisee. However, the alliance model entails reminding them that this need not – often should not – be the case. Needs will differ with the developmental stage of the practitioner, but increasingly supervisees should be able to respond to an offer of choice of focus points, and often themselves determine where the appropriate focus lies. If, in training to use supervision, a framework of possible foci is given to them (or they are encouraged to create their own), they will quickly become more self-directing. (Of course, since this is an alliance, the supervisor does not give away his right and responsibility to challenge or offer a differing perspective, within their working agreement.)

Action

Skills for encouraging *action planning* can also be taught specifically before being incorporated in supervision practice.

Practising 'doing supervision'

To enable participants to juggle with the responsibilities of setting up working agreements, 'doing supervision', monitoring learning aims and reviewing, we encourage practice 'for real' with a partner or in threes (which allows for an observer/commentator). Where time is limited, live peer practice between course sessions can be taped and used for identifying particular skills or tracking the course of a specific piece of supervision work. The tape can also include feedback and comments from the supervisee and observer, if there is one.

The learning cycle

Box 3.4 is a reminder that all practical learning results in change.

Box 3.4

A Learning Cycle

With each new skill the cycle moves from

unconscious incompetence to

unconscious competence

self-conscious incompetence to ⟶ self-conscious competence to

Each new enterprise we approach requires us to develop some new skills and to weld them into skill combinations which amount to new abilities. In addition, we may need to weld old skills into new combinations and even make some old favourites redundant. (For instance, while learning to ride a bike, we have to become used to not planting our feet on the ground.)

The learning cycle suggests that before approaching a new enterprise we are in a comfortable state of *unself-conscious incompetence*. However, having seen others 'do it' – riding a bike or counselling others – we move into *self-conscious incompetence*. Choice point – to go on, and almost certainly make a fool of our- seslves to some degree, to choose gracefully not to proceed or to pretend (or rationalise) that it's not worth doing.

Having decided to proceed, we have to learn new skills, and to experience feeling *self-consciously incompetent*. These feelings are enhanced or softened by the learning culture set up by our trainer or supervisor.

With luck and good management – starting riding on the grass, allowing someone to hold the saddle – we come through with only minor traumas and eventually reach the point of *conscious competence* – 'Look – no hands!' And with practice we can stop thinking about it and weave in and out of the traffic – *unconscious competence*.

Supervision is an almost infinite set of minor learning cycles. It is easy to feel as foolish at the start of each new cycle of learning and to discount our now uncon- scious abilities and wisdom. The trouble is that because interpersonal skill is so close to our identity and sense of self, we can feel very foolish if we get it wrong. So, never discount your unconscious competencies and remember, there is usually some pain on the road to gain, and that gain can be extraordinarily satisfying.

Adapted from Inskipp and Proctor (1993)

Changes that are to do with the way we are with other people can be uncomfortably close to the bone if they call in to question our sense of self. For experienced practitioners, especially, changing may mean acknowledging shortcomings of which they were previously unconscious. Self-conscious incompetence is very painful. That is why it is so important to allow for free choice on a course and why time is well spent in helping people identify what is 'in it for them' in learning to become a competent supervisee or supervisor. This means acknowledging and accepting reluctance, incomprehension and resentment.

However, like supervisors, educators and trainers are also in an advocacy relationship for the 'off scene' stake-holders – employers, professional colleagues and, most particularly, patients, clients, or whatever. While accepting and understanding reluctance, they also have a responsibility to speak for the obligation to offer our best service. Becoming competent at offering and using opportunities to reflect on practice can be both personally and professionally rewarding.

In summary

This supervision alliance model spells out aspirations and tensions which will be inherent in non-hierarchical (or co-operative) supervision, wherever it is practised. The training programme outlined is extensive. It can be offered in progressive modules which need to be adapted for specific contexts. Experience suggests that the learning opportunity offered is of use in many settings other than clinical supervision.

For some trainers, and some participants, aspects of it might be quite alien and unhelpful. However, any training which results in the good use and provision of the kind of clinical supervision advocated in this book will necessarily have to address, in some way, appropriate attitudes and skills, and offer frameworks which make clear the intentions behind the complex task of clinical supervision.

References

British Association of Counsellors (1992) *Codes of Ethics and Practice for Counsellors* London: British Association of Counsellors.

British Association of Counsellors (1995) *Codes of Ethics and Practice for Supervisors* London: British Association of Counsellors.

Cutcliffe J R and Proctor B (1998a) An alternative approach to clinical supervision: Part One. *British Journal of Nursing* 7(5), pp280–285.

Cutcliffe J R and Proctor B (1998b) An alternative approach to clinical supervision: Part Two. *British Journal of Nursing* 7(6), pp344–350.

Cutcliffe J R, Epling M, Cassedy P, McGregor J, Plant N and Butterworth T (1998a) Ethical dilemmas in clinical supervision 1: need for guidelines. *British Journal of Nursing*. 7, 920–923.

Cutcliffe J R, Epling M, Cassedy P, McGregor J, Plant N and Butterworth T (1998b) Ethical dilemmas in clinical supervision 2: need for guidelines. *British Journal of Nursing*. 7, 16, 978–982.

Egan G (1994) *The Skilled Helper* (4th edition). Pacific Grove, California: Brookes/ Cole.

Gilmore S (1973) *The Counsellor-in-Training*. Englewood Cliffs, New Jersey: Prentice Hall.

Gilmore S and Fraleigh P (1980) *Communication at Work.* Oregon: Friendly Press.

Hawkins P and Shohet R (1989) *Supervision in the Helping Professions.* Buckingham: Open University Press.

Heron, J (1990) Helping the Client. London: Sage.

Inskipp F and Proctor B (1987) *Skills for Supervising and Being Supervised.* Audio tapes with workbook. Alexia Publications, 2 Market Terrace, St Leonards-on-Sea, E. Sussex TN 38 0DB.

Inskipp F and Proctor B *The Art, Craft and Tasks of Counselling Supervision.* Part 1. (1993, 1995) *Making the Most of Supervision.* Part 2. (1995) *Becoming a Supervisor.* Cascade Publications, 4 Ducks Walk, Twickenham, Middlesex TW1 2DD.

Morton-Cooper A and Palmer A (2000) *Mentoring, Preceptorship, and Clinical Supervision.* Oxford: Blackwell Science.

Rogers C (1952) *On Becoming a Person.* London: Constable.

4 An alternative training approach in clinical supervision

John R. Cutcliffe

Editorial

This chapter focuses on training practitioners to become supervisees rather than supervisors. It examines the drawbacks to training practitioners to become supervisiors and some of the principal problems that are facing the widespread introduction of clinical supervision in nursing practice. It then provides an argument that illustrates the advantages of training practitioners to become supervisees. It suggests a possible structure for this training and considers ways that it could be evaluated.

We feel that students, trainees and learners as aspirant healthcare practitioners should be exposed to the practice and theory of clinical supervision early on in their training. Once such foundations are in place, they serve as the building blocks upon which more sophisticated and advanced supervision practices can be built. We also believe that early exposure to high quality supervision will imbue the practitioner with a desire to continue to receive supervision throughout his or her career.

Current issues in clinical supervision training

Clinical supervision continues to be one of the central nursing issues within the National Health Service (NHS) (Cutcliffe and Burns, 1998). The National Health Service Management Executive (NHS ME, 1993), the UKCC (1995) and the King's Fund (1995) all advocated the implementation and use of clinical supervision for all practitioners. Recent literature has reiterated this point of view, with Bond and Holland (1998) asserting the need for all practitioners in all clinical areas to receive supervision. It is reasonable to say that many nursing researchers, academic nursing departments and self-governing (NHS) trusts have responded to this need and clinical supervision is being increasingly incorporated into nursing strategies within faculties, departments and directorates (Farrington, 1995).

Given the continued attention that clinical supervision in nursing receives, it is worth examining briefly how the need for this practice originated. The argument for formalised support mechanisms for nurses in the form of clinical supervision was pioneered by Professor Tony Butterworth in the early 1990s

(Butterworth, 1991, 1992). Additionally, reported work from other professions was beginning to influence thinking in nursing (Butterworth *et al.*, 1996) and supervision models from counselling and psychotherapy were starting to be incorporated into nursing practice (Proctor, 1986; Hawkins and Shohet, 1989). Subsequent to these developments, according to Bishop (1994) the significant factors to emerge from the UKCC Code of Professional Conduct (1992a) and The Scope of Professional Practice (UKCC, 1992b) are the individual's increased accountability combined with the demise of traditional support systems, which make clinical supervision essential. Furthermore, the findings of the Allitt enquiry (Clothier *et al.*, 1994) emphasised the need for safe and accountable practice. Clinical supervision within nursing was then endorsed by the Chief Nursing Officer of the Department of Health (D of H, 1994) who considers it to be fundamental to safeguarding standards, the development of expertise and the delivery of quality care.

Alleged benefits

Ultimately, the central purpose of clinical supervision is improvement in client care and this can be regarded as the principal benefit. At the same time, it is also alleged that clinical supervision brings about benefits for clinicians. These are described in Table 4.1.

Current attempts to research these alleged benefits centre on the three components suggested by Proctor (1986), these being normative (organisational, professional ethics and quality control), restorative (support for staff) and formative (education and development). Indeed initial findings from Butterworth *et al.*'s (1997) multi-site study, which explored several questions of clinical supervision, provided some evidence to suggest that receiving clinical supervision benefits the recipient, in particular in the realms of reducing emotional exhaustion and depersonalisation. Furthermore, qualitative and anecdotal evidence exists that suggests clinical supervision can improve client care (Paunonen, 1991; Booth, 1992; Timpson, 1996; Cutcliffe and Burns, 1998).

Table 4.1 Alleged benefits of clinical supervision for clinicians

---

- Increased feelings of support and feelings of personal well-being (Butterworth *et al.*, 1996).
- Increased knowledge and awareness of possible solutions to clinical problems (Dudley and Butterworth, 1994).
- Increased confidence, decreased incidence of emotional strain and burnout (Halberg and Norberg, 1993).
- Higher staff morale leading to a decrease in staff sickness/absence, increased staff satisfaction (Butterworth *et al.*, 1996).
- Increased participation in reflective practice (Hawkins and Shohet, 1989).
- Increased self-awareness (Cutcliffe and Epling,1997).

The introduction of clinical supervision in practice

As indicated above, many self governing (NHS) trusts have already begun to implement clinical supervision. This introduction is evidenced in the anecdotal accounts that proliferate in current nursing literature (Halberg and Norberg, 1993; Barton-Wright, 1994; Coleman, 1995; Everitt *et al.*, 1996; Fisher, 1996; Fowler, 1996a; 1996b; McGibbon, 1996; Morcom and Hughes, 1996; Wilkin *et al.*, 1997; Wright *et al.*, 1997). Examination of these papers indicates that there is no one singular method of implementation. However, it is clear that the one commonality all these attempts share is that any training that is provided is centred on equipping and enabling individuals to become supervisors not supervisees. Whilst this approach has benefits, it also has major drawbacks which warrant further consideration.

The drawbacks of training nurses to be supervisors

Clinical supervision is a specific skill. Whilst some of the interpersonal skills utilised in supervision may be transferable from nurse or counselling training, it goes far beyond basic interpersonal skills and has its own unique set of skills. Consequently, there is a need for specific clinical supervision training. Yet there is no standardised minimum quality and no widely accepted definition of what constitutes clinical supervision training. Within Butterworth *et al.*'s (1997, p17) multi-site study it is reported that the respondent sites had offered a wide variety of training opportunities:

Courses and training ranged from 6.5 days to 1 day, most commonly 2–3 days.

This cross-sectional view of clinical supervision training reflects the experience of the author. His contact with self-governing (NHS) trusts, higher education institutions and individuals who offer clinical supervision training privately, indicated a wide range of practices and desired outcomes, all under the general heading of clinical supervision. Yet the diversity in the quality of the training may well have a detrimental effect on the quality of supervision provided. Cutcliffe (1997) argued that there is a need to examine if a correlation exists between the level or intensity of supervision training given and the extent of positive outcomes in terms of benefits to clients and clinicians. The author suggests it is not unreasonable to postulate that if a nurse receives insufficient or inappropriate training in supervision, then the quality of the supervision they provide is unlikely to be capable of producing measured change indicating improvement in the supervisees' mental well-being or improvements in the care they provide.

However, enabling all potential supervisors to attend quality supervision training presents many logistical problems. High quality training is likely to be relatively lengthy and expensive when compared to the other options, such as in-service training. Smith (1995) reported that a director of patient care and nursing estimated that it would cost around £100,000 to implement clinical supervision based on the calculation that each nurse in her hospital would receive two hours of supervision per month. It is unclear whether or not these calculations take into account the cost of training the nurses to become supervisors, so this could be considered as a conservative estimate. Admittedly, a counter argument exists that suggests £100,000 is not really very much as it represents the cost of employing an NHS trust chief executive for a year (Smith, 1995). This problem is exacerbated if Regional Health Authorities do not provide additional funding to pay for the training and/or pay for additional nurses to ensure the wards are staffed whilst the training occurs. Furthermore as we operate in a climate where economics play an ever increasing role in determining the strategic planning of trusts, the real and reasonable position of these organisations is to say we cannot afford to release large numbers of staff to undertake extensive, intensive and expensive training courses. Especially if there is a paucity of empirical data that conclusively supports the assertion that clinical supervision will benefit both clients and staff.

Problems with implementing clinical supervision in nursing

In addition to the absence of a plausible economic option for trusts, the culture of the NHS does not yet have the infrastructure necessary for the widespread uptake of clinical supervision. Some of the problems relate to the limited understanding of clinical supervision practice. How can managers be expected to facilitate the equipping of nurses to the necessary extent if the nurses themselves do not have this understanding? Fowler (1996a, p382) supported this argument, suggesting:

> Nursing and health visiting does not, as yet, have a culture of clinical supervision for qualified nurses ... If we have little or no experience of being supervised ourselves, how do we clinically supervise others?

Smith (1995) stated that feedback from the NHSE conference on clinical supervision upheld this viewpoint. Conference participants argued that a cultural shift was necessary in order to move the clinical supervision agenda into the whole organisation, and that crucially, clinical supervision may be needed but it also has to be wanted. Bishop's (1994b) survey of nurse's attitudes towards clinical supervision indicated that only 0.2 per cent of the *Nursing Times'* estimated readership responded to the questionnaire. Whilst workload pressure and slow circulation rates may account for some of this very low response rate, a distinct lack of interest in clinical supervision must also be considered as a reason (Bishop, 1994a). Furthermore less than half of this sample (46 per cent) had clinical supervision up and running. Therefore it is reasonable to suggest that there are many nurses who do not want clinical

Table 4.2 Reasons for resisting clinical supervision within nursing

---

- A tradition and culture that discourages the public expression of emotion.
- The perception of clinical supervision as yet another management monitoring tool.
- The perception of supervision as a form of personal therapy.
- A continuing lack of clarity regarding the purpose of supervision.
- Resistance itself is an unavoidable component of the process of change (Wilkin *et al.*, 1997).

---

supervision at this time. Such resistance has many reasons for its existence and these are described in Table 4.2.

The author argues that when considering the resistance to clinical supervision, there is a crucial point that needs attention, and that is the apparent continuing lack of clarity regarding the purpose of supervision in nursing. Examination of the current literature highlights two separate perspectives on the purpose of clinical supervision. One view appears to conceptualise clinical supervision as an opportunity for more experienced nurses to monitor, educate and support less experienced nurses in how they do practical skills. This would create the need for all supervisors to be more 'expert' in the particular speciality of nursing than the supervisee. **Alternatively, there is another view that appears to conceptualise clinical supervision as an opportunity to help and support nurses to reflect on their dilemmas, difficulties and successes, and to explore how they reacted to, solved or achieved them. This view posits supervision as a forum for considering the personal, interpersonal and practical aspects of care so as to develop and maintain nurses who are skilled and reflective practitioners.** This situation creates the need for supervisors to be effective at supporting nurses in self-monitoring, identifying difficulties in practice and finding the proper place to make good the deficit, not necessarily to be more expert in the particular nursing speciality. This pivotal difference is seldom spelled out in the nursing literature and consequently it is not surprising that a sense of confusion exists for many nurses. Confusion concerning the purpose appears to create a resistance, and nurses appear to be unsure what they are entering into.

The author has stated previously that despite this resistance some trusts and educational institutions have made real progress in the implementation of supervision and such endeavours should be applauded. If these efforts are combined with systematic review and action research that produces evidence supporting the link between receiving supervision and improved client care/ positive outcomes for staff, then this resistance may begin to decline. However, such change will take time and may be somewhat parochial. The author argues that whilst such implementation should be encouraged, what is needed is a radical shift in the emphasis of training staff in the practice of clinical supervision. An alternative approach is needed, one that features training nurses to be supervisees, and it is this alternative approach that warrants further examination.

Alternative approaches to training

It is interesting to note that feedback from the NHSE conference on clinical supervision (Smith, 1995) argued that training was necessary but that creating special courses should be avoided. The first point of this statement certainly supports the author's argument that clinical supervision is a specific skill, yet the second point perhaps casts some doubt on this issue. Surely, if clinical supervision is a specific skill, does that not denote the need for specific training? However, perhaps there is an argument here for providing a standardised training, a training that could be available to all nurses. If all nurses are to be become familiar with the practice of clinical supervision, and if clinical supervision should be a part of every nurse's career (McLoughlin, 1995) then there may be merit in examining how other common training requirements for nurses have been met.

All qualified nurses share a commonality in that they undertake a period of training before qualifying. Given that there is an identified need for some form of training for clinical supervision and that all nurses have a common experience prior to becoming qualified, the logical solution to this problem is to incorporate clinical supervision training into pre-registration nurse training. However, the crucial difference of this training is that student nurses would be trained to be supervisees and not supervisors. This has many advantages, which will be discussed later. However, it also addresses the problems identified above, in that this form of clinical supervision training reduces the need for lengthy and costly post-registration clinical supervision training. The author is not suggesting that training student nurses to be supervisees removes the need for post-registration training, but a common foundation, used in nurse training, establishes the framework on which future supervision experience can be built. It sets in place, for the future, cohorts of new practitioners who can use supervision well, even if the supervisors were limited in their knowledge and application of supervision. Additionally, it would provide fertile foundations which act as the blocks of material needed for training supervisors, consequently new supervisors can build on their training and experience as 'good' supervisees rather than starting from scratch.

Perhaps what this method of training would do most is change the climate from the bottom upwards. Whilst it does not meet the training needs of those nurses who are already qualified, it reduces the amount of time that future nurses would spend in post-registration supervision training since they would already possess the basic understanding and experience of clinical supervision. Consequently, post-registration training in clinical supervision would be shorter, thus saving a great deal of money. Additionally the supervisee training would be relatively straightforward to standardise so that each nurse education centre provides at least the same minimum quality of training, thus addressing the problem of the wide diversity evident in current supervision training.

Table 4.3 Advantages of training student nurses to be supervisees

---

- The creation of greater equality and intentionality in the working alliance.
- The increased awareness and understanding that supervision is something for the supervisee.
- The sharing and agreeing of values, ground rules, terms and aims between the supervisee/supervisor and the organisation.
- A sense of comradeship between peers, a greater sense of team cohesion as counteraction to a culture of divide and rule.
- The development of basic intrapersonal skills (e.g. reflecting on practice, choosing issues, asking for and using help appropriately) in a less personally threatening forum.

Training student nurses to be supervisees

Advantages of supervisee training

In addition to the substantial reduction in training costs, and the possible standardisation of supervisee training, this approach brings additional advantages. The author lists these advantages in Table 4.3 and then discusses them in more detail.

The creation of greater equality and intentionality in the working alliance

Clinicians' resistance to supervision includes justifiable concerns that it is another management monitoring tool (Wilkin *et al.*, 1997) and consequently the locus of control (Rotter, 1972) remains very much with the supervisor. This position can be understood further when consideration of current training methods suggests supervisees will be entering into the supervision with little (if any) idea of what to expect. The current training is aimed at enlightening nurses on how to supervise, not on how to be a supervisee. If students are equipped to become supervisees, they are placed in an empowered position. The awareness and experience of the supervision process during their training could enable them to realise they are not 'done unto' during supervision. There is more equity in the distribution of power. Hawkins and Shohet (1989) suggested that evaluation within supervision is a two way process where both parties have the opportunity to give and receive open, honest, constructive feedback. Inskipp and Proctor (1989) argued that there is a joint responsibility for the supervision, and thus supervisees need to be active in seeking the right sort of supervision for themselves. If subsequent supervision moves away inadvertently from support, development, growth, and education and becomes custodial, punitive, or disabling, the students' knowledge and experience of the process could enable them to deal with this more effectively and seek help in bringing the supervision back within the defined boundaries. The intentionality is increased in that both supervisor and supervisee are aware of the reasons for their time together. Hawkins and Shohet (1989) pointed out that this intentionality helps supervisees become more proactive in gaining the support they need. Thus the supervision becomes a shared responsibility, a purposeful, deliberate, conscious act of support, education and development aimed at facilitating client care, and ceases to be an ambiguous and amorphous concept.

The increased awareness and understanding that supervision is something for the supervisee

Current introduction of clinical supervision may well be viewed by nurses as yet another imposition from nursing hierarchies. If supervision is seen as serving the organisation, not the client or the clinician, then it is understandable that resistance exists. In order for this resistance to be counteracted nurses need to discover that clinical supervision is primarily for them and their clients, not something for the supervisor, and certainly not something primarily designed as a tool for the management of the organisation. By making supervisee training an integral component of nurse education, students would be acclimatised to the experience of supervision and encounter the benefits for themselves. This argument is supported by Bishop (1994a) who reported that 98 per cent of nurses who had previously participated in peer review expected to benefit from clinical supervision. There appears to be a phenomenon whereby the experience of receiving quality clinical supervision rapidly removes miscomprehensions, anxieties, and resistance. Fowler's (1995, p37) study also corroborates this argument. He examined post-registration nursing students' perceptions of the elements of good supervision, and suggested that a key finding from stage three was that:

> All students wanted to see evidence of supervisors putting themselves out and helping the student build on their knowledge base.

Students who had experienced supervision felt it was for them, and wished to see evidence of this in the behaviour of the supervisor. Whilst the sample size in this study (50 students from two courses) represents only a fraction of the population of nursing students, it provides a valuable insight into the world of students. This increased awareness that exposure to supervision generates also addresses the issue raised in the first part of this paper, that of confusion concerning the purpose of clinical supervision and the subsequent resistance this confusion creates.

Ritter *et al.* (1996) described a model of supervision provided to undergraduate general nursing students who undertook clinical placements on psychiatric wards. The model incorporates Schon's (1987) work on reflective practice and coaching, whereby students are helped to identify and articulate their experience on their own behalf and in their own way, in other words it makes attempts to be supervisee led. Ritter *et al.* (1996, p155) stated,

The model of clinical supervision enables students to choose to demonstrate their understanding by turning up to the supervision with something quite different from what the supervisor asked for.

The students who became self-directed in their own supervision appear to have grasped that it is for them. Whilst this model appears to be a move towards training supervisees as it has an element of being supervisee led, it is still driven and guided by the supervisor. It is only when the supervisee has some understanding of the process and structure of the supervision that it becomes more completely supervisee led and consequently that supervisees acknowledge that supervision is for them. How much more would the students benefit from this supervision if they began their placement already equipped with an understanding of what clinical supervision is for and what it is to be a supervisee.

The sharing and agreeing of values, ground rules, terms and aims between the supervisee/supervisor and the organisation

If all student nurses are provided with the same supervisee training then this can create a commonality in the perception of the roles and tasks of supervision and how these can be distinguished from similar roles and tasks. White (1996) submitted that the term clinical supervision has yet to be universally distinguished by practitioners from preceptorship, individual performance review or personal therapy. He goes on to suggest that debriefing and the opportunity to reflect on clinical incidents was universally welcomed by the students in his study. Therefore whilst students may be unclear of the values, ground rules, and terms of supervision prior to receiving supervision, participation in the practice of supervision produced a joint ownership. Once more, the value of providing students with experience of being a supervisee during nurse training is illustrated. Supervisee training exposes the student to the process of negotiating ground rules, and the need for this explicit contracting is identified by Proctor (1988) who stated,

> If supervision is to become and remain a co-operative experience which allows real rather than token accountability, a clear – even tough – working arrangement needs to be negotiated.

Additionally an awareness of the aims of supervision is increased. The student can start to appreciate how supervision contributes to client, clinician and organisational need as a result of the increased self awareness that clinical supervision can bring (Cutcliffe and Epling, 1997). When given supervisee training the students can begin to appreciate their need for development and importantly the personal responsibility they have for their own development. Students can begin to see how clinical supervision affects the way they deliver care and consequently, the quality of care they provide. Similarly, such improvements in care will probably be part of the organisation's philosophy and/or strategy and thus both student and managers can see how the aims of supervision also contribute to meeting organisational need.

A sense of comradeship between peers, a greater sense of team cohesion as counter-action to a culture of divide and rule

It is reasonable to suggest that traditionally nurses have been encouraged to contain their emotions and keep a lid on things. Many anecdotes exist of nurses crying in the sluice room having just dealt with yet another emotional traumatic interpersonal situation. Such repression can only bring about a sense of isolation and inadequacy. Especially if the nurse believes that her peers regard her as someone who cannot cope because she weeps or lets off steam. Faugier (1992, p27) also pointed out that nursing has a system loaded against the development of continued learning, fuelled by: 'the threat of losing position or face before junior or untrained members of staff.'

For continuing learning to emerge from reflective practice, a culture of safety and honesty needs to be systematically developed. Supervisee training could begin to eradicate debilitating and restrictive attitudes. What better way to begin to change the culture than by introducing students to the practice of reflection, of being open, of being able to recognise and express the impact of emotionally charged experiences, all of which are encouraged within well set up clinical supervision? The increase in self-awareness brought about by participating in supervision (Faugier, 1992; Cutcliffe and Epling, 1997) enables trainees and nurses to realise when they need to express emotion and obtain support, and importantly that such processes are healthy. Furthermore that such processes are an integral component of each nurse's professional life. It encourages them to realise that 'mistakes' are usually opportunities rather than marks of failure. The sense of a shared experience, of participating in a common, widespread phenomenon, creates a collective sense of cohesion. Additionally the support experienced in supervision enables the nurse to think 'I am cared for by these people, I am not on my own, I belong to this team.'

The development of basic intrapersonal skills (e.g. reflecting on practice, choosing issues, asking for and using help appropriately) in a less personally threatening forum

Training students to be supervisees creates an environment where the student will need to enter into reflective practice, self-examination of learning needs, and practising being assertive. Yet all this can occur in a forum where there is no punitive presence, since the underpinning essence of supervision is support. Students who experience this support in supervisee training, and conceptualise that in order to support one needs to listen actively and empathise (Burnard, 1989), become arguably more capable of providing support. Butterworth

(1992) hypothesised that students who are trained in a learning environment which encourages active listening, empathy and support will lead to qualified nurses who foster similar therapeutic exchanges between nurses and patients. This argument is supported by Cassedy and Cutcliffe (1998) who reasoned that students need to experience in counselling training the kind of empathy, genuineness and respect for their own personhood which the author wants them to be offering clients. This entire training ideology of nurturing qualities is captured by Connor (1994, p37) who stated:

> Qualities are not developed by just practising skills or writing essays. They develop through the sum total of the learning experience and they are more likely to develop if there is intentionality in the learning process through ongoing structural experiences of reflection, reviewing and objective setting.

A suggested structure of supervisee training in nurse education

One possible structure for this training is as follows.

Year One: Teaching would be provided on the theory of supervision. It would include: definitions of supervision and delineation from related concepts; models of supervision; a historical overview of its inception; how the processes of reflection and self-examination are interwoven with supervision; roles of supervisees/supervisors; ground rules and boundaries; the process of contracting; giving and receiving feedback; and ethical issues in supervision.

Year Two: Following early clinical placements students would have a minimum of one hour per month supervision, using material they have recorded in their personal learning journals. The particular format of this supervision, (i.e. one to one, group) would be determined partly by the human resources available, and partly by the number of students on each course. In addition to the benefits of receiving the supervision, at the end of each module, placement or term, feedback could be given to the student on their use of supervision. How evident was it that the student participated in the roles, responsibilities and expectations of a supervisee? Have they taken responsibility for the actions, reflections and learnings? Did they appreciate their own needs for support?

Following this the student would complete a case study which would include the participation in and influence of supervision. Students would need to illustrate their active participation in supervision and how this influenced their client care and personal/professional development. This would include a written piece of work, but could also include audio or video taped sessions of their practice.

Problems with training students to be supervisees

This alternative approach to training is not without problems. One argument against the idea centres on the issue that this process will have to be experiential, with students using material from their clinical practice as a source of learning (Schon, 1984). However, since students are at an early stage of their training, they may have insufficient critical incidents or clinical material to bring to the clinical supervision session. Clinical supervision would not be relevant until you have some clinical practice. Another problem might be that students at this early stage in nurse training are too inexperienced to have an awareness of what they do not know or what they need to know. Individuals would only gain an awareness of their deficits once they had faced clinical situations and found themselves lacking. There is also the issue that trained supervisees could produce feelings of anxiety and disempowerment in their subsequent supervisor. Such new practitioners will be able to use supervision well and will not require such highly trained supervisors. However, being faced with a supervisee who knows more about the process of supervision may be unnerving. Supervisors may well be anxious that they are unable to deal with the issues the supervisee raises.

In reply to these arguments, there is a case for first training students in the theory of supervision and then exposing them to the process. This is the same way that students are taught the theory of interpersonal communication skills prior to these skills being utilised in a clinical environment. Therefore the experiential component of this training would only commence after a student has been on a clinical placement. As the student accrues more experience they will access more material that can be brought into the supervision. Yet the theory would already equip them with reasons why the processes that occur in supervision are necessary. The possible anxieties and feelings of disempowerment for a new supervisor are not exclusive to those individuals providing supervision to trained supervisees. The same feelings could well be present for any supervisor as Hawkins and Shohet (1989, p33) declared: 'Suddenly becoming, or being asked to be a supervisor can be both exhilarating and daunting.'

Additionally, if supervisors are equipped with information about the supervisee training, it can both inform and challenge their existing supervision practice.

Another problem would be incorporating this training into an already cramped pre-registration nurse training curriculum. Whilst the author acknowledges this issue, he still feels the need to construct the argument for including training to become a supervisee at this early stage in each nurse's training. The specific infra-structure of nurse training curriculums can then be debated widely, and the argument this paper puts forward could then be included in those debates.

Evaluating supervisee training in nurse education

Butterworth *et al.* (1996) highlighted that initial attempts to evaluate supervision centre on the three components suggested by Proctor (1986), these being normative (organisational and quality control), restorative (support for staff) and formative (education and development), and they provide a format for this evaluation (Butterworth *et al.*, 1997). It would be logical for evaluation of supervisee training to follow a similar format. However, the authors feel that evaluation in the normative category needs to be refined to ensure that the distinction between the supervisors' and supervisees' responsibility for overall normative development is clarified. This category needs to reflect their shared responsibility for learning, the internalising of professional ethics and standards of practice, and their shared responsibility for learning and developing competent practice. Crucially comparisons would have to be made between a control group of students who receive no supervisee training and a group of students who do receive supervision training, measured in terms of Butterworth's multi-centre study.

Normative

Quantitative research into this component would centre on audit data concerned with rates of student sickness/absence and student satisfaction levels. In particular, do students find they are more satisfied with their training if they have supervisee training? Qualitative data could include supervisee preparation. Additionally, in their case study (see above) students would be required to cite an instance where supervision has helped them with an issue of evaluating good practice or making an ethical decision, thus addressing the shared normative responsibility in supervision.

Restorative

Quantitative research into this component would centre on measurement of student stress levels, coping levels questionnaires and burn-out inventories. In particular how supported and listened to do students feel on a course that provides supervisee training? How does being on a clinical placement and receiving supervision training compare to being on a placement that does not have this training, i.e. does the training make it easier for the student to meet other educational criteria? Qualitative data would include identifying what being supported and listened to felt like on a course providing supervision training, i.e. how does the training for supervision increase the students' confidence, well-being and creativity in a way that contributes to their meeting other educational and practice criteria?

Formative

Research into this area would centre on evaluating observed performance, perhaps in the form of audio tape records, video tape records, or observations of clinical practice. This method of evaluation has already been used on Thorn training courses (Gamble, 1995). This could also include the case study assignment which could provide qualitative evidence of the benefits of receiving supervisee training. i.e. comparisons between students' experiences of clinical problems and how these were addressed. In addition, in the case study, trainees would be expected to include particular incidences of how supervision had affected subsequent understanding and practice.

Conclusion

Clinical supervision is considered by the Chief Officer of the Department of Health to be fundamental to safeguarding standards, the development of expertise and the delivery of quality care and it is reasonable to say it is here to stay. It allegedly brings significant benefits to clients and clinicians, and recent research has produced both quantitative and qualitative evidence that supports this argument. Many trusts have already made attempts to introduce the widespread implementation of clinical supervision with most developments being concerned with equipping clinicians to be supervisors not supervisees. This presents several logistical and financial problems, and currently neither the infra-structure nor culture are in place throughout nursing that would facilitate its widespread and effective uptake. However, an alternative method of tackling this problem would be to include supervisee training within the CFP component of diploma nurse education and within the first two years of undergraduate nurse education. Training student nurses to be supervisees has several alleged advantages. These are:

- a substantial reduction in training costs and time;
- a possible standardisation of training;
- the creation of greater equality and intentionality in the working alliance;
- the increased awareness and understanding in students that supervision is something for them;
- the sharing of values, ground rules, terms and aims between the supervisee/supervisor and the organisation;
- a sense of comradeship between peers in a culture that is often described as having a sense of divide and rule, and a greater sense of team cohesion;
- the development of basic intrapersonal skills (e.g. reflecting on practice, choosing issues, asking for and using help appropriately) in a less personally threatening forum.

An educational model would include both theoretical and experiential components with the theory preceding the experience, thus addressing some of the arguments raised against supervisee training. Evaluation of this training would be carried out using a format similar to the format used by Butterworth *et al.* (1997) when they evaluated the impact of receiving supervision. Finally, the idea of supervisee training is supported by Butterworth (1992, p12) who states: 'Introduction to a process of clinical supervision should begin in professional training and education, and continue thereafter as an integral part of professional development.'

This chapter is based on the papers that were originally published in the *British Journal of Nursing*: Cutcliffe J R and Proctor B (1998) An alternative training approach in clinical supervision, Part One. *British Journal of Nursing* Vol.7, No.5, p280–285 and Cutcliffe J R and Proctor B (1998) An alternative training approach in clinical supervision, Part two. *British Journal of Nursing* Vol.7, No.6, p344–350

References

Barton-Wright P (1994) Clinical supervision and primary nursing. *British Journal of Nursing* 3, 1, pp23–30.

Bishop V (1994a) Developmental support: For an accountable profession. *Nursing Times* 90(11) pp392–394.

Bishop V (1994b) Clinical supervision questionnaire. *Nursing Times* 90, 48, pp40–42.

Bond M and Holland S (1998) *Skills of Clinical Supervision for Nurses*. Buckingham: Open University Press.

Booth K (1992) Providing support and reducing stress: a review of the literature. In Butterworth T and Faugier J (eds) *Clinical Supervision and Mentorship in Nursing*. London: Chapman and Hall.

Burnard P (1989) The role of the mentor. *Journal of District Nursing* 8, 3, pp8–17.

Butterworth T (1991) Setting our professional house in order. In (Salvage J (ed.) *Working for Change in Primary Health Care* London: King's Fund Centre.

Butterworth T (1992) Clinical supervision as an emerging idea in nursing. In (Butterworth T and Faugier J (eds) *Clinical Supervision and Mentorship in Nursing* London: Chapman and Hall.

Butterworth T Bishop V and Carson J (1996) First steps towards evaluating clinical supervision in nursing and health visiting: I. Theory, policy and practice development. A review. *Journal of Clinical Nursing* 5, pp127–132.

Butterworth T Carson J White E Jeacock J Clements A and Bishop V (1997) It is good to talk. Clinical supervision and mentorship. An evaluation study in England and Scotland. Manchester: The School of Nursing, Midwifery and Health Visiting, The University of Manchester.

Cassedy P and Cutcliffe JR (1998) Empathy, students and the problems of genuineness. *Mental Health Practice* 1, 9, pp28–33.

Clothier C, MacDonald C and Shaw D (1994) *Independent Inquiry into deaths and injuries on the children's ward at Grantham and Kesteven General Hospital during the period February to April 1991* (Allitt Inquiry). London: HMSO.

Coleman M (1995) Using workshops to implement supervision. *Nursing Standard* 9, 50, pp27–29.

Connor M (1994) *Training the Counsellor: an integrative model*. London: Routledge.

Cutcliffe J R (1997) Evaluating the success of clinical supervision. *British Journal of Nursing* 6, 13, p725.

Cutcliffe J R and Burns J (1998) Personal, professional and practice development: clinical supervision. *British Journal of Nursing* 7, 21, pp1318–1322.

Cutcliffe J R and Epling M (1997) An exploration of the use of John Heron's confronting interventions in clinical supervision: case studies from practice. *Psychiatric Care* 4(4), pp174–175, 178–180.

D of H (1994) CNO Letter 94(5) *Clinical Supervision for the Nursing and Health Visiting Professions*. London: HMSO.

Dudley M, Butterworth T (1994) The costs and some benefits of clinical supervision: an initial exploration. *International Journal of Psychiatric Nursing Research* 1, pp34–40.

Everitt J Bradshaw T and Butterworth T (1996) Stress and clinical supervision in mental health care. *Nursing Times* 92, 10, pp34–35.

Farrington A (1995) Clinical supervision: UKCC must be more proactive. *British Journal of Nursing* 5, 12, p716.

Faugier J (1992) The supervisory relationship. In Butterworth T and Faugier J (eds) *Clinical Supervision and Mentorship in Nursing* London: Chapman and Hall.

Fisher M (1996) Using reflective practice in clinical supervision. *Professional Nurse* 11, 7, pp443–444.

Fowler J (1995) Nurses' perceptions of the elements of good supervision. *Nursing Times* 91, 22, pp33–37.

Fowler J (1996a) Clinical supervision: What do you do after saying hello? *British Journal of Nursing* 5, 6, pp382–385.

Fowler J (1996b) How to use models of clinical supervision in practice. *Nursing Standard* 10, 29, pp42–47.

Halberg IR and Norberg A (1993) Strain among nurses and their emotional reactions during one year of systematic clinical supervision combined with the implementation on individualised care in dementia nursing. *Journal of Advanced Nursing* 18, pp1800–1875.

Hawkins P and Shohet R (1989) *Supervision in the Helping Professions.* Milton Keynes: Open University Press.

Inskipp F and Proctor B (1989) *Skills for Supervisees and Skills for Supervisors.* Audio-tapes, Alexia Pubns, 2 Market Terrace, St. Leonards, E.Sussex.

King's Fund (1995) *Clinical Supervision: An Executive Summary.* London: King's Fund.

McLoughlin C (1995) *Clinical Supervision for Nursing and Health Visiting.* London: UKCC.

McGibbon G (1996) Clinical supervision for expanded practice in ENT. *Professional Nurse* 12, 2, pp100–102.

Morcom C and Hughes R (1996) How can clinical supervision become a real vision for the future. *Journal of Psychiatric and Mental Health Nursing* 3, pp117–124.

NHS Management Executive (1993) *A Vision for the Future.* London: HMSO.

Paunonen N (1991) Changes initiated by a nursing supervision programme: a analysis based on log-linear models *Journal of Advanced Nursing* 16, pp982–986.

Proctor B (1986) Supervision: A co-operative exercise in accountability In Marken, M and Payne, M (eds) *Enabling and Ensuring.* Leicester National Youth Bureau and Council for Education and training in Youth and Community Work.

Proctor B (1988) *Supervision: A Working Alliance* (Videotape training manual). Alexia Pubns, 2 Market Terrace, St. Leonards, E. Sussex.

Ritter S Norman I J Rentoul L and Bodley D (1996) A model of clinical supervision for nurses undertaking short placements in mental health care settings. *Journal of Clinical Nursing* 5, pp149–158.

Rotter J B (1972) *Applications of Social Learning Theory of Personality.* New York: Holt, Rinehart and Winston.

Schon D (1984) *The Reflective Practitioner.* New York: Basic Books.

Schon D A (1987) *Educating the Reflective Practitioner: Towards a New Design for Teaching and Learning in the Profession.* New York: Basic Books.

Smith J P (1995) Clinical supervision: conference by the NHSE. *Journal of Advanced Nursing* 21(5), pp1029–1031.

Timpson J (1996) Clinical Supervision: a plea for 'pit head time' in cancer nursing. *European Journal of Cancer Care* 5, pp43–52.

United Kingdom Central Council for Nursing, Midwifery and Health Visiting (1992b) *The Scope of Professional Practice.* London: UKCC.

United Kingdom Central Council for Nursing, Midwifery and Health Visiting (1992a) *Code of Professional Conduct for the Nurse, Midwife and Health Visitor.* London: UKCC.

United Kingdom Central Council for Nursing, Midwifery and Health Visiting (1995) *Proposed Position Statement on Clinical Supervision for Nursing and Health Visiting*. London: UKCC.

Wilkin P Bowers L and Monk J (1997) Clinical supervision: managing the resistance. *Nursing Times* 93, 8, pp48–49.

White E (1996) Clinical supervision and Project 2000: The identification of some substantive issues. *Nursing Times Research* 1, 2, pp102–111.

Wright S Elliot M and Scholfield H (1997) A networking approach to clinical supervision. *Nursing Standard* 11, 18, pp39–41.

5   Clinical supervision

Visions from the classroom

Mike Epling and Paul Cassedy

Editorial

This chapter focuses on the development and delivery of a diploma level clinical supervision course at the University of Nottingham. It provides a brief background to the course, looks at methods of assessment on the course, and then the developmental nature of the training is emphasised. The chapter then uses data obtained from evaluation of the course to highlight emerging issues. Three key issues arising are: issues of confidentiality; theoretical orientation of the supervisor/supervisee; and the status of the supervisor in relation to the supervisee.

Aspirant clinical supervisors (and supervisees) often state that they would prefer a supervisor (or to be supervised) by a practitioner who is from the same discipline. These preferences appear to be grounded in context that only another person from the same discipline would understand what it is like to operate in that discipline, and that this person needs to be more 'expert' than the supervisee. However, an alternative argument, supported by a growing body of evidence, posits that viewing the supervisor as 'the expert' or 'more expert' in the supervisees discipline can impede an exploratory and reflective style of supervision. One in which supervisee's are helped to find their own answers and solutions (where they exist). We would reiterate that there is no one 'perfect way' to organise and conduct supervision. Nevertheless, we would encourage aspirant supervisors/supervisees to consider the cogent argument made in this chapter when choosing a supervisor.

Introduction

This chapter will concentrate on the development and delivery of a clinical supervision course, run by the authors at the School of Nursing within the University of Nottingham. An examination of data which emerged from experiential group-work teaching sessions in the classroom on the clinical supervision course will be discussed; this highlights aspects of teaching and learning and raises issues that learners bring to the course. The course consists of two modules at diploma level two, and accepts post-registration students from a wide and varied background. The course is accessed via the contracting system through local consortia or independent funding to meet the continuing need for clinical supervision training.

The course was developed in 1994. Earlier ideas were to devise a programme with the original intention of providing a supervision course which would complement a counselling course as the recognised need for supervision in counselling is well documented (Page and Wosket, 1994).

However, examination of the literature (Hawkins and Shohet, 1989; Butterworth and Faugier, 1992) pointed out that the concept of 'clinical supervision' clearly located supervision in the helping professions. Clinical supervision was no longer the exclusive activity of those primarily offering psychological interventions. The emphasis of the course developments embraced this notion of clinical supervision training and education being offered to a much wider audience and the first intake in 1995 was the authors' first experience of delivering a course, which has matured with time. The length of training in clinical supervision is a debatable point; this needs negotiation between purchaser and provider and raises the issue of: what are the essential components and elements required by the supervisee and supervisors? There is a danger that prospective supervisors could be offered too little training and that lengthy courses could be superfluous to requirements (Power, 1999). **It is the authors' experience that unless purchasers recognise the need for well-trained staff they may be offered either nothing to prepare for this role or minimal guidance and support.**

Some students report that they are providing supervision with no previous training whilst others receiving supervision comment that their supervisors have equally received no formal training for the role of supervisor. We have found that over the period of the course, these practitioners often engage in a critical examination of their previous experience, which results in a redefinition of the role of supervision. The two modules 'Making the most of supervision' and 'On becoming a supervisor' are titles which were adopted from the work of Inskipp and Proctor (1993, 1995) as the authors considered these to reflect the nature and progression of the course. The first module is designed to enhance the knowledge and understanding of clinical supervision from a supervisee's perspective on the premise that developing skills and qualities of the supervisee will make the unity, intention and purpose of supervision more therapeutic. Building on the principles of the first module, the second module is aimed at those practitioners who are providing or anticipate providing clinical supervision for others.

Course assessment

The assessment of the course is in two parts, which aims to reflect the general course content of each of the two modules. Schön (1987) called for a new way of assessing learning and to achieve this suggested that assessment might have two interrelated components: first, some assessment of the art of skilful 'doing' and second an assessment of theory underpinning this skilful doing.

Part one: Making the Most of Supervision, encourages a critical analytical review of clinical supervision in a 4000 word written assignment. Most students focus on the theoretical frameworks and operational/organisational issues of clinical supervision placing this in context of their own practice often examining issues such as implementing supervision and resistance to it. The focus of this assignment is flexible enough to meet the individual's needs and concerns about clinical supervision.

Part two: On Becoming a Supervisor is a 2000 word reflective analysis of the students' video or tape recorded clinical supervision session of themselves in the role of a supervisor. The emphasis being that the recorded session provides a means for analysing the supervisory alliance, it is not an assessment of the performance of the actual clinical supervision session. This analysis encourages students to reflect on and punctuate the clinical supervision session utilising a framework such as Heron's (1990) six-category intervention analysis for examining the interpersonal aspects of the supervisory relationship within the context of Proctor's (1986) normative, formative and restorative framework for supervision.

Developmental model for clinical supervision training

Developmental models of supervision have become the mainstream of supervision thinking; the focus of how supervisees and supervisors change and develop as they enter into and gain experience moving towards increased competence through a series of stages can provide reference points for the individual as well as the education provider. Consideration of these stages may help to externalise what is being experienced intuitively. There are many developmental models of supervision, mostly taken from the fields of counselling and psychotherapy (Russell *et al.*, 1984).

However, they do not appear to translate wholly to the nursing profession which is more diverse in its range of helping interventions. Supervision may be one of only a few safety nets for counsellors to explore and discuss their work whereas nursing has a greater variety of managerial systems to monitor practice. However a developmental model is still a useful aid for the beginning supervisor, helping to map out the processes and frameworks which encompass function and process of supervision. In terms of education this can be viewed as the themes and content of the course and the process of learning which are translations of the aims and learning outcomes at levels of competence. Most students are at the 'beginner supervisee' stage: (see Figure 5.1), learning and development model of training, in relation to receiving and providing supervision. They have developed skills through practice which are transferable, such as basic communication, listening and attending skills, but still need to further develop the specific skills of supervision to understand and facilitate reflective practice in others. In order to understand the purpose of supervision students need to critically examine various models and theoretical frameworks and the qualities of interpersonal relationships, which can enhance a meaningful and effective supervisory alliance.

The overall aim of the course is to support the view that clinical supervision is now a major issue on the nursing agenda and has enormous potential for the profession (Bishop, 1998), whilst also considering it to be an effective learning and developmental tool which all healthcare professionals can utilise to promote and maintain high standards of practice. By the end of the programme, participants will have more of an in-depth understanding of clinical supervision and enhanced competence to implement and practise. In order to achieve this, the authors have developed a training model that has four essential components and can be viewed as a learning cycle that is experiential (Connor, 1994).

Whilst the programme is designed to move through the four components in sequence, they are however integrated and revisited within the cycle of learning. The student is at the heart of the model and may enter the course with different levels of experience. The aim of the course is to develop learners to a competent level, analogous to Benner's (1984) work on Novice to Expert. Depending on the previous experience of the learner, certain course components may become more of a focus. For example some learners may have developed competent interpersonal skills and be providing supervision, but have little understanding of the theories and frameworks which may enhance the effectiveness of supervision (see Figure 5.1).

Component one. Personal development and self-awareness

Learning objectives

Learners will be able to:

- explore and clarify attitudes, values and beliefs for greater awareness and effectiveness in clinical supervision;
- develop core therapeutic qualities;
- be aware of ethical and professional issues and expectations in supervision;
- develop a personal and professional code of standards and ethics;
- facilitate reflection in self and others through active participation in supervision practice groups;
- gain confidence in appropriate self-sharing and disclosure;
- review and ensure own clinical competence and standards.

Component two. Knowledge, theory and frameworks

Learning objectives

Learners will be able to:

- critically analyse the development of clinical supervision in nursing and its recommended implementation;

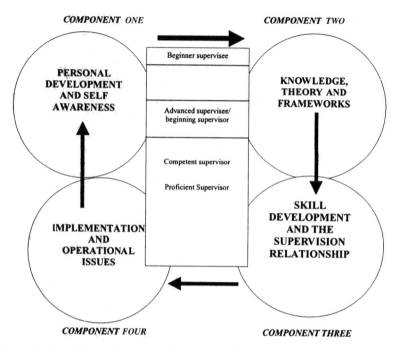

Figure 5.1 A training model for learning and development in clinical supervision

- define clinical supervision and separate from other similar activities;
- develop a working knowledge and become familiar with a core model for supervision: normative, formative and restorative (Proctor, 1986);
- become aware of other models for supervision and reflection (Kolb, 1984; Hawkins and Shohet, 1989; Johns, 1994; Faugier, 1992);
- become aware of group processes and dynamics that occur in group supervision.

Component three. Skill development and the supervision relationship

Learning objectives

Learners will be able to:

- develop a climate for an effective supervisory alliance and therapeutic process;
- develop skills of immediacy and the giving and receiving of feedback;
- learn, develop and apply a variety of therapeutic techniques and interventions consistent with the principles of supervision with individuals and groups;

- identify personal strengths and limitations in relation to skills and interventions;
- maintain a balance of support and challenge;
- regularly reflect upon supervision practice and experience supervision through active participation in supervision practice groups;
- develop confidence as both a supervisee and supervisor;
- develop the internal supervisor.

Component four. Implementation and operational issues

Learning objectives

Learners will be able to:

- set up contracts for supervision in the work setting;
- be aware of the rights and responsibilities of both supervisee and supervisor;
- be aware of responsibilities to the organisation;
- critically analyse different modes of supervision and apply to own work setting, such as group, individual or peer supervision;
- consider the appropriate environment, time and frequency for effective supervision and apply to own work setting;
- review and evaluate the effectiveness of the supervisory alliance;
- develop an awareness of the importance of research in the field of supervision.

Developmental levels

Beginner supervisee:

- recognises own need for personal and professional development;
- overcomes resistance to seeking out clinical supervision;
- understands the definitions and purpose of supervision;
- confident in the ability to recognise the benefits of supervision provided;
- develops reflective skills;
- is open to self-disclosure through increased self-awareness.

Advanced supervisee/beginning supervisor:

- needs to develop the skills of encouraging reflection in others;
- recognises the need to provide support in the development of others;
- open to constructive feedback and challenges;
- develops challenging skills and immediacy;
- overcomes anxieties of being in a position of responsibility;
- is able to identify and own personal strengths and limitations.

Competent supervisor:

- is congruent and able to trust in self;
- recognises changes to own practice and benefits to patients and clients;
- receives and continues own supervision;
- is flexible in meeting supervisee needs;
- transfers inter/intrapersonal and professional skills of helping into the supervisory relationship;
- maintains, holds and organises structures and boundaries of supervision in groups and individually;
- is able to work more holistically, more egalitarian, less reliant on status differential;
- is less prescriptive and informative, more facilitative and explorative promoting growth and challenge;
- is confident to facilitate group supervision;
- is aware of parallel process, transference/counter-transference;
- is able to make accurate, reliable observations and interpretations of supervisee's work.

Proficient supervisor:

- can work creatively with group dynamics;
- is confident supervising other disciplines within the profession;
- supervision becomes a major part of clinical role;
- implements and utilises supervisory structures which impact on organisational systems as well as individuals;
- is able to work with issues of transference and parallel process;
- has a sense of competence in own speciality and practice integrating a range of therapeutic skills providing clinical supervision for others;
- continues own professional development and lifelong learning;
- is aware of specific needs and agendas in relation to culture, gender and sexual orientation;
- is recognised and respected for role as a supervisor;
- utilises research and systematic enquiry to enhance supervision.

Teaching process and principles

The authors encourage students to participate in experiential learning (Kolb, 1984) as part of the overall strategy to develop self-awareness (Cutcliffe and Epling, 1997). To increase participation in reflective practice as suggested by Hawkins and Shohet (1989) the principles of adult student centred learning (Rogers, 1983) underpin the learning process.

The authors attempt to model and parallel the supervision working alliance in the classroom reflecting the interactional framework of the normative, formative and restorative functions of supervision as suggested by Proctor (1986).

It is intended that the quality of the teaching will parallel a climate of high support and high challenge creating an atmosphere of immediacy and self-disclosure (Connor, 1994) while an empathic understanding is communicated (Cassedy and Cutcliffe, 1998). **At every opportunity the authors facilitate the training in a style that would parallel the skills of running a clinical supervision group.** Our approaches to training have been largely adopted and adapted from the material of Bond and Holland (1998). Sessions begin with a 'settling stage' enabling learners to feel welcomed and relaxed.

Ground rules are established not only for group collaboration but also for maintaining boundaries. Students agree to avoid going back into the content of personal work during breaks and we agree to timekeeping. Settling is also about clarifying the aims and objectives of the session and establishing the order of the content; whilst there is lecture time and information giving we endeavour to deliver these as workshops or small group discussions to enable the 'energising phase'. A variety of experiential teaching methods are employed to promote an atmosphere of enthusiasm, participation and creativity utilising group facilitation skills.

Challenge and feedback are introduced early in the course as it is the authors' belief that you need to set out your stall from the onset of how you intend to work and the style of learning which will ensue; this creates respect and understanding The longer you leave or hesitate to challenge either working with an individual or a group, the harder it becomes later and raises the anxieties of all parties concerned. We are attempting to create a live experience for the students, emulating a climate of effective supervision either as a giver or receiver as the overall aim is to establish a working alliance. Activities, sessions and days are ended by the 'completing stage' of the process. Here we attempt to tie up loose ends, give students an opportunity to debrief, clarify outcomes or set goals for themselves, reflect on issues raised and summarise the content.

Developing skills in clinical supervision

It is the authors' experience that it is mainly recently qualified nurses that have developed reflective skills from the Project 2000 curricula yet most nurses lack the skills of facilitating reflection in others.

Supervision practice groups are an integral part of the course, which provides an opportunity for students to participate in clinical supervision practice during the second module of the course for one and a half hours of the teaching day per week. Students are given the opportunity to select and divide themselves into small groups of threes or fours in which supervision will be practised. The initial process encourages members to consider the varied aspects of selecting a supervisor, such as orientation, expertise and trust to mention a few. A cosy and comfortable relationship may not be challenging and someone from the same or different background may impact on the supervisory alliance. This process parallels the possibilities of selection of supervisors in practice; where possible the authors would endorse the principle of choosing a supervisor based upon the consideration of the overall aims of clinical supervision. Students are encouraged to utilise either audio- or videotape during the sessions to provide an opportunity for further reflective analysis of the supervisory alliance. Dreyfus and Dreyfus (1980) suggests that skills development should be embedded in actual clinical situations; to this end the learners are encouraged to bring real aspects of practice to the supervision practice groups. This enhances the development and practice of the skills of receiving and providing clinical supervision. The authors demonstrate live supervision with volunteers from the group in an attempt to model a session. This provides an opportunity for critique and feedback utilising the frameworks the group have explored. It is our intention to provide an example of the learning process which can be transferred into their practice groups, rather than a performance to emulate. The acquisition and development of skills in clinical supervision is of paramount importance and the authors support the notion of experiential learning, 'getting your feet wet and having a go'.

Whilst in closed groups, working on a supervision issues, other group members will provide observed critical feedback; the opportunity to experience and facilitate group supervision is also possible. One of the difficulties in utilising this approach to learning is the student's perception of experiential learning; the psychology of interpersonal relationships may feel alien and unfamiliar to some nurses depending on their previous experience and background. The nature of clinical supervision inevitably raises the need to focus on human relationships. We remind students that this is not counselling, but it focuses on self-development with the intention to raising self-awareness in order to understand the supervisory alliance. Learning needs to feel accessible to all disciplines which is non-threatening yet is challenging, the gentle introduction of experiential learning early in the course encouraging student participation helps to facilitate an atmosphere whereby students feel more comfortable with this approach to learning. Students' evaluations have consistently valued the opportunity to practise supervision and whilst the use of recording equipment is initially anxiety provoking, overcoming this is outweighed by the benefits of practice and feedback.

Group supervision

Whilst approaches and models for clinical supervision will vary according to a wide range of factors, the authors have encountered many instances of students reporting that it is the intention of their employers to develop clinical supervision in groups. Most students accessing the course are from general nursing backgrounds and have limited experience and/or education in group work approaches. Students undertaking the clinical supervision course are therefore exposed to the concepts of group dynamics in order to develop a better understanding of group processes and to aid the critical analysis of the pros and cons of group supervision as suggested by Inskipp and Proctor (1995).

To meet the needs of students embarking on the rather arduous task of group supervision, the authors have included sessions in the course which encompass the participation in and examination of group dynamics, processes and tasks. The giving and receiving of clinical supervision in groups is not primarily concerned with the issue of studying the dynamics of the group participants; however, the dynamics of being a participant within group supervision carries more complexity which needs to be acknowledged.

Bond and Holland (1998) consider many of the parameters of group supervision and give examples of what it is and what it is not.

They offer a definition of group supervision as:

> Three or more people who form a fixed membership group and have planned, regular meetings in which each person gets the chance for an in-depth reflection on their own practice and on the part they as individuals play in the complexities and quality of that practice, facilitated in that reflection by the other group members.
>
> (Bond and Holland, 1998, p.173)

Issues emerging from the classroom

Data has emerged from classroom activities that were originally planned to focus on group work processes and dynamics in relation to clinical supervision. This became a small-scale study, which highlighted several important factors which students brought to the course.

What emerged and was striking was the concordant and consistent level of agreement across the different cohorts in relation to some of the statements ranked. The information was extracted from a seventeen-statement ranking order form, which was devised by the authors to reflect some of the issues of clinical supervision to encourage students to participate in a group activity.

This information was collated over a two-year period and included six different cohorts with an average number of 20 students in each cohort.

The authors suggest that the data strongly reflects the concerns and issues which have been discussed in previous literature on clinical supervision, particularly in relation to:

- issues of confidentiality in clinical supervision;
- theoretical orientation of the supervisor and supervisee;
- the status of the supervisor in relation to the supervisee.

The statements in Table 5.1 were drawn from the literature to act as a vehicle in which the students would be encouraged to participate in a group work exercise in relation to group supervision and group dynamics. The statements were originally in a different order and have now been included according to rank order of importance according to six different groups' results. The groups were not aware of previous groups' ranking.

Table 5.1 Descriptive statistics showing the maximum/minimum scores including the mean and standard deviation for each ranked statement. Statements are in rank order (1 = most agree and 17 = least agree).

Statement	Mini-mum	Maxi-mum	Mean	Standard Deviation	Rank Order
Confidentiality is assured and agreed.	1.00	2.00	1.1667	0.4082	1
Members should provide support for one another.	2.00	7.00	3.5000	1.8708	2
The goals of supervision are explicitly formulated.	1.00	10.00	4.1667	3.5449	3
A written contract for supervision is completed.	3.00	9.00	4.8333	2.3166	4
Member's feelings should be considered during supervision.	3.00	10.00	5.5000	2.5884	5
Members should challenge one another's practice.	6.00	10.00	8.0000	1.2649	6
Time is allocated for each member by the supervisor.	5.00	13.00	8.0000	3.5214	7
The supervisor should direct the focus of the group.	5.00	15.00	8.0000	3.7947	8
Supervisees should be allowed to express negative feelings.	4.00	13.00	8.1667	3.1885	9
Supervision groups should be of closed membership.	2.00	13.00	8.3333	4.6762	10
Time should be allowed to facilitate personal issues if they emerge.	6.00	16.00	10.3333	3.3267	11
Each member should have the opportunity to facilitate supervision.	6.00	14.00	10.3333	3.3862	12
The supervisor should be an expert practitioner.	8.00	15.00	11.5000	2.2583	13
Supervisees should be of roughly equal experience and status.	10.00	16.00	13.3333	2.1602	14
Supervision notes should be maintained by the supervisor.	12.00	17.00	14.5000	2.0736	15
Supervisor and supervisees should share the same theoretical orientation.	14.00	16.00	14.8333	0.7528	16
The supervisor should be a manager.	16.00	17.00	16.8333	0.4082	17

Example of teaching and learning: group work exercise

The group work exercise involves half of the group sitting in a circle with the ranking form (see Table 5.1). The task is to consider the list of statements and come to a consensus of opinion. These are ranked accordingly, 1 being the most important and 17 the least important. They are encouraged to work as a total group and dissuaded from voting; the importance of total group consensus is reaffirmed. The other half of the group is briefed separately in relation to the task of the students who will be ranking the 'supervision statements'. This half of the group are also given a form (see Table 5.2), including description statements in relation to observable behaviour of individuals within groups.

The observer group sits behind the students involved in the group ranking exercise in order to observe a student's behaviour on the other side of the circle.

The students on the outside of the circle are in effect 'fish-bowling' the students on the inner circle and making observations of an individual's behaviour using a behaviour analysis sheet as a guide.

Once the inner group has completed the task of ranking the statements in relation to group supervision, the observer joins the observed to feed back his or her observations of how that particular student performed in the group.

The exercise works on several levels: it encourages discussion on the principles and practice of group supervision whilst participating in group processes, and provides a workshop in which the students have the opportunity to observe group dynamics and provide feedback to colleagues.

Confidentiality

Confidentiality is assured and agreed ranked as the most important aspect of clinical supervision, perhaps reflecting the students' possible distrust of disclosing information to potential supervisors. Issues of confidentiality often arise in discussion with students and are of such concern that anecdotal reports of resistance to the uptake of supervision by potential supervisees may be attributed to the unclear boundaries of confidentiality and the accountability of each of the participants in the supervisory relationship. The rank

Table 5.2 Some examples taken from the behavioural observation statements

---

Behaviour analysis sheet: examples of behaviour observation statements

---

Group task behaviours

- Initiating : Proposes aims, ideas, action or procedures;
- Summarising : Pulls data together, so group may consider where it is;
- Clarifying : Illuminates or builds upon ideas or suggestions.

---

order highlights this, as five of the six course intakes ranked this consistently as being the most important statement. Issues of confidentiality have been discussed by numerous authors. 'A contract of ground-rules should be negotiated at the start of any supervisory relationship to protect both the person giving and the person receiving supervision' (Hawkins and Shohet, 1989). Recent literature by Cutcliffe *et al.* (1998) examined the need to develop agreed working principles in relation to ethics and the dilemmas of confidentiality. This has highlighted the complexities and ambiguities of the supervisory relationship incumbent with the accountability of the nurse's role in relation to the professional bodies and the law. It is clear that confidentiality is not only of concern to the supervisees but supervisors are equally uncertain when it comes to the rather murky boundaries of confidentiality.

The supervisory relationship must have a strong confidential ethic to encourage a trustworthy and safe environment in which nurses can discuss practice in an open and honest manner, which may include self-disclosure. If this environment is not available and the limits and boundaries of confidentiality are not fully understood within the supervisory relationship, both parties will be less likely to explore the more risky elements of unsafe or unprofessional practice or to disclose emotions or feelings which may place the supervisee in an otherwise vulnerable position. Tschudin (1992) addresses the ethics of confidentiality by suggesting that we ask ourselves two questions:

- What is meant by confidentiality?
- What is confidential material?

By answering the first question, the answer to the second question will largely become apparent. Students are encouraged to discuss and engage in the initial stages of creating a contract for supervision as part of the clinical supervision practice groups. Kohner (1994) believes it is vital that the extent and limits of confidentiality are clarified and agreed with an understanding reached about what does and does not fall within the scope of clinical supervision. She further concludes that a contract of ground rules should be negotiated at the start of any supervisory relationship to protect both the person giving and the person receiving supervision.

An example of a clinical supervision contract is suggested by Bond and Holland (1998), which embraces the concepts of confidentiality considering the boundaries roles and responsibilities of the supervisor and supervisee.

This is a good starting point for students to refer to in order to develop their own working agreements for the supervisory relationship which we encourage in the initial stages of the formation of supervision practice groups.

Theoretical orientation and status of the supervisor and supervisee

Students ranked this statement consistently low, perhaps indicating that the supervisor and supervisee do not necessarily need to be from the same background. The theoretical background and orientation of the supervisor may be particularly important specifically in relation to the formative and normative function of clinical supervision. However, the ability to choose an appropriate supervisor may not be an option for many nurses if supervision is structured and implemented by management. Whilst nurses undertaking the clinical supervision course are encouraged to be reflective and to promote reflection within their supervisees, many nurses report the urge and tendency to act as expert advisor and problem solver. This tendency seems to have a relationship to status and orientation; if the supervisor is of higher status or indeed also more experienced than the supervisee the expert advisor pattern of interaction seems to emerge which has been characterised by Holloway and Poulin (1995) as the 'teacher–student' function. French and Raven (1960) refer to this process of advising as exerting expert and legitimate power where the supervisor provides information, opinions and suggestions based on professional knowledge and skill. Communication is largely controlled by the supervisor thus emphasising the hierarchy of the relationship; when the supervisory alliance is more equally matched in perceived expert power a decreased amount of advising may result.

In the authors' experience of supervising supervisors, it has been frequently reported by supervisors that the tendency to act in the role of expert advisor diminishes when their own orientation and experience is different from that of their supervisee. Some of the supervisors have reported that the role of being an expert can get in the way of supervision. The tendency to encourage a more exploratory and reflective style of supervision is almost forced by the virtue of not having a similar orientation to that of the supervisee.

The supervisor may not be the expert 'knower' in relation to the supervisee's clinical speciality and to rely on the 'teaching of' rather than encouraging the 'reflection on' will continue to reinforce the status of the 'teacher–student' roles thus reducing the supervisee's capacity for reflection and problem solving. This status position may continue to develop if nurses are unable to let go of the notion of clinical supervision being implemented in a hierarchical manner. Parallels from the supervision alliance may be drawn from the Japanese title 'Roshi' (Zen teacher or master) and 'Inka', the term given by the Zen master to a disciple who has completed his training and is now considered qualified to guide others. Zen stresses self-inquiry and independence of spirit; the teacher who, instead of liberating students, makes them dependent upon him has surely failed both his students and his Zen. Part of the problem here is that people may invest the teacher with an almost divine aura. It is assumed that anyone in the role of Zen master must be a person of deep spiritual insight and compassion and that such a person can do or say no wrong. Such misconceptions should be rejected and the aspiring trainee would be wise to maintain some of his or her natural scepticism. These analogies are worthy of reminding us as teachers and students embarking on the journey of clinical supervision that clinical supervision is a developmental process whereby the confidence and competence to supervise others unfolds gently rather than being forced or thrust upon the unwilling.

Should the supervisor be a manager?

This statement was consistently ranked as the least important aspect of clinical supervision. Nurses undertaking the course frequently report that the development of their clinical supervision structures has been imposed from the top down rather than grown organically out of practice. Whether it is the framework in which supervision takes place, group, individual or peer, or it is hierarchically structured with higher grade nurses supervising lower grade nurses, the discussions in many areas of clinical practice have been few or the options have not been considered. **Many nurses have reported their suspicions to the authors that lip service is being paid to the implementation of clinical supervision and particularly the implementation of group supervision being based on economic principles rather than evidence of good practice.** Nurses may resist entering into a supervisory relationship if they perceive it to be a management led initiative and it is imposed upon them with little ownership of the way they may provide or receive clinical supervision. The course encourages a high degree of supervisee ownership of 'bringing your own agenda to supervision'. The King's Fund (1994) stated 'Clinical supervision must not become yet another imposition from managers or academics.' Skoberne (1996) suggests the ideal supervisor is a person who possesses the necessary professional skills and knowledge to fulfil the role of enabling and supporting the supervisee to grow into an effective practitioner in ways that are unique and meaningful also creating a relaxed and trustful atmosphere. As yet many managers still need to develop clinical supervisory skills and the evidence from course records would bear out that the uptake of clinical supervision training from those above G grade or ward managers' level is still minimal. There needs to be a clear recognition and delineation of competing agendas and roles for managers as supervisors.

Whilst we would not endorse managers as clinical supervisors based on the grounds of organisational structure alone, to exclude managers from developing supervisory responsibilities would be tantamount to cutting out experienced staff undertaking a rewarding role which is to enhance quality care.

Supervision and training in the wider context

As providers of education in clinical supervision we believe that training and education does make a difference and can influence practice; hopefully the implementation and take-up of clinical supervision increases as a result of undertaking the course. Our personal hopes and visions are that clinical supervision becomes a cornerstone of practice, organised systematically with regular protected time that is valued by the participants and of value to patients. Overcoming resistance to the uptake of clinical supervision and converting the sceptical and non-believers perhaps sounds rather zealous, but the authors believe that the perceived benefits of clinical supervision is spreading. Those who are not involved are starting to ask themselves why not; it is becoming 'wanted' rather than 'needed' and the cultural acceptance of clinical supervision is creeping into practice. It is not yet the cultural norm but hopefully rooting itself permanently to quality care. We know of examples where previous students have been charged with the responsibility of implementing clinical supervision either in directorates or in some cases across the whole of a large trust as a condition of undertaking the course. The results of course follow-up evaluations received from past students show that the course prepared them to both receive and provide supervision in groups and on an individual one to one basis.

There are numerous reasons why the uptake of clinical supervision is still patchy; as course providers we are considering ways forward for the course to be more influential in the uptake of clinical supervision in practice.

We are considering future assessment strategies for the course to be linked with evidence of receiving and/or providing clinical supervision in the practice setting over a period of time, which could be verified and would ensure that students are practising what they have learnt. Unlike other courses such as communication or counselling skills training which have many transferable skills, learners can possibly see that they are utilising these, or parts of it, in a variety of settings.

In respect to clinical supervision, it is different, it needs to be implemented fully; you are either doing it or not. Students will know that they are not providing supervision if they are providing *ad hoc* support to colleagues without due respect to the aims, function and purpose of clinical supervision. Similarly they will fully understand that what they are receiving, is or is not clinical supervision, and should be able to help the uninformed supervisor to redefine the nature of supervision.

The possibility of a database including 'willing supervisor' profiles could offer choice and opportunity for those wishing to receive supervision. We could see that educational providers could have a role to play in this process and that the continuing development of supervisor competence could perhaps be monitored by the development of supervisor registers in conjunction with participating purchasers. This could encourage networking within directorates or trusts and possibly across them. As clinical supervision becomes implemented more widely, some supervisors may have responsibility for the supervision of numerous staff. This raises the question of supervisors not only receiving clinical supervision for their clinical practice but receiving supervision for their role as supervisors. The educational needs of those 'supervising the supervisors' is possibly as yet an unmet demand, bearing in mind that there may be future need for the possibility of requiring more than one supervisor for the complexity of the care provided.

For example healthcare staff may be offering counselling as a major part of their delivery of care in specialities where counselling is not the core business. The specialist midwife who provides counselling for complicated ante-natal care, or the nurse therapist who provides group therapy, may need more than one supervisor to support the specialist role as well as mainstream care.

The UKCC (1996) has clearly stated that it wants to see a component of pre- and post-registration training dedicated to preparing practitioners to *receive* clinical supervision. However little guidance has been given with regard to the prerequisite level or the kind of training necessary to *provide* effective clinical supervision. Wright (1992) compared the supervisory role of nursing to that of a consultant in medicine and suggested that a supervising nurse would not only need to have advanced standing as a practitioner but would need to be educated at least to master's degree level. **Whilst the authors recognise that practising supervisors should meet a minimum prerequisite for supervising others we would argue that Wright's suggestion of a master's degree level of education would presently preclude many potentially 'good enough' supervisors from undertaking this role.**

There is much debate about clinical supervision training and education, mostly regarding when, for how long and where it should take place, be it in preregistration, post-registration, 'in-house', or whether it is offered at diploma, first degree or master's level. We would suggest that these issues are primarily a reflection of the developments and changes which are taking place both in practice and nurse education, and will change again over time.

It would seem wise to have the foresight to prepare nurses at a pre-registration level to be effective supervisees with the capacity for reflective practice, and it makes sense for trusts to provide in-house training for staff who are unprepared for taking on the role of supervising others. As course providers we are currently experiencing a very mixed picture of staff accessing our course: some are receiving and providing supervision, yet many more have heard clinical supervision but have never experienced it or previously reviewed relevant literature. Currently the course is providing education and training primarily for those who are at the 'beginning stage' (see Figure 5.1), as supervisees who will most likely become supervisors once they have completed the course developing as competent supervisors.

Some may become 'proficient' but it is our belief that this happens over a longer period of time with increased experience and responsibility for supervising others. It is a maturation process that cannot be taught within the confines of a curriculum which sets out to meet the more immediate needs of preparing practitioners to embark on something for which they have little previous experience. Courses aimed at developing 'proficient supervisors' may be required for some or it may be a future need as competent supervisors increasingly take on the role of supervising others. Many authors have commented on the need to be first an expert practitioner, and second with a 'good enough' experience of clinical supervision oneself (Hawkins and

Shohet, 1989; Sharpe, 1995; Carroll, 1996). The need to be an expert practitioner prior to undertaking the role of supervising others is considered later when discussing theoretical orientation and status of the supervisor.

As providers of a course in clinical supervision the authors would suggest that the complexities of the supervisory relationship demand the need for designated training for supervisors and that previous experience of supervision itself is not sufficient to prepare for this role.

Presently the current climate of training and education in clinical supervision is diverse. It is always contentious and perhaps rather arbitrary to put a figure on how many days or hours should be spent on training, as the quality of the training will have as much bearing on the outcome as the length. Whilst we have not undertaken a full scale study of these two correlates, the course we provide is continually evaluated by the students which presently indicates that we are meeting current needs. There is always room for growth, change and developments and the course should mature in tandem with the complexities of changes in practice.

Conclusion

There is presently a need for courses on clinical supervision to feature both within pre-registration and specialist post-registration curricula in a much more robust manner. This requires an investment of time and the skilled facilitation of learning which embraces experiential methods providing the opportunity to practise, and not as isolated didactic lectures within an already crowded and competing timetable. The reflective practitioner has become synonymous with clinical supervision. Schön (1987) called for 'practice-led' curricula to enable a more reflective approach to practice. We would support the concept of learning by 'doing' and analysing that 'doing'. This approach to learning facilitates the development and improvement of the skills of supervision through observed critical feedback combined with self-evaluation.

This chapter has outlined the authors' learning and developmental model of training which has been built upon our visions generated from the classroom as well as our personal experiences of providing and receiving clinical supervision. The curriculum has matured and grown in tandem with consideration of the learners' perceptions, evaluation and feedback encompassing practice issues as they change and develop. We believe it is essential that supervisors use a developmental model to make reference to the process and stages of learning. We believe this also applies to ourselves as course facilitators, to map our personal skills, development and course curricula in an ongoing way.

References

Benner P (1984) *From Novice to Expert: Excellence and Power in Clinical Nursing Practice.* Reading, MA: Addison-Wesley.

Bishop V (1994) Clinical supervision for an accountable professional. *Nursing Times,* 90(39), pp35–37.

Bishop V (1998) *Clinical Supervision in Practice: Some Questions, Answers and Guidelines.* London: Macmillan.

Bond M and Holland S (1998) *Skills of Clinical Supervision For Nurses.* Buckingham: Open University Press.

Butterworth T and Faugier J (1992) *Clinical Supervision and Mentorship in Nursing.* London: Chapman and Hall.

Carroll M (1996) *Counselling Supervision: Theories Skills and Practice.* London: Cassell.

Cassedy P and Cutcliffe J R (1998) Empathy, students and the problems of genuineness. *Mental Health Practice.* 1, 9, pp28–33.

Connor M (1994) *Training the Counsellor.* London: Routledge.

Cutcliffe J and Epling M (1997) An exploration of the use of John Herons' confronting interventions in clinical supervision: Case studies from practice. *Psychiatric Care* 4(4), pp174, 175, 178–180.

Cutcliffe J Epling M Cassedy P Mcgregor J Plant N and Butterworth T (1998) Ethical dilemmas in clinical supervision: need for guidelines. *British Journal of Nursing* 7 (15), pp920–923.

Dreyfus S E and Dreyfus H L (1980) A five-stage model of mental sctivities involved in directed skill acquisition. In P Benner (ed.) *From Novice to Expert: Excellence and Power in Clinical Nursing Practice.* Menlo Park, California: Addison-Wesley.

Faugier J (1992) The supervisory relationship. In: Butterworth T and Faugier J (ed.) *Clinical Supervision and Mentorship in Nursing.* London: Chapman and Hall.

French J R P Jr and Raven B H (1960) The bases of social power. In Cartwright D and Zander A (eds), *Group Dynamics: Research and Theory.* (2nd edition pp607–623) New York: Peterson.

Hawkins P and Shohet R (1989) *Supervision in the Helping Professions.* Milton Keynes: Open Univerity Press.

Heron J (1990) *Helping the Client.* London: Sage.

Holloway E L and Poulin K (1995) Discourse in supervision In Holloway E (ed.), *Clinical Supervision: A systems approach.* London: Sage.

Inskipp F and Proctor B (1993) *The Art, Craft and Tasks of Counselling Supervision, Part 1, Making the Most of Supervision.* Twickenham, Middlesex: Cascade Publications.

Inskipp F and Proctor B (1995) *The Art, Craft and Tasks of Counselling Supervision, Part 2, Becoming a Supervisor.* Twickenham, Middlesex: Cascade Publications.

Johns C (1994) Guided reflection. In Palmer A *et al.* (eds) *Reflective Practice in Nursing.* Oxford: Blackwell Science.

King's Fund (1994) *Clinical Supervision: An Executive Summary.* London: King's Fund Centre.

Kohner N (1994) *Clinical Supervision in Practice.* London: King's Fund Centre.

Kolb D A (1984) *Experiential Learning.* London: Prentice Hall.

Page S and Wosket V (1994) *Supervising the Counsellor.* London: Routledge.

Power S (1999) *Nursing Supervision: A Guide for Clinical Practice.* London: Sage.

Proctor B (1986) A co-operative exercise in accountability In: Marken M and Payne M (eds) *Enabling and Ensuring: Supervision in Practice.* Leicester: National Youth Bureau and Council for Education and Training in Youth and Community Work.

Rogers C R (1983) *Freedom to Learn in the 80s.* Colombus Ohio: Charles Merrill.

Russell R K, Crimmings A M and Lent R W (1984) Counsellor training and supervision: Theory and research. In: S D Brown and R W Lent (ed.), *Handbook of Counselling Psychology.* New York: Wiley.

Schön D A (1987) *Educating the Reflective Practitioner.* San Francisco: Jossey-Bass.

Sharpe M (1995) Training of supervisors. In: Sharpe M (ed.) *The Third Eye. Supervision of Analytic Groups.* London: Routledge.

Skoberne M (1996) Supervision in nursing: My experience and views. *Journal of Nursing Management* 4, pp289–295.

Tschudin V (1992) *Ethics in Nursing*. Oxford: Butterworth Heinemann.

UKCC (1996) *Position Statement on Clinical Supervision for Nursing and Health Visiting*. London: UKCC.

Wright S G (1992) Modelling excellence: the role of the the consultant nurse. In Butterworth T and Faugier J (eds) *Clinical Supervision and Mentorship in Nursing*. London: Chapman and Hall.

6 Developmental transitions towards effective educational preparation for clinical supervision

Mick Rafferty and Mick Coleman

Editorial

This chapter focuses on the development of a diploma-level clinical supervision module at the University of Wales, Swansea. It provides a background to the course, identifies the experiential learning components and the theoretical components, and looks at links with additional institutional developments, designed to expand and forward the uptake and practice of supervision. The chapter then includes reflections on the experience of educational developments in clinical supervision and uses metaphors to illustrate these reflections. The chapter also points out that despite undertaking training, not all trained supervisors take on the role of supervisor when they return to their practice setting. The chapter also serves as a logical precursor to the next section of the book.

We believe that this chapter draws attention to a particular issue in the training or preparation of supervisors, namely that even though clinical supervision has been described as a career-long activity, most current training or preparation appears to be a 'one stop' or 'one off' occurrence. We would support the point raised by the authors and would add that career long 'top up' courses or training days need to be designed, funded and provided to practitioners as a matter of urgency. We acknowledge that some ongoing development of one's supervision skills can (and does) occur as a result of receiving supervision. However, there is a case for additional, career-long training. Attendance at such training might then be linked to inclusion on a register of supervisors (see Chapter 14).

Introduction

The School of Health Science in the University of Wales, Swansea, came into being in 1992 through the amalgamation of three existing Colleges of Nursing and Midwifery. In the original structure of the School, a post was created with a specific remit for clinical developments. Immediately there was recognition that one of the main areas of development within nursing and health care was that of clinical supervision. This recognition was partly in response to the initial signs of interest occurring in the profession, but was largely driven by the experience and interest of individuals within and outside the School. Correspondingly, a decision was made to convene a curriculum planning team. Its aim was to develop educational provision to assist local services develop meaningful and effective structures for clinical supervision. The curriculum planning team consisted of a mixture of educationalists with backgrounds and experience in clinical supervision, clinicians from both acute, community settings, and service managers. In order to provide direction for curriculum development, an early function of this group was to generate a working definition of clinical supervision, which was produced in the form of a series of statements outlined in Table 6.1.

The module

The decision was taken that this initial provision would take the form of a diploma level module within the Welsh National Board for Nursing, Midwifery and Health Visiting (WNB) framework of Continuing Education. To comply with the framework it was decided that the course would consist of fifteen study days over a period of eighteen weeks. The module aim was 'to equip practitioners with the necessary knowledge, experiential understanding and organisational insights to enable them to function as clinical supervisors. The preparation should allow participants to make supervisory arrangements for themselves and organise supervisory structures for their practice' (Rafferty and Coleman, 1996).

The module was constructed around the notions of 'learning by doing' and by 'studying the doing' and consequently had a heavy experiential emphasis. The structure for the experiential learning components was loosely built on the functions described by Proctor (1986): namely the supportive/restorative, formative and normative functions. The areas of practice seen as the necessary work agenda for clinical supervision in

Table 6.1 Working definition of clinical supervision

- Supervision is a growth focused relationship which leads to safe and enhanced practice.

- The focus of supervision should be the practice of care.

- The supervisory relationship should allow practitioners to report upon their care, defend their actions and be given opportunities to reality test for appropriateness.

- Supervision should provide a balm for the bites and stings of practice.

- By connecting the practitioner with others, supervision should reduce professional isolation.

- Through raising consciousness about practice, supervision might lead to the development of practice theory.

nursing and health visiting, as well as the modes of delivery, are set out in Table 6.2.

The large group as a whole and its associated discussions were also seen as a valuable means for exploring the problems, challenges and successes of clinical supervision that inevitably preoccupied every module. This 'learning from the doing' was formalised by three evaluations at five, ten and fifteen days. The theoretical content of the module is briefly listed in Table 6.3.

The taught content of the module outlined in Table 6.3 provided a broad basic introduction aimed at helping practitioners to recognise the interpersonal, moral and contextual dimensions of clinical supervision. This emphasis was set within a wider purpose of clinical supervision: namely, that it is about helping practitioners to manage professional change, loss and transition. The

Table 6.2 Experiential learning components

Function	Focus	Structure	Agenda
Supportive / Restorative	Need for professional support and restoration	Peer exercise in pairs 7 occasions for 30 minutes	Dynamics of change, transition and loss Joys and sorrows of practice Looking at what happens when things go wrong Characteristics of helpful support How life events impact on work performance Endings
Formative	Issues of how to learn from practice events	Facilitated groups of 6 to 8 participants 8 occasions for 75 minutes	Describing practice events Reflecting effectively on practice events Identifying how to help people learn
Normative	Issues of enabling accountable practice	Facilitated groups of 3 to 4 participants 5 occasions for 75 minutes	Exploring the exercise of appropriate authority Justifying professional autonomy Understanding resistance to change Dealing with human destructiveness

Table 6.3 Theoretical content of the clinical supervision course

---

- Transactional analysis
- Systemic theory
- Change and transition theory
- Ethics
- Group dynamics
- Theory and practice of clinical supervision (contracts, use of time, ground rules, models of supervision, practice models)

---

module was formally assessed by completion of a written assignment, which emphasised the practitioners' journey of experiences and learning about clinical supervision and their plans for the future. Greater detail about the module and its initial evaluation can be found in Rafferty and Coleman (1996) and course supervisory process in Rafferty (1998).

To date fifteen modules have run. Corresponding with them have been other developments to support and expand the concept and take forward institutionalisation of clinical supervision. The plan was not to see the module as an end in itself but a beginning for all kinds of action to do with making the practice of clinical supervision a reality. Such action initiatives took the form of offering co-supervisory places, Trust-based support groups, pilot implementation projects, supervisory consultancy and research about the practice of clinical supervision and the effect of the educational preparation.

Opportunities for co-supervision

Practitioners who had completed the module could apply for training positions on future modules that allowed them to work with an experienced supervisor. This in turn provided opportunities for them to practise as co-supervisors in the module's groups. This structure enabled them to obtain skills practice, feedback and provided opportunities to learn from the practice of an experienced supervisor. The number of co-supervisors in any module has ranged from two to four practitioners.

Support groups

Two of the local trusts who had supported staff to attend the module asked for further assistance in establishing forums where practitioners could come together to work on developing clinical supervision in their settings. After contract negotiations, one group met monthly and used the group as a medium for the supervision of the work of supervisors. The other group saw its task as raising general awareness of supervision within the trust by contributing to the production of a 'standard' and a 'mission statement' for clinical supervision as well as supporting the members' attempts to introduce clinical supervision.

Pilot implementation projects

The team also had invitations to support implementation pilots within a community healthcare trust (Draper *et al.* 1999) and more recently with a professional association for practice nurses. Such support took the form of working with the supervisors and the practice and professional development officers to plan the pilot. It also incorporated structures for the systematic evaluation of these projects. Structures were also put in place for the supervision of the supervisors and the monitoring of the projects, in order to help those involved understand and deal with critical events that occurred.

Supervisory consultancy

Educationalists have also been contracted by local trusts to offer supervision with selected members of staff. This seems to have been associated with a need to assist individuals to cope with role change such as promotion.

Research

The module and its associated developments have provided a useful platform and a source of data for reports (Morris, 1999), research projects related to the educational experience (Rafferty, 1999) and the module's impact on practice (Jenkins *et al.*, 2000). It has also acted as an impetus for the generation of a conceptual model for clinical supervision (Rafferty, 2000). This conceptual model for supervision is being used as the basis to guide supervisory skills rehearsal in a Level 3 module within the School's BSc(Hons) Nurse Practitioner pathway.

Study days

Part of the initiative has involved study days. These were essentially to do with introducing the concept, enabling participants to understand the functions of clinical supervision and then make links with the utility of such ideas for the participants' own practice. As well as single study days (Coleman and Rafferty, 1995), there has been a programme of two-day and three day workshops. The two-day workshops have been experiential and skills focused. The three-day workshops have been with group specific teams of colleagues. Here the approach has been about the generation of a 'common vision' of clinical supervision within that practice setting and helping them to think through an action plan for its implementation.

On top of such initiatives, since 1995 we have held three recall days, partly funded by the WNB. These served both to chart the progress of development in relation to clinical supervision and to provide participants with occasions for support and reunion. Two conferences have also been held by the School on the theme of clinical supervision. It is worth stressing that a number of practitioners have developed their own in-house training schemes for clinical supervision.

Reflections on the experience of these educational developments

Our experience of working with practitioners as well as our own experience of supervision lends support to the case for clinical supervision in nursing and health visiting. In order to provide an explanation of our conviction, it is helpful to revisit the three functions that form the basis for the experiential elements of the module.

Restorative function

Working with practitioners gives force to the fact that care work is emotional work and the emotions engendered by the work can be complex, disturbing and potentially damaging. Our experience suggests that many practitioners have to deal with the emotionality of their work alone, with little help and perhaps ability to find restorative meanings out of the often sad, perplexing and overwhelming nature of care work. **In short, care can hurt and our experience reinforces the belief that people who feel cared for are more able to care for others.**

Formative

Practice is complex. Providing nurses with opportunities to speak about their practice puts them in touch with how complex their familiar world is and how much it is 'taken for granted'. It is worth recognising that there is a relationship between a low sense of accomplishment at work and burnout. It may be regarded as somewhat obvious however that one way of 'taking this on' is by helping practitioners to make sense of the work that they do.

Normative

Professional care always involves judgements that involve risk. Providing nurses, via supervision, with the opportunity to account for their decisions and subsequent actions in an environment that is supportive, challenging and non-punitive provides the conditions where practitioners can protect themselves. **Supervision provides opportunities to rehearse the choices that are available as well as enabling practitioners to acknowledge the limits of their own capabilities and the capabilities of others.** Such a service is a principal means of protecting clients and organisations.

Phenomena worth noting

However whilst these statements reflect our beliefs and learning reinforced by the experience of the module, it also need to be acknowledged that there are phenomena (which we illustrate using metaphors) that could bedevil further implementation of supervision. These may only be local phenomena but it is possible that they may well be generalisable to a UK-wide context.

Metaphor one. The wings, the halo and the harp phenomenon

This phenomenon refers to what seems to be an expectation that supervisors have to be perfect. Such an expectation we believe leads many experienced and able individuals with highly developed clinical and interpersonal skills to avoid taking on the role of being a 'clinical supervisor'. Our hunch is that the clarity that supervision structures can give to supervision means that inevitably we will often realise that most of the time we are just 'good enough' and sometimes 'not good enough'. This needs to be understood in terms of an established social myth that nurses have to be perfect. Ultimately, acknowledging that each of us is imperfect and learning to become comfortable with this awareness is one of the tasks of being a supervisor and hopefully facing this fact will begin to enable many able individuals to act in this capacity.

Metaphor two. The rabbit in the headlight phenomenon

This is another way of describing the concept of 'learned helplessness' which appears to affect many nurses in relation to the problems they encounter in their work. Again, the resistance that nurses can exhibit to the inevitable personal challenge that is involved in clinical supervision can be seen as the result of a common coping strategy. This is characterised by 'frozen inaction' or 'we can't do anything about it', employed to avoid difficult, painful and challenging issues. Effective supervision breaks the illusion of 'powerlessness' and reinforces accountability to act. But as this means action rather than inaction, we can well understand how a profession affected with such a degree of 'learned helplessness' would balk at the challenge that clinical supervision presents.

Metaphor three. The can of worms phenomenon

This refers to the recurring fear that a practitioner is going to bring something to supervision that is troublesome and dangerous. The fantasy then is that the supervisor will be left 'holding the baby' or potentially damaged by it. Another aspect of this phenomenon is the fear that supervisors will not be able to cope with the issues brought to supervision. It is a feature of supervision that practitioners may bring troublesome issues. The function of supervision is to enable such issues to be considered in a constructive and healthy fashion. However, if supervision is not in place, then the question is how might such issues be considered and what could be the consequent damage to patients, the organisation and practitioners themselves? Supervision can be about opening 'cans of worms' but in a way that leads to appropriate and thoughtful action.

Metaphor four. The 'it will rock the boat' phenomenon

Another way of explaining the problem of finding resources or the will to support clinical supervision is that this is a covert way to maintain the status quo. Clinical supervision, which is inevitably about change, also is inevitably about creating another way of seeing things i.e. 'Super Vision'. This other way of seeing things inevitably challenges established hierarchical structural and practice norms. This tension needs to be faced in order to challenge any covert practices.

Metaphor five. The 'nobody knows what it is about' phenomenon

Despite the level of attention that has been placed within the nursing profession on clinical supervision, many course participants claim that their colleagues are mainly ignorant about what 'it really is'. One interpretation of this could be that some nurses don't read, however, another interpretation is that this represents a widespread non-acceptance that it is possible to have helpful, growth focused and sustaining relationships as a matter of course in our work. If true then this represents a serious problem in healthcare organisations.

The need for curriculum reform

As part of the evaluation process of the module, which has included a course-monitoring group, supervisor's supervision and research initiatives (Jenkins *et al.*, 2000; Rafferty, 1999), a curriculum review is at present occurring. This review is attempting to address some of the following issues:

• The course aims are to prepare supervisors when in reality we have some evidence that the number of students on the course who go on to function as a supervisor is low. A factor that seems to enable the transition of students to become supervisors appears to be that they are based in settings where there is an organisational commitment to making it happen. Attendance at a course, by itself, does not make it happen. A painful aspect of being involved with the course is that you are inviting the practitioner in many clinical settings to go and 'bang their head against the wall'. It appears to be an uphill struggle to implement this innovation. One explanation for this is that despite all the work and the publications, general knowledge about clinical supervision in practice remains low. Another explanation, particularly in acute care, is that there are just about enough resources to do the job of care and none for this 'luxury' called clinical supervision. The legitimate need to recognise and resource 'pit head time' and the value of learning from practice in practice have still to be won.

- We believe that one of the strengths but also one of the difficulties associated with the course is that it is concerned with the 'essence and not just the trappings' of clinical supervision. By this we mean that it attempts to deal with supervision meaningfully and not just pay lip service to the meaning of the concept. The time frame of the course may well be seen as generous (fifteen study days). However, to bring about the 'new meaning' of supervision seen as necessary by Faugier and Butterworth (1993) involves a process of deconstruction, challenge and learning which to the course team makes the current time frame feel ambitious, if not constraining.

- Central to the experiential activities incorporated within the original design of the course were menus of appropriate concerns intended to address our view of the focus and remit of clinical supervision in practice. The experience of running the courses indicates that the original division of the experiential activities needs to be redrawn, because having a focus for the activities based around the functions of supervision often prevented adequate exploration of their interrelationship and were too complex a task at the typical practitioner level.

- The content of the courses has presented students with a 'smorgasbord' of different concepts and perspectives seen as valid knowledge by the original course planning team. Examples include moral and ethical thinking, group dynamics, systemic thinking, transactional analysis, change theory and crisis theory. Such a diet is often experienced by the practitioners as rich and a cause of indigestion. Whilst this indigestion often resolves itself in time there is a need to find a way of helping the students digest it more easily. This is part of a wider need not to see such courses as 'one off' or standalone 'entities'. It is now clear that courses such as this should be a point on a continuum that begins at a pre-registration level and continues to levels of advanced practice development.

The ongoing process of the curriculum review has been very difficult in terms of trying to make sense of a complex, tangled range of learning, from which we had to bring into a new pattern to go forward. On the positive side, a function of the module was to establish the case for clinical supervision in practice. We feel that we have achieved this. We have also been able to determine something of the nature of appropriate practice and the kinds of challenges that complicate practice.

However, the negative side draws attention repeatedly to problems of language (jargon) and the increasingly complex 'ideas world' of supervision. These ideas, however, as identified earlier need to be conveyed at an appropriate developmental level. Another important issue is providing the kind of supervisory experience which was a developmental challenge to the participants, without being perceived as an assault on self. The danger is that individuals can be forced to face elements of awareness about themselves and their practice that they were neither intellectually or developmentally equipped to deal with.

We were also increasingly confounded by having to meet so many different developmental needs, from 'tell me what supervision is?' to 'help me examine my supervisory practice of other supervisors'.

Health and education organisation's problems in creating the macro structure for clinical supervision seemed also to rest in not being able to see further than the supervisee/supervisor relationship. This is because of the lack of models, which sets this professional relationship within a wider developmental and organisational context.

The clear message that comes from these reflections about the module is that it has taken us a considerable amount of time to gain clarity and certainty about the aim(s) and purpose(s) of education for clinical supervision. It is now obvious that what the module intended to achieve and prepare participants for was unclear. We now see that the module was a product of its time. The service and educational understandings that were once relevant now have to be rethought.

Conclusion

If clinical supervision is meant to be a 'career-long' concept then it is important that preparation should mirror the developmental stage of the practitioner. Preparation for clinical supervision should not be a 'one-stop shop' occurring at one stage of the practitioner's journey from beginner to expert. The new structures need to be built on partnership between practice and education in order to encompass the principle of 'life-long learning'. They also need to model appropriate structure and process for clinical supervision itself in both service and educational settings.

Figure 6.1 outlines a possible structure for addressing these issues. It is built on a model of six stages within an individual's career path starting at pre-registration and continuing to advanced level practice. At each stage there would be a preparatory educational input and supervision experiences. These experiences not only set the model for the educational process but also establish an appropriate practice model for each stage. For example, professional transitions are not confined to the move from student to qualified nurse. Transition experiences are career long. Undertaking educational preparation to become a clinical supervisor of other supervisors also needs to be robust enough to provide a model for the practice. The boxes in each stage begin to establish the tasks and processes related to clinical supervision activity

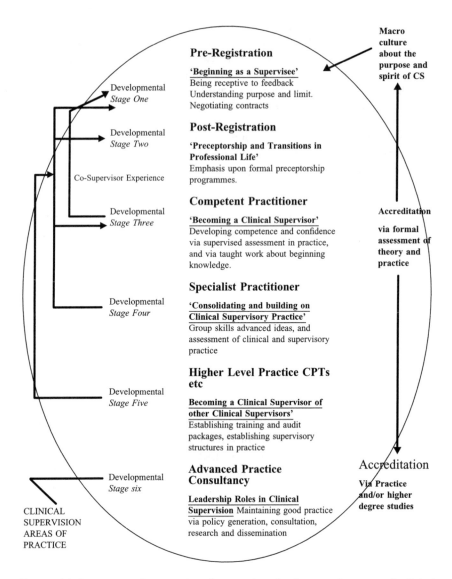

Figure 6.1 A structure for ensuring the ongoing developmental nature of clinical supervision throughout a practitioner's career (SHS (UWS) CS INFO. GROUP 1. (MC.EJ.IL.MR)MARCH 7, 2000)

appropriate at that level. The lines between the stages identify the patterns of supervisory practice appropriate within the educational preparation and within practice. For example, an individual at Development Stage Four (whose key task is 'Consolidating and building on Clinical Supervisory Practice') would be involved as a clinical supervisor for individuals in Stages One, Two and

Three. An individual in Developmental Stage Three would obtain experience as a co-supervisor of individuals in Development Stage One and Two, with the co-supervision being with an individual at Developmental Stage Four.

The boundary around the model is designed to point up the need for a macro culture pertinent to all levels of supervisory development that is congruent with the knowledge, ideals, philosophy and spirit of this type of professional relationship.

The exact specification with regards to the knowledge, skills and experience at each level is the next task of the curriculum review. We feel confident that we have the stories of such experiences in ourselves and in the practitioners that we work with.

References

Coleman M and Rafferty M (1995) Using workshops to implement clinical supervision. *Nursing Standard* 9(50), pp27–29.

Draper B Koukos C Fletcher P Whitehead A Reynolds F Coleman M and Rafferty M (1999) Evaluating an initiative: clinical supervision in a community health trust. *British Journal of Community Nursing* 4(10), pp525–530.

Faugier J and Butterworth T (1993) *Clinical Supervision: A Position Paper.* School of Nursing Studies, University of Manchester.

Jenkins E Rafferty M and Parke E (2000) Clinical supervision: What is going on in West Wales? Results of a telephone survey. *Nursing Times Research* 5(1), pp21–37.

Morris L (1999) Definition and the case for clinical supervision. *Assignment* 5(2), pp4–10.

Proctor B (1986) Supervision: a co-operative exercise in accountability. In Maken M and Payne M (eds) *Enabling and Ensuring* National Youth Bureau for Education and Training in Youth and Community Work, Leicester.

Rafferty M and Coleman M (1996) Educating nurses to undertake clinical supervision in practice. *Nursing Standard* 10(45), pp38–41.

Rafferty M (1998) Clinical Supervision. In Barnes E, Griffiths P, Ord J, Wells D. (eds) *Face to Face with Distress* London: Butterworth Heinemann.

Rafferty M (1999) A study of student responses to an educational preparation for clinical supervision. *Development of Professional Practice – Occasional Papers (WNB)* April 1999 (3), pp14–18.

Rafferty M (2000) A conceptual model for clinical supervision in nursing and health visiting based upon Winnicott's (1960) theory of the parent-infant relationship. *Journal of Psychiatric and Mental Health Nursing* In press.

Part II

7 Implementing clinical supervision in a NHS community trust – sharing the vision

Jenny Bennett, Bob Gardener and Fiona James

Editorial

This chapter outlines how a group of practitioners (lead professionals) facilitated the widespread implementation and development of clinical supervision within a NHS community trust. Drawing on the experiences of health visitors, general nurses and community psychiatric nurses, the authors describe the phases or stages of this implementation process. Furthermore, they describe their particular roles involved in the implementation and use case examples of the introduction of clinical supervision into each practice discipline. The chapter concludes with reflections on the implementation process and identifies some of the barriers to introducing clinical supervision.

The widespread introduction of clinical supervision within the NHS is not a development that can be introduced using a 'quick fix' technique. We believe that in order to bring about the widespread introduction, a shift in culture throughout the NHS, may be required: a shift towards a culture that welcomes and encourages the examination of one's practice, the ventilation of any feelings, openness and transparency within practitioners, and views such endeavours as supportive, necessary and enabling.

Introduction

This chapter describes how a group of three lead professionals underwent the task of facilitating the implementation and development of clinical supervision within our community health care trust. Our organisation is a community trust, including several community hospitals, which serves a wide geographical area with both rural and urban locations with a population of 370,000.

Our roles as lead professionals were new within our organisation and were part of the Quality and Professional Development Directorate, which took the lead on the clinical governance agenda. We had specific responsibility for the facilitation of professional and practice development within our nursing disciplines of community hospital nursing, mental health nursing and health visiting.

A central aspect of the role of lead professional for the first two years of the post was the promotion, implementation and development of clinical supervision. We were to focus on our own nursing disciplines but also to forward recommendations for the long-term strategic implementation of clinical supervision throughout the organisation.

Our implementation plans were guided by:

- *National picture* – responding to national policy documents on the health service and the development of nursing which highlighted the need for lifelong learning and the role of clinical supervision in providing a quality service (UKCC, 1996; Department of Health, 1997, 1998).
- *Local picture* – within our organisation a comprehensive nursing review had recently been conducted guided by *Vision for the Future* (Department of Health and NHSE, 1993). All nursing disciplines identified a role for clinical supervision in supporting clinical practice and a major recommendation was to plan for its introduction.

Throughout this chapter we therefore describe how we worked in our own nursing disciplines to facilitate the implementation of clinical supervision. This involved working with community mental health teams, health visitors working within primary health care teams and the wards/departments of community hospitals.

Planning

Following our appointment as lead professionals we allocated time to enable all three of us to have a full discussion and debate on clinical supervision. This was guided by our experience of clinical supervision, our own beliefs about its value and limitations, discussions with other colleagues and the literature on clinical supervision. As a group we had a shared belief in the value of clinical supervision in improving the quality of services we provide. We debated the role, purpose and function of clinical supervision and adopted the three interactive elements of educative, supportive and personal management and monitoring, as the primary functions of clinical supervision as derived from Proctor's model (1986). This common understanding and agreement on the function of clinical supervision was essential in enabling us to share a vision of how we could facilitate the implementation and development of clinical supervision and communicate this to others.

We used the knowledge and understanding we had gained during our discussion to produce a project plan. The stages of the rational planning process, described in Table 7.1, guided the production of our project plan.

Through this process we were able to identify the practical tasks we would need to undertake and the personal, professional and organisational issues we would need to address. We set ourselves clear objectives with time scales for review. A central tenet supporting the project plan was for us to openly

Table 7.1 Identified stages of the planning process

- What are we trying to do?
- What is the best way of doing it?
- What are we going to have to do?
- In what order?
- What resources will we need?
- Let's review it: is it going to work?
- Who is going to do what and when?

express our enthusiasm for and belief in clinical supervision, inspiring others to be involved in developing a true shared vision of the potential of clinical supervision in enhancing the quality of clinical practice. A shared vision has been shown to be an important element in achieving successful organisational change (Kouzes and Posner, 1995). We would be seeking to develop relationships that encouraged others to become actively involved and inspired. Bass and Avolio (1994) and Guastello (1995) describe how this approach can 'transform' work areas to become more productive and more responsive to change.

Kohner (1994) in her discussion on introducing clinical supervision highlighted the need for all staff locally to be involved in the process of planning for its introduction. We wanted to engender a style that encouraged commitment and used the strengths and creative ideas of practitioners. Therefore our approach to the implementation and development of clinical supervision was to encourage its introduction from the practitioner level in the first instance and was underpinned by the following principles:

- To build on the good practice that was already taking place within the organisation with respect to clinical supervision.
- To provide information, advice and support to practitioners that would facilitate individual areas to make informed decisions with regard to the implementation and development of clinical supervision.
- To respond enthusiastically to the positive requests from individual areas within our organisation with regard to their desire to implement/develop clinical supervision.
- Where available, to work alongside clinical leaders in individual areas to develop their knowledge base and experience, promoting local ownership and their role and strengths as change agents.
- To use a flexible approach that was responsive and sensitive to practitioners' level of knowledge, experience and professional confidence.

Using the above as our guiding principles we reflected on what our roles as leaders and facilitators in the implementation process should involve. We identified the following key elements:

- Change agent: To act as key change agents with a formal responsibility for advising on the implementation and development of clinical supervision. Our leadership style would promote ownership and commitment by individuals in local areas, building on their strengths and talents.
- Partner: To work alongside practitioners and managers to meet shared objectives.
- Educator: To organise and deliver informal and formal training on the role, function and benefits of clinical supervision.
- Advice and support: To develop a resource library on clinical supervision and respond to managers' and practitioners' requests for information and support.
- Communicator: To ensure managers and practitioners are informed of the local and organisational developments regarding clinical supervision.
- Networking and co-ordination: To promote the sharing of good practice across the organisation and the sharing of strategies to overcome difficulties.

Establishing a baseline

One of our first tasks on the project plan was to establish what clinical supervision was already taking place within our individual nursing disciplines and what practitioners' knowledge, thoughts and attitudes were regarding clinical supervision. We devised a comprehensive questionnaire, based on the issues identified in a review of the relevant empirical literature, in conjunction with the clinical audit and research team, and sent this to all practitioners in our disciplines. In total 377 questionnaires were distributed and there was an overall response rate of 55 per cent. This was an encouraging response and reflected a positive attitude towards clinical supervision which was evident in the qualitative sections of the questionnaire. The questionnaire covered areas such as baseline provision, practitioners' level of knowledge and understanding and their views as to how clinical supervision should be developed further. The results highlighted an overall lack of knowledge and experience with regard to clinical supervision and therefore a high level of training needs. However, within community mental health teams clinical supervision was established, though its purpose and content was in need of review. Guided by the results we devised a flexible introductory training package on clinical supervision and decided to meet with all areas to give them the opportunity to be informed of clinical supervision and take part in its implementation.

Sharing the vision

We therefore visited individual areas and were enthusiastic to inspire others in our belief that clinical supervision had a valuable contribution to make in improving the quality of service we provide. We initially targeted receptive clinical leaders or teams that we had identified through meetings during our induction as lead professionals or by direct interest that we had received. **Working with individuals that had a positive interest enabled us to initiate a change process and these areas were able to act as motivators and role models for others.**

Whilst we had a desire to share our enthusiasm, it was important that during our initial meetings with individuals we actively listened to their beliefs and opinions about the functions of clinical supervision, the implementation process and their expectations of us. This proved essential to the development of shared and realistic implementation plans. Time was spent discussing and clarifying all aspects of clinical supervision. It was important that there was a shared understanding of the aims and functions of clinical supervision and its impact upon their practice and development. Our approach in supporting the development of local implementation plans was to empower them to reflect on their current situation and be enthusiastic about what could be achieved. Their central role in the implementation process was reinforced and we informed them that we were available to provide them with help, advice and formal training. When discussing the implementation process there was open and honest communication regarding the difficulties that could be encountered.

Case study examples

Below are three examples that illustrate the implementation process in action in each of our respective disciplines. As discussed previously, to support this work we provided awareness raising sessions across the organisation. These sessions were organised around individual areas' work patterns so that they were accessible to as many practitioners as possible. We also provided more in-depth supervisee' and supervisor's training as requested. The provision of a formal clinical supervisors' course for practitioners from all nursing disciplines was then purchased from a local university and following on from the success of this, a contract was agreed for them to provide further courses.

Example one. Health visiting

The results of the baseline questionnaire highlighted that the majority of health visitors within the organisation did not give or receive clinical supervision. Of those that did report being involved in the process of clinical supervision, the results of the questionnaire suggested that there were different interpretations of the term amongst health visitors, including confusion with mentorship and child protection supervision. It was identified that there was a need to clarify and clearly define what is meant by the term clinical supervision and its aims and objectives, with 62 per cent of health visitors reporting that they had only an average knowledge of clinical supervision and 20 per cent reporting having a poor knowledge base. However, overall health visitors were positive about the concept of clinical supervision and welcomed its introduction into practice.

Within the organisation, health visitors worked in widespread geographical areas and many were based within individual primary health care teams. Initial discussions with health visitors across the district raised several key issues and concerns. These included how clinical supervision could be organised and resourced within each geographical area in addition to who would co-ordinate this, as for many areas there wasn't a designated team leader or health visitor with a practice development role. There was also a debate as to which health visitors would become clinical supervisors of others and whether one-to-one, group or peer supervision would be the most appropriate model for health visiting. There was also the issue that no one was trained as a clinical supervisor. Reflection on these discussions highlighted that there was a diversity of opinions amongst health visitors as to a strategic way forward in health visiting and that there was no easy solution to these questions.

Returning to the principles that we had set in our initial discussions as lead professionals, and a certain level of pragmatism, proved to be the way forward. We wrote to all health visitors offering them the opportunity to be a pilot site for clinical supervision with support and individual training. One group of health visitors who worked together in a clinic setting came forward requesting to undertake peer group supervision. Within this group one health visitor did have previous experience of clinical supervision and a further health visitor had previously received some training. Two morning workshops were spent exploring the concept of clinical supervision, models of reflection, contracting and documentation and how to conduct a group session. The health visitors were keen to proceed and began meeting on a monthly basis with regular review. Their continued interest and motivation was key to the success of this pilot.

Simultaneously, four health visitors from different geographical locations were invited to attend the external clinical supervisor's course. Nominations were requested from individuals who would be prepared to undertake this role after completion of the course and act as a champion for clinical supervision in their area. These health visitors formed a supportive group and it was arranged for them to receive group supervision from an external supervisor for six months following the course. This gave the health visitors valuable experience in receiving clinical supervision and proved to be very successful in building up their confidence, particularly in group supervision. During this six months, we organised supervisee training workshops in each of the geographical locations and conducted them alongside these four health visitors. The aim of these sessions was to support them in facilitating their colleagues' knowledge of and interest in clinical supervision and to encourage other health visitors to either receive clinical supervision or to attend supervisor training. The result of this was very positive as health visitors wanting to receive supervision approached the four clinical supervisors and they have set up both one to one and group clinical supervision, depending on what was requested, with a small number of health visitors in their area. In addition, the clinical supervisors continue to meet for peer group supervision.

Through individual health visitors beginning to set up clinical supervision arrangements on either a one-to-one or group basis, more health visitors are becoming aware of the purpose and benefits of clinical supervision and are either requesting supervision or attending clinical supervisor training. The implementation is therefore an incremental process but it is evolving flexibly with participation from health visitors and in response to local needs.

Example two. Community hospitals

This section describes three examples of how ward nurses have introduced clinical supervision. They illustrate that a diverse approach to the implementation of clinical supervision was taken within community hospitals

It is important to note that prior to implementing clinical supervision in the community hospitals, a selection of nurses from community hospitals attended a leadership course. This acted as a catalyst for discussion on clinical supervision. These nurses identified that they would need to experience clinical supervision before being able to develop clinical supervision in their ward and day hospital areas. Monthly one-to-one external clinical supervision was subsequently purchased by the organisation for a fixed period of six months. Several of the nurses who had experienced the external clinical supervision put forward formal plans to implement clinical supervision into their wards and day hospitals. They adopted different approaches according to their view of local needs as shown by the following examples.

One ward manager decided to supervise all the qualified nurses on their ward for a fixed period of time and then review the whole process. As lead professionals we made the ward manager aware of the constraints of hierarchical supervision, and the ward manager put forward a logical reason for this approach. The ward manager felt it was a starting point, as initially there were no clinical supervisors available and it would be a good way to demonstrate to ward nurses that dedicated time was available for them to reflect on their practice. The longer-term aim was to train nurses from the ward to become supervisors thus ultimately removing the hierarchical structure.

The second example involves a manager from another community hospital who allocated supervisors to all nurses. The rationale for this approach was in the manager's words 'to get clinical supervision started in our hospital'. As lead professionals we discussed and challenged this approach, making the manager aware that it was important that nurses should be actively involved and own the implementation process. However, the manager continued with this approach, and we advised that they should consider reviewing progress at an early date.

In the third example, a ward manager encouraged and supported two nurses from the ward to receive clinical supervision from the lead professionals. In time one of the practitioners went on to facilitate group supervision for four ward colleagues. This approach to implementation has proved successful and it continues to meet.

Example three. Community Mental Health Team

The Lead Professional for Mental Health Nursing met with all the community mental health teams (CMHT) within our organisation. The following is a brief outline of the discussions with one specific team, which highlights the issues facing the majority of the teams. The key discussion points were guided by the results of the questionnaire, and the discussions occurred within meetings with the lead nurse within the CMHT and with all the CMHT nurses.

On a positive note, the majority of nurses reported that they were receiving clinical supervision on an individual basis, at a monthly interval. Whilst there were nurses who reported they were not receiving clinical supervision on a monthly basis, this was the frequency they were aiming for.

There was a history of clinical supervision taking place within the CMHT and it was valued and seen as 'much needed'. However, there were issues raised by the lead nurse and the nurses within the CMHT as to the way clinical supervision was organised and carried out.

The lead nurse within the CMHT who has designated management responsibility for all the nurses provided clinical and management supervision within one session, dividing the time between both areas. This structure of provision had developed in an unplanned way and was a response to a rapid increase in the number of nurses working within the CMHT, who needed both types of supervision.

The nurses expressed a positive view of the clinical supervision they received from the lead nurse. However there was confusion between clinical and management supervision and concern that the sessions were dominated by management issues.

Other issues that arose out of the discussions were that prior to commencement of clinical supervision there had been no contract drawn up between the clinical supervisor and supervisee, and that in the subsequent session little or no documentation was used. It was also apparent that there was no choice of clinical supervisor.

The lead nurse within the CMHT was motivated to further explore the issues raised by the discussions and the results from the questionnaires. I therefore continued to meet with the lead nurse providing written information and offering guidance about the issues that had been raised. The lead nurse after discussion with the nurses from the CMHT decided to implement the following changes:

- To hold clinical supervision separately from management supervision.
- Management supervision would be termed caseload management.
- The lead nurse within the CMHT would continue to be clinical supervisor for all the nurses but it had been openly acknowledged that there could be potential conflict in a line manager providing clinical supervision.
- The supervisee would be responsible for setting the agenda within the clinical supervision sessions. The lead nurse had provided all nurses with

a booklet in which to document the sessions. This was their property and they were encouraged to use it in support of their professional portfolio.

- A contract would be drawn up based around the discussions that had taken place as to the aim and function of clinical supervision. Sample contracts were available to the team.

At the time of writing no formal evaluation has been carried out as to the effects of these changes. There have been positive verbal comments from the lead nurse and by some of the nurses from the CMHT, especially that the changes have allowed them to focus and reflect on their issues with regard to clinical practice.

In implementing these changes the lead nurse within the CMHT has been able to promote clarity as to the function of clinical supervision and caseload management and as to how they both support the nurses in their demanding role. The lead nurse dealt positively with the change process and educated his manager as to the need for and benefit of the changes made.

Finally two other points raised are worthy of mention. First, whilst most nurses had experience of clinical supervision, very few had received training. Second, some nurses identified a need for 'specialist' supervision to enable them to practise a specific therapeutic approach i.e. cognitive behavioural therapy.

Reflections on the implementation process

There are relatively few studies that specifically discuss the local implementation of clinical supervision (Fowler, 1996). Authors have generally highlighted specific areas that need considering and/or potential problems that need to be overcome (Devine and Baxter, 1995). Below are our reflections on the process of facilitating the local implementation of clinical supervision. Our aim during the first year of the implementation process within our organisation was to develop a culture that supported and valued clinical supervision. To add clarity on this we have divided our discussion into the separate areas of ownership, developing an organisational approach and barriers to change.

Ownership

The importance we gave to the need for practitioners to own the implementation process, to value and want clinical supervision has proved to be successful. In areas where there are identified clinical leaders motivated to promote clinical supervision the process of implementation has moved forward. We have positive examples of areas where clinical supervision is now happening on a regular basis and is valued by practitioners. An example is given in Box 7.1.

We now need to build upon this success, sharing the good practice and positive experiences of clinical supervision with other areas. At an organisational level we are considering how we identify and develop future clinical leaders to progress the implementation of clinical supervision in areas where

Box 7.1: Clinical supervision. A ward manager's reflections

It has taken a long time and a lot of work to get clinical supervision up and running on our ward. Prior to my arrival as ward manager, my predecessor and the ward staff had put a lot of effort into the topic. Some staff had been on courses to learn about it and the lead professional had been involved for several months, first in an educative role, then in a supportive role, leading some group supervision.

Despite all of this there was a degree of apprehension about taking on the issue. People felt that they still did not know enough about it. In many ways it was like learning to ride a bike. They had had the theory, they had seen other people do it, but there was still some reluctance to actually have a go. It took some bravery to get on and try but the staff did so, deciding to offer supervision to each other. At the same time the G grades in our local community hospitals took the initiative to buy in the services of an outsider to provide supervision for themselves.

With two very different models (peer and external supervisors) there have been strikingly similar outcomes. Almost everybody who has had access to clinical supervision has said the same thing, that they have been surprised at how much benefit they have got from the process. Also it is a bit like riding a bike in that the more you try to break down and explain it the more complicated it appears. As long as you have some knowledge about safety, when and how to apply the brakes etc. then the best way to learn is to actually have a go. It is not as hard as it seems.

Personally I have worked through some very complex and troublesome situations in my sessions. They have helped me to focus on and resolve some problems, which I believe would otherwise have caused me far bigger head-aches. Were it not for my one hour per month of supervision, the same problems would probably have caused me many times more hours of work and hassle, so it has saved me time and helped me to work more efficiently. In a nutshell, clinical supervision has enabled me to work smarter, not harder.

A Ward Manager

minimal supervision is taken place. The need to maintain local ownership will remain important as will the need to work in partnership with the managers of the service.

Developing an organisational approach

As discussed in our reflections on ownership, in the first instance we were keen to promote individual practitioners' understanding of clinical supervision and their role in developing supervision locally. We became acutely aware that this needed to be supported by an organisational approach to clinical supervision. Practitioners have an important role in developing clinical supervision but they also need the support of managers and the organisation to do this. As we worked with practitioners they raised this issue. For example, practitioners were keen to know that they were entitled to clinical supervision and questioned whether there was an organisational policy to support this.

They were also requesting standard guidelines for issues such as setting up contracts between the supervisor and supervisee and the documentation of clinical supervision sessions.

Throughout the first stages of the implementation process we worked with practitioners' line managers on an individual basis but we also led a formal session for managers on their role in supporting clinical supervision and the difference between clinical supervision and management supervision. The implementation of clinical supervision was seen to need a 'partnership approach': to be successful, both managers and nurses would need to see its value and be committed to its development. In order to promote an organisational strategy for clinical supervision including the provision of resources to ensure that the implementation moved forward, we produced an interim report after twelve months in post. The report detailed current progress with the implementation process and put forward recommendations for a future organisational approach to implementation, including resource and training implications. Together with the Director and Assistant Director of Nursing, we presented the report to the senior management board and the senior nursing and professional advisory groups.

As a result of this process and significant background work, we have made progress in promoting practitioner involvement and local implementation supported by an organisational approach. We now have a written validated clinical supervision policy in addition to guidelines on the aims and function of clinical supervision, the role and responsibilities of supervisors and supervisees and the use of documentation. Importantly we have agreement on the need to draw up contracts prior to commencing clinical supervision that cover the issues of confidentiality and information that needs to be disclosed/shared and the need for regular review. We have also set up a clinical supervision steering group that includes senior management and practitioner representation to strategically take forward the implementation of clinical supervision. We are formulating a five year implementation plan and through the clinical supervision steering group progress will be monitored. We will continue to empower local areas to develop implementation plans, and as they report on progress this will inform our continued planning.

Barriers to change

Implementing clinical supervision has involved a change process. As with any change process, as lead professionals we were aware that we might encounter barriers to change and resistance. Our leadership approach within our disciplines has aimed to minimise barriers and resistance and has promoted a positive approach.

Our approach of sharing a vision of the potential of clinical supervision for nursing practice and promoting practitioner involvement enabled practitioners to be committed to receiving clinical supervision and finding realistic ways to achieving its implementation.

It would be unrealistic to suggest that we are not encountering barriers. Examples of barriers to change that lead professionals and practitioners have identified are summarised in Box 7.2. These have ranged from individual factors to wider organisational issues.

Box 7.2: Examples of barriers to change

- Resources: e.g. lack of clinical supervisors
- Individual resistance: e.g. some practitioners expressed that they did not need it
- Workload factors: e.g. high caseloads, shortage of qualified nurses
- Concurrent change: e.g. other practice developments taking place
- Lack of knowledge: e.g. high level of training needs

We have openly recognised these barriers to change and through our ongoing discussions and support within the lead professional team we have developed the following strategies for addressing them:

- Developing supportive relationships with practitioners which encouraged them to identify potential problematic areas and develop creative approaches to deal with them.
- The use of informal and formal training sessions in an environment that allowed practitioners to openly express their beliefs and concerns regarding clinical supervision.
- Developing implementation plans with individuals and their areas that were realistic, achievable and encouraged an incremental approach.
- Building on success and empowering practitioners to motivate their colleagues.
- Our use of self to provide ongoing positive support and encouragement through time of resistance and change.

Conclusion

The implementation of clinical supervision should not simply be seen as a task that needs staff to be trained and then to do it. Clinical supervision should be seen as part of the framework that enables nurses (and others) to provide a quality service. It needs to be introduced into the culture of the organisation, one that promotes individuals to maximise their strength, promotes autonomy and encourages reflection. In order to achieve this culture, managers and practitioners need to work in partnership and the organisation needs to be committed to being a learning organisation that aims to facilitate lifelong learning (Haire, 1997). Planning for the implementation of clinical supervision therefore needs to include a long-term goal of aiming for it to become a routine and valued practice.

References

Bass B M and Avolio B (1994) *Improving Organisational Effectiveness Through Transformational Leadership*. London: Sage.

Department of Health and NHS Management Executive (1993) *Vision for the Future: The Nursing, Midwifery and Health Visiting Contribution to Health and Health Care*. London: HMSO.

Department of Health (1997) *Modern and Dependable*. London: Department of Health.

Department of Health (1998) *A First Class Service: Quality in the new NHS*. London: Department of Health.

Devine A and Baxter T D (1995) Introducing clinical supervision: a guide. *Nursing Standard*, 9, (40), pp32–34.

Fowler, J (1996) The organisation of clinical supervision within the nursing profession within the UK. *Journal of Advanced Nursing*, 23, pp471–478.

Guastello S (1995) Facilitative style, individual innovation and emergent leadership in problem-solving groups. *Journal of Creative Behaviour*, 29, pp225–239.

Haire C (1997) Life-long learning, *Nursing Management*, 3 (9), pp24–25.

Kohner N (1994) *Clinical Supervision*. London: Kings Fund Centre.

Kouzes J M and Posner B Z (1995) *The Leadership Challenge: How to keep getting extraordinary things done in organisations*. San Francisco: Jossey-Bass.

Proctor B (1986) On being a trainer. In Drydrew W and Thorne B (eds) *Training and Supervision for Counseling in Action*, pp49–73. London: Sage.

UKCC (1996) *Position Statement of Clinical Supervision for Nursing and Health Visiting*. London: UKCC.

8   Implementing clinical supervision

A personal experience

Denise Hadfield

Editorial

This chapter reports on the experiences of a former clinical supervision co-ordinator and her attempts to implement clinical supervision within a medium sized NHS trust. It includes the background to this development, the particular plan of action produced to introduce supervision and highlights the training which occurred. The measures taken to evaluate the effects of introducing supervision are described and the author outlines the next steps which were planned.

In keeping with the 'practice development' literature, attempts to introduce clinical supervision within NHS trusts appear to be most successful using a 'normative/re-educative' approach. Collective ownership of the development is encouraged whereby practitioners are encouraged to become key players (or change agents) in the change process. Consequently, the widespread introduction of clinical supervision is not experienced as yet another 'top down' imposition.

We believe that the enabling underpinning philosophy of clinical supervision dovetails well with 'bottom up' approaches to practice development, in that both endeavours appear to be concerned with empowering practitioners and increasing awareness. It is perhaps no surprise then that 'bottom up' or 'normative/re-educative' approaches to practice development have been used to introduce clinical supervision.

Introduction

The following account is intended to guide the reader through my own experiences of implementing clinical supervision within a medium sized NHS trust. It is not intended as an academic analysis, rather one example of the practicalities of building a framework for implementing clinical supervision. It provides a 'real world' commentary of this endeavour, including all the twists and turns.

This chapter describes the process of introducing, at the time, a somewhat extraordinary concept to many practitioners. Despite their relative unfamiliarity, it was envisaged that the practitioners would enlist their commitment to the implementation process and the subsequent changes brought about in their clinical practice. The origins and *a priori* thinking essential to the building of the infrastructure necessary for the introduction and continued practice of supervision will be made clear. Further, an outline of the plans for the future will be provided: plans that contain the aim that, in time, purposeful clinical supervision will become an ordinary and fully integrated activity for all practitioners.

Background

Stockport Healthcare NHS Trust is co-terminous with Manchester, Tameside and the High Peak and has a population of approximately 350,000. Originally, the trust was a large District General Hospital, which in 1993 split into two trusts, Stockport Healthcare and Stockport Acute NHS Services. Stockport Healthcare Trust comprises six directorates, Primary and Public Health, Children's Services, Mental Health, Disabilities, Care of the Elderly and Maternity. For some of the acute services, such as Mental Health and Children's Services, accommodation is shared with Stockport Acute Services Trust. Care of the Elderly services is located in two satellite hospitals. Primary and Public Health services are incorporated within health centres and clinics throughout Stockport.

My first encounter with clinical supervision was in 1985. I had recently returned from H.M. Prison 'Styal' to Stockport Psychiatric services in order to take up the post of ward sister on an acute admission ward. This sojourn reawakened my interest in the 'talking therapies' and I began training as a counsellor. I had no idea nor experience of clinical supervision yet was instructed to choose a suitable supervisor. I was aware that the majority of my colleagues could not fill the bill due to their lack of knowledge, understanding or experience of clinical supervision. However, there was someone who worked within the services who was interested in family therapy who I felt might be able to challenge me sufficiently and encourage me to explore my assumptions and practice. We agreed that we would concentrate on the process of the work (as I now understand it) and not the content. We still see each other now for supervision and this relationship has been instrumental in shaping my values and beliefs regarding clinical supervision.

Since 1985, I have received and provided regular clinical supervision and it is an everyday aspect of my practice whatever the setting. During the past fourteen years, I have chosen supervisors and been chosen by supervisees ranging from nurses to doctors, social workers to occupational therapists and from teachers to priests.

In December 1994, the Director of Nursing for Stockport Healthcare NHS Trust invited a group of interested nurses to consider how clinical supervision could be developed within the trust. This was motivated by the substantial review and recommendations regarding clinical supervision (Butterworth and Faugier, 1994; Department of Health, 1994). I was already a member of a 'think tank' for Mental Health considering clinical supervision. With approximately one thousand nurses and six directorates across three sites with dozens of health centres and clinics, introducing and implementing regular, effective, and consistent clinical supervision was clearly not an easy task. A smaller steering group was formed and I was nominated to organise an 'in-house' conference to ignite the idea of clinical supervision and begin raising awareness.

Introducing clinical supervision

The conference was held in March 1995 and was attended by more than two hundred nurses and managers. Professor Tony Butterworth provided the keynote speech and as a result we were invited to tender for inclusion in the Department of Health/National Health Service Executive funded Triple Project Plan (latterly It *is* good to talk), an evaluation study in England and Scotland (Butterworth *et al.* 1997).

It became clear that in order to drive the implementation trust-wide a focus and lead for the development was required. For this purpose, I was given a half-time secondment for a three-year tenure, to lead and co-ordinate the implementation of clinical supervision funded by the trust.

The Trust's understanding of clinical supervision is described in its bespoke definition: '*Clinical supervision is a clinically focused partnership, encompassing reflective practice, critical analysis, self-audit and support, with the ultimate intention of safeguarding the well being of the patient/client.*'

Clearly clinical supervision was understood as a clinical and professional activity incorporating many different aspects of professional concern within an equally supportive and challenging relationship, designed to ensure quality and effectiveness. Clinical supervision therefore would be separate from, yet complementary to, existing systems of supervision within the trust, such as line management, individual performance review and appraisal. The context being process and supervisee-led rather than outcome driven.

Stockport Healthcare Trust, like other similar trusts, had resource and staffing problems and a 'fire fighting' culture, that is where demands create re-activity rather than reflection and pro-activity. Thus, the cost of implementation had to be absorbable. In order to develop accountability, clinical supervision implementation would be a long-term project and require a developmental approach as described by Hawkins and Shohet (1993). A strategy for implementation was designed with a ten-year life span though the initial commitment was for only three years. I believed once clinical supervision was established and successful then the trust would remain committed to it. My brief was to 'drive it or drag it' so consequently the field was wide open, which prompted voracious reading of the subject to learn how to do it. At that time, there was a paucity of useful literature providing advice on the 'how' of clinical supervision rather than the 'what'. The useful literature available originated from psychoanalysis, counselling and psychiatry. I realised that although I could relate to and work with these philosophies,

I suspected many nurses I would be working with might question their relevance.

At this point I was not only responsible for the strategic lead, developing protocols and standards, selling the 'product', designing and providing training, audit, and evaluation, not to mention changing the culture to enable clinical supervision to 'take off'. I also had two weeks in which to recruit staff from the two paediatric wards identified for the evaluation project and find suitable clinical supervisors, train them and protect the security of the research field. The priority was the evaluation project and an expectation that the experience of setting up the research on two acute wards, with staff who had never heard of clinical supervision, would be invaluable, and would inform trust-wide implementation.

The evaluation project had a fixed term. However, I was keen that clinical supervision would have a longer 'shelf life' and that the systems established would integrate easily with the trust-wide project. Eventually after much explanation and persuasion enough nurses volunteered. The supervisees were chosen randomly and as the supervisors would be required to commit more time than the supervisees, two specialist nurses, one home care sister and a night sister were chosen by the leaders of the project. These choices provided some impartiality and enabled twenty-four hour access to clinical supervision. This was an important aspect of the project when I was 'selling' the notion that clinical supervision is for all, irrespective of clinical setting.

Only one day of training was available for the four supervisors due to time restrictions and this training focused on theory, specifically functions (Proctor, 1991), types (Hunt, 1986) and a model (Hawkins and Shohet, 1993). I was aware of using my own supervisor skills and experiences to contain and allay their understandable anxieties. Clinical supervision was something of an extraordinary activity for these trainees and they were apprehensive. We therefore decided to meet monthly as a group. The group allowed ongoing access to support and supervision of the new supervisors. Such a system of support and supervision was one of a number of recommendations included in the evaluation report (Butterworth *et al.*, 1997). It was also apparent that by discussing theory, anxiety increased. Consequently, emphasis was placed on skills development to help build confidence in the supervisors, and also on incorporating further training into the groups.

Schon (1987, p30) provides a helpful analogy of the experienced jazz musician employing reflection-in-action. He suggests, 'They listen to one another, to themselves, feel where their music is going and adjust their play accordingly.'

This epitomises the atmosphere and learning created through involvement in the research. These novice supervisors were experimenting with clinical supervision as practice and I was experimenting with project management and creating change.

Butterworth *et al.*'s (1997) evaluation project recommended a minimum of forty-five minutes for each session but I had reservations about this. It seemed likely that the supervisees felt as anxious about clinical supervision as the supervisors did. Clinical supervision relies on an effective relationship with engagement between the supervisor and supervisee. Anxiety and demanding schedules might reduce commitment to an activity that, at that time, had few known benefits. Of a possible nine monthly sessions, only half may be managed half due to sickness, leave and low staffing levels. The Senior Nurse Manager was committed to the project and had given written permission for the time to be taken. However, I had some doubt that all the nurses involved would be able to give themselves the necessary permission. Consequently, sessions were forty-five minute fortnightly. **This would allow some sessions to be missed without too much detriment to engagement and by increasing frequency and time it might encourage a momentum allowing speedier absorption into ordinary practice.** This would enable commitment to clinical supervision beyond the Evaluation Project. Quiet private rooms had to be found so that sessions could be conducted off the clinical areas, and we negotiated the use of offices.

An implementation strategy for trust-wide implementation was required. Agreements with managers and facilities were needed in order to ensure that clinical supervision took hold. In addition, the implementation had to be amenable to audit and evaluation. There was an expectation of yearly reports for the Director of Nursing and the Board, as this would constitute some evidence of ongoing commitment.

Action plan

- To introduce clinical supervision by raising awareness and developing a common understanding of clinical supervision by all nursing specialities.
- To provide advice and support to managers on the impact of this development within their areas of responsibility.
- To establish working parties within each directorate who would agree protocols and standards, following consultation with their colleagues.
- To establish a system of preparation, support and monitoring of clinical supervisors.
- To develop strategies for audit and evaluation.
- To co-ordinate the successful implementation of the Triple Project Plan (Evaluation Project).

Raising awareness

Agreements were reached with Senior Nurse Managers for roadshows and seminars to be held during the day, at night and at the weekend in each directorate. In addition, invitations were procured to unit, manager's and senior ward sister/charge nurse meetings, handovers and staff meetings. It was intended to capture as many nurses as possible and to build interest generated by the conference held four months previously. This allowed promotion of clinical supervision, discussion leading to a shared understanding, demonstration of the trust's commitment and access to willing volunteers. It was at this point that the Maternity Directorate disengaged from the trust-wide project to concentrate on developing their statutory supervised practice, leaving five remaining directorates.

The Primary and Public Health Directorate had commissioned training for a group of health visitors, district nurses and school nurses based on a manager's interest from further educational study. This training was arranged for the end of 1995 and I was given a place. It was anticipated that the trust training would begin in 1996. This training would provide ideas for the nature and content of the trust training.

Advice and support

Before training could begin, alliances with clinical managers needed to be forged and working parties established. Discussions with senior nurse managers allowed agreements to be reached regarding introduction and development of clinical supervision in their areas. These included the level of responsibility managers should have for clinical supervision, and the resource implications. The Director of Nursing had agreed objectives with each of the senior nurse managers, which included the facilitation of clinical supervision. This ensured a corporate approach whilst, at the same time, fostered a collaborative relationship. Clinical supervision in the trust would be practitioner-led yet, facilitated and supported by the trust and its managers, thus utilising the principle of valuing all participants in the change process, in order to facilitate engagement (Spradley, 1979).

Working parties

Following the consultative discussions with the senior nurse managers' working parties were established in each directorate. Each working party included myself as advisor, the senior nurse manager and representatives of each grade of nurse (qualified), from both day and night, inpatient and community settings. Terms of reference were agreed and each working party existed from six to twelve months. Tasks of the group included:

- discovering and obtaining pertinent literature;
- selecting literature for, and developing an introductory pack, for their colleagues;
- agreeing and proposing a definition and philosophy of clinical supervision;
- setting standards for supervision activity;
- agreeing criteria for selection of clinical supervisors;
- formulating a consultation document for every qualified nurse within the directorate;

- amending document following consultation;
- accepting as policy and disseminating.

To inform the process of achieving a consensus and to provide additional educational material, money was made available to each group. Small libraries of clinical supervision texts were made available to allow access within the directorate spanning the twenty-four-hour/seven-day week.

A consistency of standards and policy was achieved across the trust, without sacrificing local and practitioner ownership, by encouraging contribution from the working parties from each of the five directorates. In addition, members of the working parties, especially the senior nurse manager, became knowledgeable opinion leaders within the directorate and effective advocates. This partnership promoted collaboration and was essential to enable practitioner and manager colleagues to work together in a spirit of creativity and innovation (Morton-Cooper and Bamford, 1997). The working parties also produced the first wave of trainees for clinical supervisor training.

Training

The design of the training was dependent on a number of factors. First there was the necessity of getting clinical supervision going, second, the cost of the training, and third, providing appropriate content that prepared the trainees and allowed ability and confidence to develop. Within the training, Kolb's experiential learning cycle (1984) was promoted as a possible practice model for clinical supervision. This model struck a chord with the practitioners. It was pragmatic and I believed would appeal to trainee supervisors irrespective of speciality, grade or even discipline. Since the use of a problem solving approach was familiar to some practitioners, utilising Kolb's model would 'sit comfortably' with existing approaches and additionally, it wouldn't require a great deal of psychological mindedness in order to make it work. It was also apparent that this six-day course would be too costly for the trust, therefore, a modified version would be more appropriate. It was clear that the needs of trainee supervisors were common to all directorates and professions.

A further advantage of attending this training was that I was able to negotiate that this cohort of trainees act as the directorate working party (and they continue to meet as a steering group for the directorate). It also yielded three trainees who had an interest and some experience in training: thus a Training Team emerged and has developed to be able to manage and provide the training, which would be crucial to the longer-term implementation.

It was also important that when trust-wide implementation reached critical mass, a co-ordinator might no longer be viable. The co-ordinator was replaced by a network of identified individuals, usually individuals who had been involved in the working party and who were enthusiastic advocates of clinical supervision. These link co-ordinators had the necessary expertise to maintain the structures built within the trust and would enable the continued roll-out of clinical supervision. The link co-ordinators would take on the liaison responsibilities within their own directorates, which would include maintaining a supervisor and supervisee database, arranging nominations for training, allocations and arbitration. Each directorate had its own link co-ordinator by 1997. For time and cost required for the training team and link co-ordinators, agreements were reached with the senior nurses for each directorate to resource dedicated time for this role. For the trainers an average of six days a year was negotiated and for link co-ordinators, time allowed ranges from one to three days a month: a commitment from the managers of the trust to facilitate clinical supervision effectively. It also provided local ownership which encouraged the practitioners, whether involved or not, to accept clinical supervision as a part of the directorate's professional activity, by providing 'in-house access'. This would create developmental opportunities for staff within the trust and further foster the sense of ownership and collaboration.

Consequently, the training team designed a three-day generic course, which would be available five times a year and be delivered by the co-ordinator as lead trainer and one of the co-trainers. The content would include contracting, Kolb's model (1984), skills development, ethical and professional dilemmas, managing the process and supervisor self-awareness. A variety of training

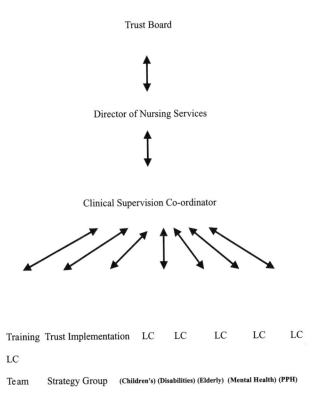

Figure 8.1 Communication and implementation framework

techniques would be used including didactic teaching, open and controlled group discussions, small groupwork and role-play, with an emphasis on building confidence.

Each cohort of trainees was divided into smaller groups which would meet monthly after training, with a more experienced supervisor as facilitator. It was envisaged that supervisees would self-nominate to become a supervisor and attend the training (given the support of their managers). They would be able to self-select against the criteria agreed within the directorate and explained in the clinical supervision policy. The supervisee's intentions would also be discussed with the co-ordinator. In the beginning the criteria for selection of supervisors couldn't be strictly applied, as there was a paucity of available and willing supervisors, consequently the majority of the first wave supervisors completed the training before receiving supervision themselves. However, the criteria could be enforced after a number of courses had been held.

Taking into account the anxiety generated by supervision and the cost implication, the newly trained supervisor would only be expected to take on one supervisee. When confident, the supervisor would be expected to take on a further supervisee or a small group of supervisees or if able a group of supervisors. **This system avoids the risk of supervisors feeling overwhelmed by this extension to their role and therefore gives the space and time to incorporate this new learning and practice into their everyday work.** A further advantage was that there was a steady manageable stream of one to one and small group supervision activity that could be absorbed into existing resources (see Figure 8.2). There are and have been exceptions to this – staff who are already expert in supervision and those who have more capacity.

The one-day training that the evaluation project supervisors received was clearly not enough and after nine months a further day was arranged which built on the abilities and confidence gained in the monthly groups. The

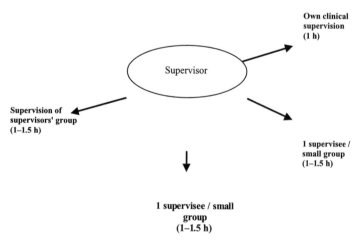

Figure 8.2 Supervisor activity model

content was determined by the supervisors and used video-taping of skills work, reflecting the increase in confidence and the ownership of their own development as supervisors. Transferring this learning into the trust-wide implementation meant supervisors were offered yearly update sessions. The content would be determined by the supervisors and delivered by the training team, and would allow further development, monitoring of standards of supervisory practice and importantly, encourage networking and collaboration.

By the spring of 1996, we had a training strategy, which would prepare, develop and monitor supervisors. This strategy is outlined in Figure 8.3. The funding by the trust (co-ordinator) and the directorates (time) further developed the collaborative nature of the implementation process.

Evaluation

According to Bishop (1998), the comprehensive strategy of audit and evaluation of the implementation used by the author produces results that are more meaningful and useful due to the comprehensive strategy being operated.

Interim and final reports of the evaluation study (Butterworth *et al.* 1997) were utilised to inform continuing implementation. Training and update sessions were evaluated, and are still consistently positive. Waiting lists have been audited regularly, formally by questionnaire and informally by link co-ordinators. That results showed that if the prospective supervisees are given information at regular intervals regarding delays, then commitment to clinical supervision is not adversely affected.

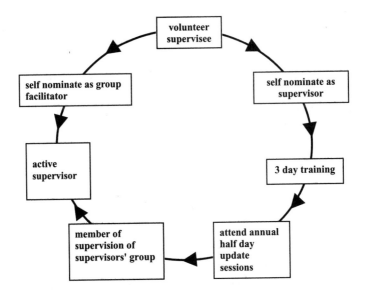

Figure 8.3 Supervisee and supervisor development strategy

Specific audits have also been carried out between 1997 and 1998. An audit within the Elderly directorate gauged activity and was able to resolve some of the flaws highlighted in the results, such as the difficulties in matching suitable supervisors with supervisees, and sickness interfering with the regularity of sessions.

Advice on methodologies of audit was sought from the North West Surveys and Research Unit, which is part of the Regional Research and Development Directorate, and this helped the author construct a questionnaire. The Primary and Public Health directorate utilised a modified version of this to gain an accurate picture of clinical supervision within the directorate and also gain some understanding of its perceived effects.

As the focus for post-graduate study a selection of the original evaluation project respondents were asked to participate in a further research project attempting to investigate any possible effect clinical supervision might have had on their clinical practice. It was anticipated it could also provide additional information, which would add to evidence already collected in the original study (Hadfield, 2000).

The most recent evaluation, conducted in the summer of 1998, was a further collaboration with the School of Nursing, Midwifery and Health Visiting at the University of Manchester. The Manchester Clinical Supervision Scale (see chapter 15) was designed specifically to measure the effects of supervision on supervisees, supervisors, and the quality of care provided. This was a direct consequence of the qualitative data collected by the evaluation study (Butterworth *et al.*, 1997) and provides much needed quantitative data. During the validation of the scale, 180 questionnaires were sent out to supervisees and supervisors of which 124 were returned. The results showed that clinical supervision sessions were regular although some reported that it was still difficult to make the time, due to clinical demands. Clinical supervision was experienced as useful and was perceived as a benefit to improved practice.

From the beginning of the implementation process in 1995, each yearly review, audit, internal and external evaluation contributed to building a body of evidence for the trust board. The results informed the discussions with the trust board in the summer of 1998. This evidence was instrumental in securing their commitment and permanent funding for the co-ordinator post for two days a week. The board also agreed that other healthcare professionals could join the clinical supervision development programme if they wished.

It had always been intended to develop a framework that would embrace all disciplines within the trust. The development of clinical supervision and mentorship for doctors gives scope for integration in the future recommended by Thomas and Reid (1995). However, some reluctance to this idea within the trust board meant that a proactive marketing campaign wasn't possible. Although as the 'word of mouth' reputation of clinical supervision increased, tentative conversations began with a number of interested individuals from community dentistry, psychologists, podiatrists and occupational and speech Therapists. As individuals, resources and management support would be required. These individual practitioners were keen; their professional leaders were not. It was difficult therefore to take hold of it in a constructive way. However by autumn 1998 we had our first occupational therapists as clinical supervisor trainees with full support of their professional and clinical managers.

Progress

The continuing integration of clinical supervision into accountable clinical practice is further enhanced by the integration of other disciplines. In addition to bi-annual introductory sessions for prospective supervisees and regular three-day training courses for supervisors, there is one-to-one and group supervision, supervision of supervisor groups, and yearly update sessions for all supervisors. In addition, there are senior staff nurses supervising ward sister/charge nurses, health visitors supervising Care of the Elderly nurses, children's nurses supervising mental health nurses and numerous variations and combinations. This all adds to the sense of peer collaboration and multidisciplinary practice and supports the clarity of the clinical supervisory relationship by providing intentionality, mutuality and impartiality. These are necessary ingredients for enabling supervisees to reflect on their practice.

To conclude, the implementation outlined in this chapter can only be regarded as the beginning. It is well documented that clinical supervision should be a lifelong activity and if that axiom is accepted, then the infra-structures, managerial support and organisational know-how need to be in place in order to enable this activity to occur. This chapter illustrates that the foundations of these structures are now in place, and that there is something secure on which future clinical supervision practice can be built. Which means that future practitioners, from various disciplines, will be able to benefit from engaging in supervision and consequently, improving the service that clients receive.

References

Bishop V (1998) Clinical supervision: what's going on? Results of a questionnaire. *Nursing Times* 94. 18.

Butterworth C A and Faugier J (1994) *Clinical Supervision: A Position Paper*. School of Nursing Studies, Manchester University.

Butterworth C A, Carson J, White E, Jeacock J and Clements A (1997) *It is Good to Talk. The 23 Site Evaluation project of Clinical Supervision in England and Scotland*. School of Nursing, Midwifery and Health Visiting, University of Manchester.

Department of Health (1994) *Executive Letter*. Chief Nursing Officer.

Hadfield D (2000) Clinical supervision: a user's perspective. *Journal of Child Health* Spring.

Hawkins P and Shohet R (1993) *Supervision in the Helping Professions. An individual Group and Organizational Approach*. Milton Keynes: Open University Press.

Hunt P (1986) Supervision. *Marriage Guidance* Spring pp15–22.

Kolb D (1984) *Experiential Learning. Experience as a Source of Learning and Development*. Englewood Cliffs, New Jersey: Prentice-Hall.

Morton-Cooper A and Bamford A (1997) *Excellence in Healthcare Management*. Oxford: Blackwell.

Proctor B (1991) On being a Trainer. In Dryden W and Thorne B (eds). *Training and Supervision For Counselling in Action*. London: Sage.

Schon D A (1987) *Educating the Reflective Practitioner*. San Francisco: Jossey Bass

Spradley J (1979) *The Ethnographic Interview*. New York: Holt.

Thomas B and Reid J (1995) Multidisciplinary clinical supervision. *British Journal of Nursing* Vol.4. No.5.

9 Clinical supervision in nursing and health visiting

A review of the UK literature

Annette Gilmore

Editorial

This chapter presents the results of a review of the current UK evaluative literature, commissioned by the UKCC, to inform their continuing programme of work on clinical supervision. The aim of the literature review was to assess progress with implementation and actual impact of clinical supervision on nurses and health visitors and service provision. Particular issues highlighted by the review include: availability of clinical supervision, barriers to the uptake of clinical supervision, training of supervisors, record keeping and the ongoing confusion that is maintained by amalgamating clinical supervision with managerial supervision and representing them as one entity. It concludes by reiterating the UKCC's position on clinical supervision.

Background

Clinical supervision has been widely discussed and written about since its endorsement by the Department of Health and UKCC (DoH, 1993; UKCC, 1995, 1996), as an essential means of supporting and developing staff.

In its position statement on clinical supervision the UKCC (1996) advocates clinical supervision as a means of assisting life-long learning and of enabling practitioners to maintain and promote standards of care. A further proposal is that the *Code of Professional Conduct* should influence employment contracts for staff and that one method of monitoring and maintaining standards is for registered practitioners to have access to clinical supervision (UKCC, 1995).

Many models have been developed and tailored to suit the workload of different nursing groups and health visitors (Proctor, 1986; Hawkins and Shohet, 1989; Johns, 1994; Butterworth and Faugier, 1994). Whilst the models vary in their focus and mode of delivery, each encapsulates a supportive, educational and quality assurance function. Moreover, ownership of the process belongs to the practitioner.

The literature review

When the literature review was being considered, clinical supervision for nurses and health visitors was not well developed in the UK. Further, the need for the literature review was reinforced by the findings of a qualitative inquiry. It was evident that there was a need to find out more about 'it', and as a consequence the review was commissioned. Published and unpublished work was included. In the main, evaluations concentrate on the processes of clinical supervision, giving important evidence of the focus and quality of clinical supervision provided. Models of good practice are identified which it is hoped will help practitioners and organisations in their efforts to incorporate clinical supervision into everyday practice. Progress with implementation of clinical supervision is also discussed. The sparse empirical evidence on outcomes is discussed elsewhere in the book. However, given that programmes are generally in the early stages of development and of variable quality it is understandable that, at the time the review was undertaken, there was little evidence of significant benefit.

Overview of the current provision of clinical supervision

Availability of clinical supervision

Brocklehurst (1996, 1997a,c) conducted postal surveys of trust nurse executives in three English regions. He reported that clinical supervision was available to some nurses in approximately 85–90 per cent of trusts. In the majority of cases developments were at the pilot phase with access limited to a minority of staff. Similar findings were reported from a large postal questionnaire survey of nurses in five trusts which found that 29 per cent of respondents worked within a structure whereby they had an identified clinical supervisor (Fowler and Chevannes, 1998).

Brocklehurst reported that the health authorities in his survey viewed raising awareness on clinical supervision amongst nurses in general practice as their highest priority. Limited written and anecdotal evidence suggests that there is very little progress with regard to implementing clinical supervision in nursing homes despite the call for such systems (Brocklehurst, 1997b; Masterson, 1997).

There is some evidence to suggest that access to clinical supervision varies between staff groups and types of units. In the main it is in mental health and learning disability trusts/units that clinical supervision appears to be more established (Brocklehurst, 1997a,c; Redfern *et al.*, 1997).

Similarly staff in innovative/progressive units, such as nursing development units, may have greater access to clinical supervision than other nursing units, probably because they tend to be used as test beds for new developments (Redfern *et al.*, 1997).

Barriers to the uptake of clinical supervision

The findings from the review of the literature indicate that a range of factors appear to impede the successful implementation of clinical supervision including time constraints, low priority ascribed to clinical supervision, lack of supervisors, major trust reorganisations, loss of leader/driving force and shortage of suitable accommodation for holding meetings. Some constraints appear to be initial operational problems whereas others, such as time constraints, organisational instability and loss of a leader could jeopardise the initial success of initiatives and the long-term sustainability of clinical supervision.

Time constraints

The most common problems reported with setting up clinical supervision were time constraints owing to workload, staff shortages, increased activity in contracts and trust reorganisations (Johns, 1996; Scanlon and Weir, 1997; Bishop, 1998). Time constraints also occur due to clinical supervision being ascribed a low priority (Scanlon and Weir, 1997; Johns, 1996, 1997).

There is some resistance, particularly in the acute sector, to protecting time allocated to clinical supervision (Lilley, 1996; Johns, 1997; May et al., 1997; Nicklin, 1997; Sams, 1997; Bishop, 1998). Nurses and health visitors frequently utilise their own time for meetings (Lilley, 1996; Marrow et al., 1997; May et al., 1997; Nicklin, 1997). Bishop (1998) reported that 75 per cent of community trusts and 60 per cent of mixed trusts achieve having clinical supervision during work time but only 40 per cent of trusts in the acute sector manage this. Replacement cover appears to be only considered for releasing supervisors for training and in some cases to fulfil their supervisory role (Bulmer, 1997; Lilley, 1996; Sams, 1997).

Resistance to clinical supervision

Wilkin et al. (1997) suggest that resistance is an unavoidable part of change and advocate acknowledging this as part of the process of implementation. Resistance appears to arise from lack of knowledge of the purpose and nature of clinical supervision (May et al., 1997; Sams, 1997; Bishop, 1998; Cutcliffe and Proctor, 1998). Managers are unsure of how it 'fits' with service priorities and question the time and cost needed for implementation (Bishop, 1998). Practitioners' reasons for not attending supervision include distrust of supervisor, not perceived as needed, not perceived as a high priority as well as staff shortages (Sams, 1997). There is some evidence that supervisees feel guilty about 'taking the time out' for clinical supervision (Johns, 1997; Bishop, 1998).

Active measures to overcome avoidance techniques include discussing this issue prior to commencing the supervisory relationship so that the supervisor is aware of and can challenge possible avoidance techniques in the supervisee (Wilkin et al., 1997). Johns (1996) suggests that the importance of frequency and commitment to supervisory meeting need to be reinforced. Furthermore any implementation strategy requires the commitment of time and resources for raising staff awareness with information workshops or 'roadshows' and information leaflets (Bulmer, 1997; May *et al.*, 1997; Sams, 1997; Cutcliffe and Proctor, 1998a,b). Supervisees need preparation which aims at enabling them to participate and to gain maximum benefit from clinical supervision (Butterworth *et al.*, 1997; Fyffe, 1997 and Sams, 1997). Unfortunately training practitioners to be 'good supervisees' has been largely neglected (Bulmer, 1997).

Leadership

Limited evidence indicates that success in implementing and sustaining clinical supervision is often dependent on the commitment and motivation of a single individual or small group within an organisation (Johns, 1996, 1997; Dunn and Bishop, 1998).

Shortage of supervisors

Lack of supervisors with the necessary skills is a frequently reported problem, which can result in some supervisors having to provide supervision to rather too many supervisees (Bulmer, 1997; Butterworth *et al.*, 1997; Scanlon and Weir, 1997; Bishop, 1998). The hierarchical nature of nursing appears to be a barrier in the identification and selection of suitable supervisors (Bishop, 1998). This problem appears to be bound up with introducing hierarchical systems of clinical supervision that mesh with the hierarchical structures within nursing. Senior staff, usually nurse or non-nurse line managers, in some cases become the supervisors for junior staff, particularly in one-to-one supervision. Many authors have suggested that this is inappropriate (Swain, 1995; Brocklehurst, 1997b; Bulmer, 1997; Redfern *et al.*, 1997; Scanlon and Weir, 1997; Davidson, 1998). Consequently, managers need to look beyond suggesting that clinical staff have their line manager as their supervisor.

Training more junior nurses, such as E grades, has proved successful (Bulmer, 1997). An organisational strategy is needed to identify, on a multi-professional basis, the personnel with the necessary clinical and supervisory skills (Scanlon and Weir, 1997), and such possible strategies have been outlined in the preceding chapters.

Environment

A frequently mentioned problem was inappropriate environmental conditions, which adversely affected the success of supervision meetings. These included lack of suitable accommodation in clinical areas or holding meetings too close to units, which increases the likelihood of being interrupted and distracts supervisees, who often feel uncomfortable about leaving their colleagues to get on with the work (Johns, 1996, 1997; Butterworth *et al.*, 1997; Fyffe, 1997; May *et al.*, 1997; Bishop, 1998; Dunn and Bishop, 1998). Removal of educational facilities from trust sites is quoted as one source of this problem (Bishop, 1998). However, inappropriate accommodation and being disturbed during meetings may be a transient problem, which resolves itself when a programme is well established (Scanlon and Weir, 1997).

The quality of clinical supervision

The nature of clinical supervision meetings

Trust nurse executives believe that the main purpose of clinical supervision is for the professional development and support of staff (Brocklehurst, (1997c). How supervision programmes aspire to meet these objectives varies between settings. Two principal and polarised types of supervision were identified in this review whereby the focus is either on caseload management or the meetings concentrate on an in-depth exploration of the practitioner's practice.

Focus on caseload management

One approach to supervision sessions concentrates exclusively on case presentations and general caseload issues (Dudley and Butterworth, 1994; Swain, 1995; Scanlon and Weir, 1997; Scott, 1997; Davidson, 1998). Here the focus is mainly centred on patient treatment pathways (e.g. how care could be planned differently and what options are open to the practitioner). This appears to happen because the meetings are structured with this purpose in mind rather than arising out of the supervisees' inexperience. Where one-to-one supervision focuses on case management, it appears to share similar processes and dynamics to management supervision. Limited evidence suggests that there is a tendency for this to occur where other forms of staff support and monitoring systems are absent (Swain, 1995; Scanlon and Weir, 1997; Scott, 1997). Furthermore, it appears that clinical supervision takes this format in organisations where it is perceived as being already established (Swain, 1995; Sams, 1997; Scanlon and Weir, 1997; Davidson, 1998). There is some suggestion that non-threatening issues, such as case conferences, have to be discussed during group supervision sessions because group members may not feel secure enough to share experiences (Fyffe, 1997; Johns, 1997).

Focus on needs identified by the practitioner

The literature also provides examples of where group and one-to-one sessions have a different focus. The meetings are practitioner-led and topics discussed include: conflict with nursing or medical colleagues; caring issues grounded in doubt or concern; issues arising from interactions with relatives and carers; and issues relating to the therapeutic relationship between client and practitioner

(Johns, 1996, 1997; Cutcliffe and Burns, 1998; Cutcliffe and Epling, 1997; Jones, 1995, 1997; Scanlon and Weir, 1997). In such cases the supervisor appears to be more challenging of the process of practice itself. The implementation of clinical supervision on a pilot basis in acute and community trusts appears to be more practitioner orientated (Swain, 1995; Johns, 1996, 1997; Butterworth *et al.*, 1997; Fyffe, 1997). In the acute sector roll-out of supervision programmes following a pilot also tend to be practitioner orientated (Bulmer, 1997; Roden, 1997; Dunn and Bishop, 1998).

Organisation and process factors

Supervisor training: current provision

The success of clinical supervision is greatly dependent on the supervisor (Roden, 1997; Bishop, 1998). Supervisor training is identified as crucial to the success of clinical supervision (Johns, 1996, 1997; Bulmer, 1997; Fyffe, 1997; Roden, 1997). However, where training occurs it varies in both nature and duration. Programmes are reported to range from half-day seminars to university courses (Swain, 1995; Brocklehurst, 1997a,c; Bulmer, 1997; Butterworth *et al.*, 1997; Fyffe, 1997; Roden, 1997; Sams, 1997; Bishop, 1998; Davidson, 1998). Empirical evidence is currently lacking on the efficacy of the range of preparation modes available for supervisors. Cutcliffe (1997) suggests there is a need to examine whether there is a correlation between the level of intensity of supervision training given and the extent of positive outcomes. Clinical supervision is a specific skill, so it is reasonable to expect that if a nurse receives insufficient or inadequate training, then the quality of their supervision would be incapable of producing change in the supervisee such as an improvement in the supervisee's mental well-being (Cutcliffe, 1997). Limited evidence suggests that in cases where models of clinical supervision resemble management supervision or IPR, supervisors usually have not had any training (Swain, 1995; Scanlon and Weir, 1997).

Supervisors as supervisees

Supervisors require an awareness of their own attitudes and how this might influence the supervisory relationship (Johns, 1996, 1997; Fyffe, 1997). It is proposed that supervisors should have experienced clinical supervision with an experienced facilitator (Johns, 1996, 1997; Fyffe, 1997). In the major study conducted by Butterworth *et al.* (1997) a trend towards increased psychological distress was observed in a group of supervisors who did not receive supervision. This phenomenon was not observed in supervisors who were also supervisees. Bulmer (1997) found that supervisors need continuing support after the initial training programme. Unfortunately strategies to implement clinical supervision do not always include systems for ongoing formal or informal support mechanisms for supervisors (Swain, 1995; Bishop, 1998).

Supervisory relationship

The central role of the supervisor is to work *with* the practitioner towards enabling the achievement of desirable/effective work (Johns, 1996, 1997). Supervisors need good facilitative skills (Johns, 1996, 1997, Cutcliffe and Burns, 1998; Cutcliffe and Epling, 1997; Fyffe, 1997; Roden, 1997; Scanlon and Weir, 1997; Dunn and Bishop, 1998). Johns (1997) developed a model to describe this relationship based on the core concept of 'being available'. The elements of this template of 'being available' are essentially the same as the therapeutic relationship between the supervisor and practitioner/supervisee identified by other authors (Bulmer, 1997; Butterworth *et al.*, 1997; Cutcliffe and Epling, 1997; Fyffe, 1997; Roden, 1997; Scanlon and Weir, 1997). He suggests that the following elements influence the extent to which the practitioner/supervisor is available to work with another practitioner within the context of guided reflection (Johns, 1996, 1997):

- positive regard;
- knowing the practitioner;
- responding with an appropriate helping style;
- knowing and managing self within a relationship.

Positive regard

The supervisor must believe that the supervisee has the potential to grow and develop, otherwise the supervisor cannot empower the supervisee (Johns, 1997). Equally the supervisee must be committed to the process of supervision.

Knowing the practitioner

Farkas-Cameron (1995) identified four key stages in the development process of the supervisory relationship as: (a) pre-interaction stage; (b) introductory stage; (c) working stage; (d) termination stage. A working stage is established when the supervisee and supervisor can openly relate to each other. Trust emerged as an essential requirement for disclosure in the supervisory relationships (Bulmer, 1997; Fyffe, 1997; Roden, 1997; Scanlon and Weir, 1997). Enabling a trusting relationship is viewed as dependent on the skills of the supervisor. The contract emerged as the initial process by which a trusting relationship could develop. Contracting allows the boundaries and parameters of the relationship to be made explicit. Issues of accountability and responsibility could be thrashed out (Fyffe, 1997; Roden, 1997).

Confidence in the confidentiality of the meetings is the cornerstone to building up a trusting relationship where disclosure is 'okay' (Johns, 1996, 1997; Fyffe, 1997; Roden, 1997; Scanlon and Weir, 1997).

Confidentiality and accountability

Cutcliffe *et al.* (1998a,b) reported on the dilemma of when the confidentiality of the meetings needs to be compromised as disclosures warrant being taken up by the relevant employer or the UKCC. Would failure to inform constitute an act of negligence on the part of the supervisor? In such cases the normative function of supervision is active with the supervisor encouraging the supervisee to consider his/her professional ethics and standards of practice (Cutcliffe *et al.*, 1998a,b). The supervisors' facilitative skills emerged as an important theme whereby the supervisor needs to enable supervisees to identify problems themselves and initiate corrective action with the supervisor monitoring progress. The issue remains, however, of what happens if the supervisee fails to take corrective action.

Knowing the practitioners' practice

A recurring theme is the need for the supervisee and supervisor to share a common set of beliefs and values, a common 'philosophy' so to speak (Fyffe, 1997; Scanlon and Weir, 1997). Supervisors need to understand the nuances of practice as a necessary starting point if they are to be facilitative and offer alternative views. Whether the supervisor needs to have more knowledge and skills than the supervisee seems to be dictated by the supervisee's individual needs or the mode of supervision (Bulmer, 1997; Fyffe, 1997; Johns, 1996, 1997; Roden, 1997). Bulmer (1997) found that nurses did not deem it necessary that supervisors knew more than they did. Fyffe (1997) reported that some supervisees felt that it was sufficient for the supervisor to be a nurse. For mental health nurses the criteria for picking a supervisor relates to their facilitative skills and knowledge of the therapeutic relationship between counsellor/clients rather than their professional background (Thomas and Reid, 1995; Scanlon and Weir, 1997). Other evidence suggests that peer group supervision can function with external facilitators where their expertise in group dynamics and management is required rather then their clinical expertise (Dudley and Butterworth, 1994; Johns, 1996, 1997; Sams, 1997). However, the possibility of internal supervision lacking objectivity should be acknowledged (Fyffe, 1997; Johns, 1996, 1997; Scanlon and Weir, 1997). Supervisees or supervisors may have the same 'blind spots' and/or lack vision to see other ways of doing things.

Responding with an appropriate helping style

Supervisees need to feel that the supervisor is not judging them (Bulmer, 1997; Fyffe, 1997; Roden, 1997). There is a growing body of evidence that clinical supervision can and is expected to raise supervisee anxiety/stress (Johns, 1996, 1997; Sams, 1996; Roden, 1997; Fowler and Chevannes, 1998). Sams (1996) suggests that when clinical supervision is incorporated into one's practice this new way of working will initially increase stress in the practitioner. Johns (1996) reported that ward sisters experienced stress when trying to work in new and better ways as a result of clinical supervision. Supervision didn't relieve the sources of stress but it did help them to grasp and take control of situations. In some supervisees it helped to promote assertive action, which the author asserts may in itself be stressful because of the uncertainty regarding how others might react to this new action.

These examples throw up pertinent questions. Is it an integral part of supervision that the practitioner feels stressed, especially when inexperienced in the technique? Is it an indication that the balance of support and challenge is not quite right in the supervisory meeting? If stress persists is it an indication that supervisees are not receiving the right kind of clinical supervision for them, as suggested by Fowler and Chevannes (1998)?

Knowing and managing self within a relationship

Some clinical supervisors, both nurses and non-nurses, also hold line management responsibilities (Brocklehurst, 1997a; Bulmer, 1997; Redfern *et al.*, 1997; Scanlon and Weir, 1997). This finding can be partly explained in the pilot sites where clinical supervision is introduced initially to senior nursing staff before being rolled out, and many trusts are still at this stage of development (Brocklehurst, 1997a; Bulmer, 1997; Fyffe, 1997; Masterson and Cameron, 1997). The review indicated that there is a substantial argument highlighting the difficulties of clinical supervisors also holding a managerial responsibility over the people who they were supervising. Managers who are supervisors tend to impose their agenda during supervision sessions, have problems being facilitative rather than directive and blur the boundaries between the two practices (Johns, 1996, 1997; Butterworth *et al.*, 1997; Scanlon and Weir, 1997). Scanlon and Weir (1997) also reported that line manager supervisors were perceived to lack insight into practitioners' practice.

Record-keeping

Johns (1996, 1997) advocates note-taking as an essential part of supervision. The merits of note-taking include improved continuity of sessions, enhancing the reflective skills of the supervisee, confronting the practitioner with issues that might have been defended against within an oral mode, to enable the supervisor to highlight key issues and as a reflective performance review. Johns (1997) has developed a model of structured reflection to guide reflective writing and practice. In the main few supervisees appear to keep comprehensive records (Johns, 1996, 1997; Bulmer, 1997). At the time of the review, there was little discussion regarding the legal standing of clinical supervision records apart from Dimond (1998a,b). However, more recently, Cutcliffe (2000) has examined issues of documentation in clinical supervision. He points out that there appear to be three principal discrete positions

- the supervisor records minimum data to meet the needs of audit;
- the supervisee makes extensive notes for his/her learning journal, reflective diary and
- the supervisor records headings or key words to be used as an aide memoire. He concludes with five key points:
- Decisions on what records are to be maintained in clinical supervision need to be negotiated in the initial session and made explicit in the supervision contract.
- Choosing the option of minimal records perhaps helps the supervision to steer clear of becoming too supervisor-led and avoids overlapping the boundaries of managerial supervision.
- If the supervisor feels his/her only course of action is available is to prescribe a course of action, it would be reasonable to record the details of this advice (and inform the supervisee of this possibility at the contracting stage).
- Reflective diaries and learning journals are a helpful, enabling tool designed to enhance nurses' professional development, not a covert method of eliciting incriminating evidence, and their use as an adjunct to supervision should be encouraged.
- Lastly, while some supervisors may feel the need to keep notes of key words or headings, these should be used with caution and an awareness that the supervisee should set the agenda and retain the control.

Moving forward

Sustaining momentum

The Department of Health and the UKCC have made considerable efforts to raise the profile of clinical supervision among practising nurses and health visitors. This strategy included a national workshop for trust nurse executives, a national clinical supervision conference for the profession and a multi-site evaluation research project (Butterworth *et al.*, 1996). Early in 1997 the Department of Health made available 1.6 million pounds on a non-recurrent basis to promote initiatives in nursing in the NHS in England (Action Agenda on Nursing) (Brocklehurst, 1997a). About half of the total was earmarked to help the profession move forward with clinical supervision. Likewise the UKCC, through its advisory role, actively encourages the implementation of clinical supervision to promote and maintain standards of care (UKCC, 1995, 1996).

However, clinical supervision is neither widely available nor of predictable quality. Further measures of continuing support and encouragement will be required if it is to become a reality for practitioners. A feasible model has evolved in Wales where clinical supervision projects received funding via money allocated to promote and sustain 'clinical effectiveness' initiatives. Linking clinical supervision to 'clinical effectiveness' initiatives has the advantage of ensuring the long-term sustainability of the initiative. The evidence indicates that any moves towards making clinical supervision a statutory requirement would be inappropriate in the current climate. Staff are the best ambassadors for the development of high quality and appropriate clinical supervision programmes as monitoring of quality supervision may be gauged by staff demand for it (Fyffe, 1997; Scanlon and Weir, 1997; Roden, 1997; Dunn and Bishop, 1998). However, a stumbling block is the difficulty in determining need for clinical supervision without having a reasonable level of knowledge and insight into the concept (Fyffe, 1997; Scanlon and Weir, 1997). Where clinical supervision strategies have been well planned and co-ordinated by an identified committed person or team the results are encouraging (Fyffe, 1997; Roden, 1997; Dunn and Bishop, 1998). Success appears to be influenced by thorough planning and organisation, making staff knowledgeable about the nature and potential benefits of supervision, staff ownership, attention to the training needs of supervisors and supervisees, and quality supervisors (Bulmer, 1997; Fyffe, 1997; Roden, 1997; Sams, 1997; Dunn and Bishop, 1998).

Organisational commitment

In the main, costing of clinical supervision has received little attention (Lilley, 1996; Brocklehurst, 1997c; May *et al.*, 1997; Nicklin, 1997). Few trusts include clinical supervision in their corporate agenda or business plans (Butterworth *et al.*, 1997; Bishop, 1998). It could be argued that if clinical supervision is to become part of a practitioner's everyday practice then the activity warrants no special costing. It does, however, involve building time into practitioners' workload schedules for preparing for and attending meetings. The limited consideration given to costs and staff time needed for clinical supervision may simply signal the low priority this initiative holds in cash-strapped trusts (Brocklehurst, 1997c).

Process of clinical supervision

Two categories of clinical supervision have evolved. In the first case a non-threatening approach is used whereby case conferences or caseload matters are the focus and practitioners receive support and guidance concerning how they are performing and with the development of future plans. Where 'one-to-one supervision' follows this format it is similar to management supervision for the purposes of satisfying the information needs of line managers. At another level clinical supervision aims to unravel the supervisee's practice at a micro level. In such instances the practitioner dictates the agenda.

'Clinical supervision by any other name'

The variable nature of clinical supervision meetings needs further exploration. The ultimate purpose in both cases appears to be similar but the means of achieving this are different. Since the process and content of these two systems are very different, can they both be termed clinical supervision? Can or should the same outcomes be expected from the two types of supervision? There is some evidence that these two types fulfil different needs of practitioners, each of paramount importance. Scott (1997, 1998) explored the support needs of health visitors in undertaking child abuse work as part of their practice. Interviewees identified two levels of support they required: support and guidance concerning how they were performing in their role and a need for supervision which allowed them to explore their feelings, knowledge and practice in a safe supportive environment (Scott, 1997, 1998).

Fowler and Chevannes (1998) warn against insisting on reflection as an integral part of all forms of clinical supervision. Clinical supervision is proposed as a way of 'harnessing' reflective practice, but reflective practice need not always be an integral part of the process. Reflection must involve the 'self' and must lead to a changed perspective (Atkins and Murphy, 1993; Johns, 1998; Lumby, 1998). However, an inappropriate model of clinical supervision is likely to be resisted or have minimal impact (Fowler and Chevannes, 1998). They suggest that some practitioners may not be able to cope with such intense scrutiny of themselves and their work. Furthermore, if the supervisee is inexperienced clinically then reflection may be an inappropriate and frustrating method. A more directive teaching programme may be more effective, such as preceptorship, or one which can progress into clinical supervision when the practitioner is more experienced. Hawkins and Shohet (1989) suggest that new supervisees need to start with most of the supervision focusing on the content of their work with the client and the detail of what happened in the session.

Standards promotion and the clinical supervision process

Clinical supervision is described in terms of its potential to assist practitioners to be accountable yet there is currently only limited evidence that explores how the quality control aspect of clinical supervision links with its supportive and professional development functions. Integrating reflective reviews into the clinical supervision model maintains the practitioner-led focus, yet has the potential to ensure the quality assurance or 'normative' function of clinical supervision receives satisfactory but not excessive or improper attention within the supervision space. It can be argued that through this self-regulatory framework practitioners are pro-active in taking responsibility for monitoring and maintaining their standard of practice as envisaged by the UKCC (UKCC, 1995, 1996).

Conclusion

As a result of conducting this literature review, the UKCC re-examined their position on clinical supervision and reiterated the key points identified in the 1996 position statement.

These key statements are summarised as:

Key statement 1

Clinical supervision supports practice, enabling practitioners to maintain and promote standards of care.

Key statement 2

Clinical supervision is a practice-focused, professional relationship involving a practitioner reflecting on practice guided by a skilled supervisor.

Key statement 3

The process of clinical supervision should be developed by practitioners and managers according to local circumstances. Ground rules should be agreed so that practitioners and supervisors approach clinical supervision openly, confidently and aware of what is involved.

Key statement 4

Every practitioner should have access to clinical supervision. Each supervisor should supervisee a realistic number of practitioners.

Key statement 5

Preparation for supervisors can be effected using 'in-house' or external education programmes. The principles and relevance of clinical supervision should be included in pre- and post-registration education programmes.

Key statement 6

Evaluation of clinical supervision is needed to assess how it influences care, practice standards and the service. Evaluation systems should be determined locally.

The position statement also includes the UKCC's (1996, p3) perception of what clinical supervision is, namely:

> Clinical supervision brings practitioners and skilled supervisors together to reflect on practice. Supervision aims to identify solutions to problems, improve practice and increase understanding of professional issues.

Clinical supervision is not a managerial control system. It is not therefore:

- the exercise of overt managerial responsibility or managerial supervision;
- a system of formal individual performance review;
- hierarchical in nature.

The UKCC (1996, p3) concludes by stating that it:

endorses the establishment of clinical supervision in the interests of main-taining and improving standards of care in an often uncertain and rapidly changing health and social care environment. The UKCC commends this initiative to all practitioners, managers and those involved in negotiating contracts as an important part of strategies to promote high standards of nursing and health visiting care into the next century.

Acknowledgements

The author is particularly grateful to Christopher Johns, John Cutcliffe, Mike Epling, Paul Cassedy, Jo Burns, A Masterson, A Cameron and Linda Scott for sharing some of their work before it reached the public arena. A final point to remember is that this programme of work was undertaken for the UKCC, not by the UKCC; therefore the views expressed are those of the author and are not necessarily endorsed by the UKCC.

References

Atkins S and Murphy K (1993) Reflection: a review of the literature. *Journal of Advanced Nursing* 18, pp1188–1192.

Bishop V (1998) What is going on? Results of a questionnaire. In Bishop V (eds) *Clinical Supervision in Practice, Some Questions, Answers and Guidelines*, Chapter 2. London: Macmillan.

Brocklehurst N (1996) *Clinical Supervision in the West Midlands: A Survey of NHS trusts*. Report prepared for the NHS Executive, West Midlands, Spring 1996. University of Birmingham: Health Services Management Centre.

Brocklehurst N (1997a) *Developing Clinical Supervision in Anglia and Oxford: A Regional Survey*. Report Prepared for the NHS Executive, Anglia and Oxford, June 1997 University of Birmingham: Health Services Management Centre.

Brocklehurst N (1997b) Clinical supervision in nursing homes. *Nursing Times*, 93 (12), pp48–49.

Brocklehurst N (1997c) *Clinical Supervision in Trent: A Survey of NHS Trusts*. Report prepared for the NHS Executive, Trent, December 1997 University of Birmingham: Health Services Management Centre.

Bulmer C (1997) Supervision: how it works. *Nursing Times*, 93 (48), pp53–55.

Butterworth C A and Faugier J (1994) *Clinical Supervision in Nursing, Midwifery and Health Visiting: A Briefing Paper*. University of Manchester: School of Nursing Studies.

Butterworth T Bishop V and Carson J (1996) First steps towards evaluating clinical supervision in nursing and health visiting: theory, policy and practice development: a review. *Journal of Clinical Nursing*, 5, pp127–131.

Butterworth T Carson J White E Jeacock J Clements A and Bishop V (1997) *It is Good to Talk. An Evaluation Study in England and Scotland*. University of Manchester: School of Nursing, Midwifery and Health Visiting.

Cutcliffe J (1997) Evaluating the success of clinical supervision. *British Journal of Nursing*, 6 (13), p725.

Cutcliffe J R (2000) To record or not to record: Documentation in clinical supervision. *British Journal of Nursing* 9, 6, pp350–355.

Cutcliffe J and Burns J (1998) Personal, professional and practice development: clinical supervision. *British Journal of Nursing*, 7 (21), pp1318–1322.

Cutcliffe J and Epling M (1997) An exploration of the use of John Heron's confronting interventions in clinical supervision; case studies from practice. *Psychiatric Care*, 4(4), pp178–180.

Cutcliffe J R and Proctor B (1998a) An alternative training approach in clinical supervision. Part One. *British Journal of Nursing* 7, 5, pp280–285.

Cutcliffe J R and Proctor B (1998b) An alternative training approach in clinical supervision. Part Two. *British Journal of Nursing* 7, 6, pp344–350.

Cutcliffe J, Epling M, Cassedy P, McGregor J, Plant N and Butterworth T (1998a) Ethical dilemmas in clinical supervision, part 1 – need for guidelines. *British Journal of Nursing*, 7 (15), pp920–923.

Cutcliffe J, Epling M, Cassedy P, McGregor J, Plant N and Butterworth T (1998b) Ethical dilemmas in clinical supervision, part 2 – need for guidelines. *British Journal of Nursing*, 7 (16), pp978–982.

Davidson J (1998) Snapshots from Scotland. In V Bishop's (ed.) *Clinical Supervision in Practice, Some Questions, Answers and Guidelines*, Chapter 4, London: Macmillan.

Department of Health (1993) *A Vision for the Future: The Nursing, Midwifery and Health Visiting Contribution to Health and Health Care*. Department of Health, NHS Management Executive. London: HMSO.

Dimond B (1998a) Legal aspects of clinical supervision, part 1: employer vs employee. *British Journal of Nursing*, 7 (7), pp393–395.

Dimond B (1998b) Legal aspects of clinical supervision, part 2: professional accountability. *British Journal of Nursing*, 7 (8), pp487–489.

Dudley M and Butterworth T (1994) The cost and some benefits of clinical supervision: an initial exploration. *International Journal of Psychiatric Nursing Research*, 1 (2), pp34–36.

Dunn C and Bishop B (1998) Clinical supervision: its implementation in one acute sector trust. In V Bishop's (ed.) *Clinical Supervision in Practice, Some Questions, Answers and Guidelines*, Chapter 5, London: Macmillan.

Farkas-Cameron M (1995) Clinical supervision in psychiatric nursing. *Journal of Psychosocial Nursing*, 26, pp30–32.

Fowler J and Chevannes M (1998) Evaluating the efficacy of reflective practice within the context of clinical supervision. *Journal of Advanced Nursing*, 27 (2), pp379–382.

Fyffe T (1997) *Clinical Supervision: Exploratory Study of Staff Experiences and Perceptions*. University of Dundee: Unpublished Masters in Medical Education thesis.

Hawkins P and Shohet R (1989) *Supervision in the Helping Professions*. Milton Keynes: Open University Press.

Johns C (1994) Can human caring in practice be an everyday reality for nurses? (editorial). *Journal of Nursing Management*, 2 (4), pp157–159.

Johns C (1996) Visualising and realising caring in practice through guided reflection. *Journal of Advanced Nursing*, 24, pp1135–1143.

Johns C (1997) *Becoming an Effective Practitioner Through Guided Reflection*. Open University: unpublished PhD submission, May 1997.

Johns C (1998) Opening the doors of perception. In Johns C, Freshwater D (eds) *Transforming Nursing Through Reflective Practice*, Chapter 1. Oxford: Blackwell Science.

Jones A (1995) Explaining the skills needed in clinical supervision. *Nursing Times* 10(93), pp50–51.

Jones A (1997) A 'bonding between strangers': a palliative model of clinical supervision. *Journal of Advanced Nursing* 26, pp1028–1035.

Lilley L (1996) *Clinical Supervision: Progress Report*. Unpublished report, April 1996. Kettering: Kettering General Hospital NHS Trust.

Lumby J (1998) Transforming nursing through reflective practice. In Johns C, Freshwater, D (eds) *Transforming Nursing Through Reflective Practice*, Chapter 8. Oxford: Blackwell Science.

Marrow C, Macauley D and Crumbie A (1997) Promoting reflective practice through structured clinical supervision. *Journal of Nursing Management*, 5, pp77–82.

Masterson A (1997) *The Continuing Care of Older People, UKCC Policy Paper 1.* Report prepared for the UKCC, London.

Masterson A and Cameron A (1997) *South and West Clinical Supervision Project: Progress Report.* Unpublished report prepared for the NHSE, South and West Region, University of Bristol.

May L, Williams R and Gorman T (1997) *Clinical Supervision: Evaluation of a Pilot Study.* Unpublished report, Edge Hill University College School of Health Studies, Liverpool.

Nicklin P (1997) Clinical supervision – efficient and effective? Paper presented at the British Educational Research Association Annual Conference, University of York, September 1997.

Proctor B (1986) *Supervision: A Co-operative Exercise in Accountability.* In Marken M, Payne M (eds) *Enabling and Ensuring.* Leicester: National Youth Bureau and Council for Education and Training in Youth and Community Work.

Redfern S Norman I, Murrell T *et al.* (1997) *External Review of the Department of Health – Funded Nursing Development Units*, Chapter 4. London: Nursing Research Unit, King's College.

Redfern S Norman I Murrell T *et al.* (1997) *External Review of the Department of Health – Funded Nursing Development Units*, Chapter 7. London: Nursing Research Unit, King's College.

Roden H (1997) *Clinical Supervision: The Outcomes Using a Grounded Theory Approach.* Unpublished BSc dissertation, May 1997.

Sams D (1996) Clinical supervision: an oasis for practice. *British Journal of Community Health Nursing*, 1 (2), pp87–91.

Sams D (1997) *Clinical Supervision: An Evaluation of the Implementation Process Within a Community Trust.* Unpublished report, BHB Community Health Care NHS Trust, Hornchurch.

Scanlon C and Weir WS (1997) Learning from practice? Mental health nurses' perceptions and experiences of clinical supervision. *Journal of Advanced Nursing*, 26, pp295–303.

Scott L (1997) Supervision for health visitors dealing with sexual abuse. *British Journal of Community Health Nursing*, 2 (6), pp303–313.

Scott L (1998) The nature and structure of supervision in health visiting with victims of child sexual abuse. *Journal of Advanced Nursing*, 29 (3), pp754–63.

Swain G (1995) *Clinical Supervision: The Principles and Process.* London: Health Visitors Association.

Thomas B Reid J (1995) Multidisciplinary clinical supervision. *British Journal of Nursing*, 4 (15), pp883–885.

UKCC (1995) *The Council's Proposed Standards for Incorporation into Contracts for Hospital and Community Health Care Services.* London: UKCC.

UKCC (1996) *Position Statement on Clinical Supervision for Nursing and Health Visiting.* London: UKCC.

Wilkin P Bowers L and Monk J (1997) Clinical supervision: managing the resistance. *Nursing Times*, 93 (8), pp48–49.

10 Implementing clinical supervision in a large acute NHS trust

Starting from scratch

Liz Williamson and Gale Harvey

Editorial

This chapter focuses on the attempts to introduce clinical supervision within a large NHS acute trust. It incorporates honest and open reflections which offer an insight into the thoughts, feelings and behaviours of two nurses as they tried to introduce supervision. The chapter describes the particular steps taken in this process including the pilot project, the pilot phase and the evaluation of this pilot. It also highlights the second phase of implementation and considers the future for clinical supervision within the trust.

Current evidence indicates that the practice of clinical supervision appears to be less widespread within general nursing than it is in some other specialities of nursing, e.g. mental health. Whatever the reasons for this disparity, this chapter indicates that the benefits of receiving clinical supervision are just as real for general nurses as they are for any other nurse. Despite the growing awareness of these benefits, there is still evidence that suggest a reluctance (of some) to engage in clinical supervision. Concerns appear to centre on the lack of time and resources, in addition to the degree of apprehension regarding examining one's practice in the company of another. We believe that many of these concerns are best overcome by experiencing high quality clinical supervision for oneself. Thus maybe practice development/clinical supervision co-ordinators should think of ways that these initial, embryonic experiences can be brought about.

Introduction

Back in 1996, nurses within the authors' Trust were waking up to the fact that clinical supervision was not going to go away and there just might be something in it for general nurses. This chapter will provide an insight into how implementation of clinical supervision has been approached within the Trust and also some reflections of the 'if only' kind which only come with hindsight. It is not meant to be an academic account of project planning, change management or even clinical supervision itself. It is a largely personal account of the process, the learning, the mistakes, the successes and the outcomes of our humble efforts at implementing clinical supervision – warts and all! Consequently, the chapter includes personal reflections in order to enhance the understanding and provide a truer picture of some of the difficulties of implementing supervision.

Background

Nottingham City Hospital NHS Trust is a large teaching hospital in the East Midlands. It provides general services to a population of around 500,000 people and specialist services for a much larger population. Around 1600 nurses and midwives are employed by the Trust in a wide range of specialities including renal, paediatrics, oncology and palliative care, cardiology, gastroenterology, neonates, cardiothoracics, obstetrics, sexual health, urology, burns and plastics, as well as other general and critical care services.

The initial interest in clinical supervision within the Trust in 1997 largely came about as a result of the publication of the position paper from the UKCC (1996) and also the increasing emphasis in other national initiatives, such as *A Vision for the Future* (Department of Health, 1993).

At this time, the authors were working clinically in our respective wards (general surgery and burns). The first author was also working on other Trust-wide projects and the opportunity arose to lead the implementation project for clinical supervision.

Personal reflection (first author) – the beginnings

'I had very little idea about what I was taking on, and I had no experience of clinical supervision at the time, only a little knowledge from what I had read in the literature. However, this was clearly a very valuable opportunity, both personally and professionally, and one I wasn't about to pass up. Looking back, I realise how naive I was about the magnitude of the task ahead – it is probably a good job that I didn't know as I might have been tempted to say no! I began to read as much as I could about clinical supervision and I soon began to realise the potential for nurses and nursing that clinical supervision could have. **I also realised that I would have to battle with hearts and minds and that something approaching a cultural revolution would be required for clinical supervision to become embedded in the organisation.***'*

Once a project leader had been appointed, we needed to establish what the current levels of knowledge and experience of clinical supervision were within the Trust, and also what level of priority nurses gave to its implementation. A simple questionnaire was designed and circulated widely within the Trust. The response rate of 75 per cent was heartening. The questionnaire helped to ascertain the level of understanding of clinical supervision, and the current level of activity in the Trust. It also ascertained the level of priority which general nurses within the Trust felt clinical supervision should have. Although it didn't reveal any great surprises, it was a useful, if rather crude, exercise as a starting point. Many wards felt they were already 'doing it' through formal and informal networks and appraisals systems at ward level; however, the knowledge questions demonstrated a lack of understanding as to the true nature of clinical supervision and revealed widespread misconceptions about what clinical supervision is and what it is not. Using a more formal definition of clinical supervision, only two nurses (both working in a counselling-type role) were identified as receiving 'formal' supervision. Interestingly, those who demonstrated a higher level knowledge about clinical supervision generally gave it a greater priority than those with poorer knowledge levels. Overall, there did seem to be a genuine level of interest in and priority for clinical supervision within the Trust. This gave us hope for the implementation project, whilst also raising our awareness about the lack of knowledge and misconceptions surrounding clinical supervision within the Trust back in 1997. We would have to ensure that knowledge levels increased within the Trust if we were to have any chance of long-term success.

Working group

Once the initial ground work had been completed, and the magnitude of the challenge was beginning to emerge, it became apparent that it would be neither advisable nor feasible for one person to take on the challenge alone. A working group, drawn from across the hospital, utilising what experience we did have of clinical supervision, seemed to be the best way to take the implementation project forward. The working group consisted of nurses from across the Trust – a senior nurse (practice development), a nurse manager, a nurse specialist (both of whom had personal experience of receiving supervision), a senior nurse (paediatrics), a staff nurse, a senior staff nurse (the second author) and a ward sister. Our remit at the start of the project was rather hazy and broad – to implement clinical supervision within the Trust. Easy to say; rather less easy to do! We had no pre-agreed terms of reference, so our first two meetings revolved around establishing our priorities and drawing up a work plan. Given that clinical supervision was an unknown entity within the Trust, a project to pilot a framework and approach to clinical supervision was proposed.

Personal reflection (second author) – getting involved

'What sparked my interest in clinical supervision was undertaking the NO1 Counselling course in 1996. It really helped me to see how reflective practice worked in action to increase self-awareness and knowledge and could provide a valuable tool for professional development. I was also aware of the growing interest nationally in clinical supervision and so I contacted the Practice Development to find out what was happening within the Trust. Perfect timing! A working group was being formed to begin the process of looking at clinical supervision with the eventual aim of designing an implementation project

plan. Given my interest in clinical supervision I was pleased to be asked to join the working group.'

All the group underwent a comprehensive reading programme around clinical supervision, particularly about implementation and evaluation. At the time the project started, much of what was being published about clinical supervision was rather theoretical and more focused on the 'what' of clinical supervision, rather than the 'how'. What we felt we really needed was to talk to others in the same positions, but preferably further along in terms of implementation. This opportunity arose through various conference attendances during early 1997. Particularly informative was an RCN conference in May 1997 in Birmingham, which focused almost entirely on implementation and 'real issues'. A number of the speakers had implemented clinical supervision within similar but smaller trusts, and their experiences and reflections proved extremely helpful in focusing our thinking and clarifying some lingering difficulties the group were having (mostly around who should act as supervisor and the provision of training for all involved in supervision).

It became apparent early on that we had a huge task on our hands and all the working group were already very busy people. As the senior nurse (practice development) was already fully committed on other projects, we realised that we needed someone committed to the idea and ideals of clinical supervision to assist with the project and who could dedicate his or her time to the pilot. However, at this early stage, there wasn't the level of commitment within the Trust to fund such a position, and so the proposal was put on hold.

Educational input

One of the biggest hurdles for the most of the working group to overcome was their own lack of experience and some lingering misconceptions around what clinical supervision was and wasn't. One of the ways this was addressed was through an education programme – a double module on clinical supervision offered by our local education provider, the University of Nottingham. This eight-day double module was delivered by two mental health nursing tutors, both of whom have considerable experience of giving, receiving and teaching clinical supervision (see Chapter 5). The course was very useful in providing the working group with a good grounding in the theories surrounding clinical supervision and also providing the opportunity to practise some of the skills vital for supervision. It also increased the confidence of the group that we were thinking broadly along the right lines.

Raising awareness

The first questionnaire gave us a overview of the level of knowledge about clinical supervision within the Trust. There were many misunderstandings and misconceptions identified, so one of the first tasks we charged ourselves with was to raise the levels of awareness and understanding about clinical supervision. We decided to start with a 'big splash' to get the ball rolling and looked around for a suitable speaker. One of the working group had recently met Brigid Proctor, and, given her 'special' place in the world of clinical supervision through her model of supervision (Proctor, 1986), she seemed the ideal candidate. She very kindly agreed to speak to a special evening session of the Nursing Forum in October 1997. The forum was set up in February 1996 as an informal meeting of nurses and midwives within the Trust to discuss and debate current and interesting topics in nursing and health care. Brigid gave a very informative overview of her vision of what clinical supervision was, and two of the working group also spoke – one presented her experiences as a 'receiver' of supervision, and one presented the findings of a small research dissertation on perceptions of clinical supervision within a small team of specialist nurses. The forum was very well attended and extremely successful in helping to raise awareness and even start the conversion process for some of the 'non-believers'!

Members of the working group also attended ward and directorate meetings to spread the word about clinical supervision, informing people of issues involved, such as why it was important, and what the purposes and benefits were. This double-handed approach was vital in raising awareness about clinical supervision and really putting it (and keeping it) on the nursing agenda. At this time, there were many lingering doubts about the benefits of supervision and real concerns about the time and resource commitment necessary to implement clinical supervision.

Drawing up the framework

Taking into account the level of knowledge about clinical supervision at the time, the working group decided to develop a framework for clinical supervision (see Figure 10.1). This allowed us to illustrate the principles and benefits of, and commitment for, clinical supervision, in an broad, overarching philosophy/statement of intent, which would allow individual needs of supervision to be developed and met, and thus had a 'bottom up' rather than 'top down' approach. This framework/philosophy approach was used instead of the more usual formal policy statement and content, which can be rather dry and off-putting for many nurses. The type of supervision adopted was very firmly in the consultation supervision mode, as opposed to managerial supervision (van Ooijen, 2000), which many nurses were already getting in the form of formal, annual appraisals. The framework clearly articulated what clinical supervision should be, and importantly, what it is not. The framework clearly separates clinical supervision from appraisals, disciplinary matters, or any other 'management' issues. Confidentiality between the supervisee and supervisor is stressed, within agreed boundaries (e.g. Code of Professional Conduct). The mode of supervision offered during the pilot was one-to-one – this was primarily a reflection of the lack of experience of most of the pilot supervisors: the skills required for good group supervision are more advanced

- Every nurse and midwife should have access to clinical supervision.
- There will be a high degree of supervisee choice – of supervisor, and of the content, form and frequency of sessions.
- Various forms of supervision are offered, one-to-one is the most common but group, peer and network forms of supervision are also offered, according to the needs of the supervisee(s) and the availability of skilled supervisors.
- Clinical supervision is clearly separate from appraisals, disciplinary, grading or other 'management' issues.
- All supervision participants will agree a written contract of what is expected from both parties, including confidentiality (and the boundaries), record keeping, frequency, cancellations, etc.
- The specific contents of the supervision session will be kept strictly confidential between the supervisee and supervisor. Even if the boundaries have been overstepped, the supervisor will encourage and support supervisees to take action themselves.
- Supervision sessions should be given priority by all staff, not just those directly involved in that particular session, to ensure that sessions go ahead.
- Nurses who would like to be supervisors must fulfil the criteria for supervisors and obtain the agreement of their line manager.
- All those involved in supervision must undergo a period of preparation specific to the role, for either supervisor or supervisee.
- Reflective practice is essential to clinical supervision: all those involved are expected to develop and use these skills.
- Each supervisor should decide how many individuals they can supervise, according to their existing workload. Inexperienced supervisors should not supervise more than two nurses.
- All supervisors must also receive their own supervision, the format to be decided by the individual.
- Records of these sessions will be kept by the supervisor, using the supervision record/audit form. These will be used only for evaluation purposes, and will not include any specific details about the session.
- Supervisees will be encouraged to keep their own records of supervision. These notes will be used only to inform the supervision process and could be included in the nurse's professional profile. Care must be taken to ensure patient and colleague confidentiality is not compromised.

Figure 10.1 Nottingham City Hospital NHS Trust framework for clinical supervision

(e.g. managing group dynamics). The importance of record keeping was stressed, including a written contract between supervisee and supervisor; the role of reflection, and ongoing records of supervision, progress, actions etc., were included.

Consultation process

The framework was widely circulated for comments; we received disappointingly few replies, illustrating perhaps that the implementation of clinical supervision wasn't as high a priority for nurses as previously indicated or that people still lacked sufficient knowledge to feel able to comment. We continued to spread the word with attendance at ward and sisters' meetings and slowly the interest started to grow into something more tangible. Some wards and individuals started to come forward with expressions of interest in being part of the pilot. The senior nurse managers gave the go-ahead following a presentation of the framework and project plan.

Funding and project co-ordinator

At this point in the project (late 1997), the authors obtained some funding for the clinical supervision implementation project from Trent NHSME, as part of the Action Agenda for Nursing initiative (NHS Executive, 1997). This enabled us to appoint a part-time project co-ordinator; the second author was already part of the working group and had already demonstrated her interest in, and commitment to, clinical supervision. The second author started her secondment in November 1997 with the express aim of co-ordinating the pilot phase and the subsequent evaluation. Appointing a co-ordinator was a turning point for the project, as we now had someone who could dedicate three days a week to the pilot project. It was crucial to establish a point of contact for the nurses within the Trust, and especially those in the pilot areas. Through extensive reading, consultation and networking, the second author was able to establish a level of knowledge about clinical supervision previously lacking within the working group and the Trust as a whole.

Personal reflections (second author) – co-ordinator role

'Being part of the working group for nine months had only served to increase my enthusiasm and firm belief in the very real and positive potential which clinical supervision had for nurses. The opportunity of the secondment came along at an ideal time for me professionally and gave me the chance to work across the Trust on a very exciting, if rather daunting, new development. It allowed me to use and put into practice some of the theories and knowledge I had gained during my degree studies, in particular change management and professional issues. It also enabled me to use my knowledge and enthusiasm to influence and inform an important professional development.'

The pilot project

To enable us to pilot the framework, we asked for six wards or departments to volunteer for the pilot project. We were looking for a wide range of clinical specialities and team set-ups. The areas which came forward for the pilot were a gynaecology ward, a general medical ward, a paediatric ward, a specialist ward (burns), an oncology ward and a group of specialist nurses (breast care) – some had volunteered themselves, and some had been nominated by their manager. From each of these areas, four registered nurses volunteered or were put forward to be the first cohort of supervisees. 'Clustering' or concentrating the supervisees together in this way (rather than drawing them from across the Trust and thus 'diluting' them) enabled the pilot areas to experience the impact of clinical supervision on the clinical area and on those not taking part in the pilot. For the supervisors, we looked to those nurses who had completed the double module on clinical supervision at the local university. This only gave us eight supervisors so we asked for additional volunteers to undergo in-house training to take on the role of supervisor. It was crucial for our 'philosophy' of supervision that we were able to offer supervisees a real choice of supervisor, not just another (more senior) nurse from within their ward team.

Following a literature review, criteria for being a supervisor were devised as part of the framework. They were not applied rigidly in the early stages of the project; they were intended to demonstrate the skills and qualities required to be a supervisor to prospective supervisors. This enabled the pilot supervisors to 'self select', thus ensuring willingness, commitment and a certain level of motivation.

In-house training for supervisors and supervisees

One of the most important parts of the framework and our 'philosophy' was that everyone should undergo some form of preparation for the role they would play within the pilot project, a factor which came across strongly in the literature and conference presentations. Because of the resource implications, it could have been overlooked or scrimped on. Fortunately, because of the external funding we had received, we were able to develop an in-house programme for both supervisees and supervisors, and to buy in expertise in the form of a trained facilitator from the local school of nursing to deliver and facilitate the training. Howard was known already known to members of the working group because of his reputation in the field of supervision and we had no doubt that he would be invaluable in helping to get the pilot off to a good start through a comprehensive preparation and training programme.

The programme consisted of two days of 'shared' learning where the supervisees and supervisor together explored the models, types, concepts and realities of clinical supervision. Skills required for reflective practice, issues around documentation, and agreeing contracts were also included. We chose this joint approach for a number of reasons. First, neither group had any experience of clinical supervision, nor a reasonable level of knowledge about it; thus, their initial learning needs were very similar. Second, it gave the two groups the opportunity to get to know each other and thus facilitate the process of choosing a supervisor. Finally, by learning together, there was a shared sense of purpose between supervisees and supervisor – there was no fear of 'hidden agendas' between the two groups. The supervisors did undergo an additional day's preparation, concentrating on the skills they would need for supervision, and three short follow-up sessions, where potentially difficult situations were explored and discussed, in the weeks following the course.

The programme ran twice during early 1998 and the evaluations of those attending the programme were very positive. There were a few negative feelings about the pace of the sessions, particularly from nurses who are used to a more didactic approach to teaching, and those who are used to 'rushing around'. The facilitative nature of the workshop, as well as the very nature of clinical supervision, meant it was vital for nurses to have the time during the programme to think and reflect more deeply than they normally do. The reasons for the deliberately slower pace is now made much more explicit; as a consequence, participants are more prepared and there are now very few negative comments about the pace.

Once the training had been completed, all the supervisors were asked to complete a 'directory' so that supervisees could choose a supervisor. This directory consists of information about clinical (and other relevant) experience, and includes a section for the supervisor to identify what he or she can bring to supervision. All the supervisees were asked to nominate two to three possibilities; these were then communicated to the co-ordinator, who ascertained if those supervisors were still 'available'. None of the new supervisors took more than two supervisees during the pilot; most had just one supervisee. This was to ensure that none of them felt overloaded with their new responsibilities and enabled them to concentrate their efforts on improving their skills with just one or two supervisees.

The pilot phase

The pilot commenced in March 1998 and ran until December 1998. The supervisees were asked to choose a supervisor and then arrange monthly meetings of an hour's duration. This meant that supervisees and supervisors could meet around nine times, which should allow sufficient time for the working alliance between the two to have developed and be functioning effectively. The first hurdle to overcome was getting the supervisees to choose a supervisor. We very much wanted the pilot project to mirror 'real life' as much as possible, and it was important that the project was able to 'run itself' without too much outside interference. One of the most important aspects of the philosophy we had developed was that it should be supervisee-led. However, in order to maintain these 'rights' for supervisees (in terms of type, content, and choice of supervisor), certain 'responsibilities' must also be met – to choose a supervisor, to arrange and attend sessions, to choose the topic for reflection and discussion at each session, etc. It soon became apparent that for some of the supervisees and supervisors, there was considerable stress when taking on supervision for the first time, as discussed by van Ooijen (2000). Some supervisees were reluctant to choose a supervisor and asked for someone to be nominated for them. It was recommended that the supervisees should make contact with their chosen supervisor and arrange a preliminary meeting prior to contract setting. The aim of this was for both parties to make a brief assessment as to whether they felt they could work together. It was intended to be very informal and unstructured, possibly over a coffee.

The authors made it clear that we were there for support and information if needed by any member of the pilot project but otherwise we would let the project run on its own. The authors needed to know if the relationships would be self maintaining and wanted a true evaluation of the experiences without interference from them.

Evaluation

The Trust framework recommended that supervisees arrange for monthly meetings of about 60 minutes. The number of meetings that supervisees and supervisors actually had during the pilot varied from one to nine with an average of six in the nine month period. The few supervisees who 'got off to a bad start' never recovered from this and didn't allow the working alliance with their new supervisor to develop.

Despite the recognised difficulties in evaluating clinical supervision and its effects (Carson, 1998; Dooher *et al.*, 1998; Bond and Holland, 1998), an evaluation of the pilot was required to establish how the implemented framework of clinical supervision impacted on practice and practitioners. This evaluative research took place in the form of a self-administered quantitative questionnaire with a space for comment after each series of questions.

An evaluation of the direct experience of clinical supervision and the perceived effect this had on the participants and their practice was required, so a questionnaire was constructed, using a self-report format comprised of groups of statements. Respondents were asked to consider each statement and then agree or disagree with it, using a Likert scale (a rating scale of strongly agree to strongly disagree – Polit and Hungler, 1995). Issues covered by the questionnaire were formulated following an extensive review of the literature. Twenty-two supervisees remained at the end of the pilot (two had left the Trust) and all of them completed a questionnaire.

The primary aim of the review was to evaluate the perceived benefits of receiving clinical supervision by those involved in the pilot. The significant investment of implementing clinical supervision in a large NHS Trust necessitates a well-planned execution and a comprehensive evaluation. This evaluation highlighted a positive perception of clinical supervision with improvements in personal and professional development.

All patients are entitled to high quality care (DoH, 1998) so nurses must continuously update their skills and knowledge. This process was highlighted in the evaluation as a number of nurses claimed that the process of clinical supervision helped them to identify their strengths (82 per cent; n=18), identify training needs (68 per cent; n=15), improve standards of care (64 per cent; n=14) and gain knowledge through the process of reflection (77 per cent; n=17).

The opportunity to reflect on practice was valued highly and an overall commitment to the process of reflection can be seen throughout the study. Clinical supervision provides the time and opportunity to reflect on practice in a supportive environment. Thirty-two per cent (7) of the supervisees claimed that they were even inspired to write a reflective diary following the pilot.

The change in nursing over the last decade from a predominantly task-orientated mode of caring to a more holistic, individualised approach has led to an increased need for support in helping to maintain effective, therapeutic relationships with patients (Playle and Mullarkey, 1998). Emotional support in matters relating to patients/clients was highly valued with 59 per cent (n=13) stating that clinical supervision did provide this support. An increase in confidence was perceived by ten of the nurses (45 per cent) as an outcome of receiving supervision.

Support is also required in professional working relationship with colleagues and managers and the chance to discuss and receive such support was very notable with 82 per cent (n=18) stating that clinical supervision had provided this.

The in-house training programme for supervisees evaluated well and experiences during the pilot highlighted the need to prepare supervisees for their new role. Elements of the training course were considered 'useful' or 'very useful' by 100 per cent (n=24) of the pilot sample and included '*a definition and outline of clinical supervision, reflective practice, responsibilities, skills and qualities of supervisee and supervisor.*' Only one respondent in the evaluation claimed that the two-day training provided by the Trust did not prepare her/him adequately for the role of supervisee.

The combined training programme was preferred by the majority of the group (82 per cent n=18). Two respondents indicated a strong desire to have separate training. A further comment was made by one of these respondents that this '*would have allowed time to clarify fears and anxieties away from the supervisors.*'

Anxiety undoubtedly exists regarding the role of supervisee within the clinical supervision relationship and in particular record keeping of the supervisory process. Such concerns regarding record keeping are not uncommon (Cutcliffe, 2000). This was always highlighted on the training days in discussion times. Despite this high level of anxiety a large increase in personal record keeping occurred during the pilot. Beforehand, only 18 per cent (n=4) respondents maintained a record of their practice; after the pilot, 82 per cent (n=18) acknowledged writing some sort of record. This ranged from discussion headings only to a detailed account of supervision. This could be due to the emphasis placed on this aspect in the training or perhaps to heightened professional awareness from receiving supervision.

Feedback from respondents leaves us in little doubt regarding the skills and qualities of a good supervisor and how fundamental to the process of clinical supervision the supervisor is. According to the respondents, the ideal characteristics for the supervisor to possess are honesty, being approachable, trustworthiness and the ability to be non-judgemental. This response mirrors that of supervisees in the study by Bulmer (1997) and is understandable bearing in mind the nature of the working alliance. Good interpersonal skills were identified as essential for the supervisor to possess and were seen as fundamental in helping the supervisee reflect on practice. Eighty-one per cent (n=18) of the supervisees felt that they had been supported to reflect on practice in their clinical supervision sessions.

The right of a supervisee to choose a supervisor should be stressed as this may determine the success of the clinical supervision relationship (Bond and Holland, 1998). Seventy-seven per cent (n=17) of the supervisees in the pilot would not have wanted a supervisor allocated to them and 91 per cent (n=20) said they would not have wanted their manager. Only one respondent chose a supervisor with whom he or she worked. Three respondents said they would prefer it to be someone they knew. This contrasts to many examples quoted throughout the literature where senior nurses are supervising junior colleagues in wards or units (Kohner, 1994; Devine and Baxter, 1995; McGibbon, 1996). In our experience, supervisees particularly valued being able to choose their own supervisor.

A cultural change is required to ensure the success of clinical supervision, with priority given by all the team to allow nurses to attend a supervision session. If lack of support from colleagues and managers is evident, nurses may feel guilty and be more likely to cancel their supervision session. Ten supervisees said that they felt guilty leaving their ward or work area to receive supervision and only 41 per cent (n=9) felt that their colleagues had a good understanding of clinical supervision. This again highlighted the need for ongoing awareness raising and education throughout the Trust in all aspects of supervision theory and process.

Interestingly after the pilot 59 per cent (n=13) of the supervisees and 50 per cent (n=6) of the supervisors felt clinical supervision should be mandatory, possibly reflecting the perceived benefit from the process and the importance they now assigned to it. It may also be that they felt that colleagues would be more supportive if supervision was mandatory.

This evaluative research was completed in April 1999 and made a number of recommendations for the future of clinical supervision within the Trust (see Figure 10.2).

The second phase

Following the completion of the pilot project, there still wasn't an overwhelming push to introduce clinical supervision, despite the positive evaluation from the pilot supervisees and supervisors. There were still many concerns about the time and resource commitment necessary, which some nurses perceived as prohibitive. Despite these reservations, the next phase to roll-out clinical

Organisational

- Maintain a high profile of clinical supervision within the hospital after a successful hospital pilot.
- The implementation of clinical supervision should proceed to other areas in the hospital and expand in the pilot areas.
- Feedback sessions regarding the pilot to all areas involved. By raising the profile again in these areas, it should support those already involved and offer others the chance to update their knowledge and to question the hospital framework and commitment to clinical supervision.
- An ongoing programme of awareness sessions regarding clinical supervision accessible to all staff within the Trust. This will ensure that staff are up to date regarding the hospital framework for clinical supervision and the larger nursing perspective.
- Include a brief introduction to clinical supervision on the Hospital Induction Programme to inform new staff about the hospital framework for clinical supervision.

Training

- Supervisees should complete the section of the questionnaire on the perceptions of clinical supervision pre-training so that a more useful comparison can be made after experiencing clinical supervision.
- More active support must be available to supervisees, immediately after training, in setting up and establishing a supervisory relationship.
- Discuss with Nottingham University the possibility of teaching pre-registration student nurses the theory, process and outcomes of clinical supervision, which will help address the long-term change of culture regarding clinical supervision.
- Training should continue for both supervisees and supervisors.

Figure 10.2 Recommendations from the evaluation

supervision was given the go ahead. Almost all the recommendations from the pilot evaluation were actioned. The plan for roll-out across the Trust in 1999 continued the centralised, tiered approach, expanding on the approach taken during the pilot, with a small number of wards joining in, in stages, and the training and co-ordination maintained centrally, through the co-ordinator. The second author's secondment was extended during this period. The training and preparation programme was reviewed – a one-day course for clinical supervision was introduced and facilitated by the authors, which everyone attends, prior to becoming a supervisee, or to find out more about clinical supervision. Those who opt to take on the role of supervisor undergo a further two-day preparation programme.

The third phase

A number of factors led us to completely review this approach in late 1999. First, this meant that the continued roll-out would be slow, if thorough. Second, there was now an ever increasing interest within the Trust and many more areas, and individuals were asking for supervision. It soon became obvious that demand (for supervision) was outstripping supply (for training and supervisors). The second factor was the publication of *Making a Difference* in July 1999 (Department of Health, 1999). During debates about the document and the implications and subsequent priorities for the Trust, clinical supervision was made one of three priorities for 1999/2001 (along with competencies and leadership) as the focus for the nursing strategy. This meant that we needed to radically review how we were going to meet the needs for supervision within the Trust, whilst still maintaining the quality of the provision, in terms of preparation, choice of supervisor and on-going support for all those involved. Finally, a centralised approach meant that many nurses didn't have a real opportunity to be involved in developing supervision within the Trust and this could discourage individual and directorate responsibility for taking supervision forward.

Directorate/divisional training and co-ordination

The model for taking clinical supervision forward within the Trust has now

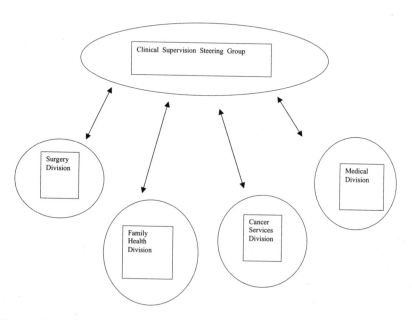

Figure 10.3 Directorate/divisional model for clinical supervision within the Trust

changed from a centralised one to a divisional model (see Fig. 10.3). The framework, philosophy and valuable lessons learnt from the evaluations have been devolved to five divisions, each with between 100 and 300 registered nurses. Steering groups have been set up in each division to identify local training needs and strategies, monitor uptake of supervision, audit and evaluate progress and standards, and provide training for supervisees.

A Trust-wide steering group continues, with our involvement, but with a different remit. This group includes a central core of experienced supervisors who now deliver the in-house training programme for new supervisors. Gradually, as the divisional groups increase their confidence and experience, they will also take over supervisor training, as well as supervisee. The steering group produces training packs and teaching aids which the divisional groups can use and adapt as necessary. This maintains standards across the Trust whilst allowing individual directorate needs to be met.

The future

Given the current level of interest in, and enthusiasm for, clinical supervision within the Trust, we now feel that we have passed the point of no return. Many of the nurses who receive supervision cannot now imagine doing without it. Quite a change from three years ago when only two nurses in the Trust could say the same! The struggle is by no means over. The ongoing debate about time and resources still continues and will go on whilst the divisional groups find their feet. There is still a great need for more research and evidence about the benefits of clinical supervision, especially in terms of improvements in patient care. Without good leadership and a sense of responsibility at all levels of the nursing profession, clinical supervision could still falter. However, instead of a few nurses on a working group, we now have over 300 nurses receiving supervision who don't want it to go away. A much more powerful voice!

A final reflection (both authors)

'Because of how the clinical supervision project has evolved, our central function in the ongoing implementation is no less relevant or useful. Given our strength of feeling for clinical supervision, and the sense of ownership of the project, this could have been a difficult time for both of us. However, these feelings are more than outweighed by the prospect of others taking clinical supervision to a whole new level of influence and importance within the Trust. Working together on a project like this has been a huge learning experience for both of us. We were able to share our knowledge and experiences, increase our own self-awareness, and motivate each other through those days when it felt like we were in a minefield! We were able to use theories of change management to begin the cultural change necessary to

implement and embed clinical supervision within the organisation. Absolutely key to the current and ongoing success of the project has been leadership skills – of those at the 'top', within the working group and at all levels of the profession – this has been a fundamental change in the way in which nurses think and work at the City Hospital and we are very glad to have been a part of it.'

References

Bond M and Holland S (1998) *Skills of Clinical Supervision for Nurses*. Buckingham: Open University Press.

Bulmer C (1997) Supervision: how it works. *Nursing Times*, 93 (48), pp53–54.

Butterworth T, White E, Carson J, Jeacock J, Clements A and Bishop V (1997) *Clinical Supervision and Mentorship: It is good to talk. An Evaluation Study in England and Scotland*. Manchester: School of Nursing, Midwifery and Health Visiting, University of Manchester.

Carson J (1998) Instruments for evaluating clinical supervision. In Bishop V (ed.) (1998) *Clinical Supervision in Practice: Some Questions, Answers and Guidelines*, pp163–178. Basingstoke: Macmillan/*Nursing Times*.

Cutcliffe J R (2000) To record or not to record: documentation in clinical supervision. *British Journal of Nursing* 9, 6, pp350–355.

Department of Health (1993) *A Vision for the Future: The Nursing, Midwifery and Health Visiting Contribution to Health and Healthcare*. London: HMSO.

Department of Health (1998) *A First Class Service: Quality in the New NHS*. London: HMSO.

Department of Health (1999) *Making a Difference: Strengthening the Nursing, Midwifery and Health Visiting Contribution to Health and Healthcare*. London: HMSO.

Devine A and Baxter T (1995) Introducing clinical supervision: a guide. *Nursing Standard* 9, (40), pp32–34.

Dooher J, Fowler J, Phillips A M and Wells A (1998) Evaluating the benefits of clinical supervision. In: Fowler J (ed) *The Handbook of Clinical Supervision: Your Questions Answered*, pp147–159. London: Quay Books.

Kohner N (1994) *Clinical Supervision in Practice*. London: King's Fund Centre.

Lucas S, Jones A, Glover D (2000) NT Open Learning: Part 8 – Implementation Problems. *Nursing Times* 96 (11), pp49–52.

McGibbon G (1996) Clinical supervision for expanded practice. In ENT *Professional Nurse*, 12 (2), pp100–102.

NHS Executive (1997) *Action Agenda for Nursing*. Leeds: HMSO.

Playle J F and Mullarkey K (1998) Parallel process in clinical supervision: enhancing learning and providing support. *Nurse Education Today* 18, pp558–566.

Polit D F and Hungler B P (1995) *Nursing Research: Principles and Methods* (5th Edition). Philadelphia: J.B. Lippincott.

Proctor B (1986) Supervision: a co-operative exercise in accountability. In Marken M, Payne (eds) *Enabling and Ensuring*. Leicester: National Youth Bureau and Council for Education and Training in Youth and Community Work.

United Kingdom Central Council for Nursing, Midwifery and Health Visiting (1996) *Position Statement on Clinical Supervision for Nursing and Health Visiting*. London: UKCC.

Van Ooijen E (2000) *Clinical Supervision: A Practical Guide*. Edinburgh: Churchill Livingstone.

Part III

11 Clinical supervision

My path towards clinical excellence in mental health nursing

Paul Smith

Editorial

This chapter focuses on the practice of clinical supervision within mental health nursing. The author, a community psychiatric nurse, demonstrates how receiving clinical supervision helped him develop skills and knowledge, improved the care he delivered to his clients and helped him maintain his own well-being. He achieves this by drawing on specific examples of problems and issues that were encountered in his practice and subsequently taken into supervision.

We believe that this chapter offers a good illustration of the particular worth and value that exists in having a significant other provide an 'outside' view of one's practice. Not just any other, but a person in whom the supervisee has trust, confidence and faith. A person who, in partnership with the supervisee, can create the necessary and sufficient environment and relationship that helps bring about the development of the supervisee. Perhaps this chapter also implicitly alludes to the importance of finding a supervisor with whom the supervisee feels he/she can work, and thus highlights the importance of being able to select one's supervisor rather than having a supervisor imposed upon him or her.

Introduction

In this chapter I am going to attempt to demonstrate that clinical supervision is effective in developing skills and knowledge, improving care delivered to patients and maintaining the health and clinical effectiveness and health of the supervisee. I hope to achieve this by describing my experience of clinical supervision, using specific examples of problems or challenges I faced in my own clinical practice. These examples have been selected to typify the range of issues that have cropped up in my practice as a registered nurse in the field of mental health but had supervision been available while I was working as an RGN the issues would have been similar. The examples are loosely arranged in three, chronologically correct, stages. They include:

- My introduction to supervision whilst studying for a post-registration diploma titled 'Understanding Therapeutic Relationships' which was run by clinical psychologists within the NHS Trust and validated by the Nottingham Trent University.
- My experience of supervision provided by a nursing colleague as I worked on the same inpatient unit for people with enduring mental health problems.
- My role as staff nurse in an acute, GP attached Community Mental Health Team.

I will also draw attention to some of the practical disadvantages that can occur if certain principles are overlooked, again using real situations from my own practice.

My approach is not overly academic but is descriptive and discursive, but hopefully can be scholarly and persuasive nonetheless. My gratitude goes to my supervisors, who here remain anonymous, for the love, patience and support they have shown me. I hope and believe that they would agree with me when I suggest that at least some of the time spent in providing my supervision has resulted in valuable (and even measurable) gains for the people we claim to care for.

Early experiences of clinical supervision

For the first six years of my nursing career I was not given clinical supervision in the form I recognise as relevant and necessary today. As a student nurse (RGN, 1984 syllabus) I was allocated to registered nurses whilst on clinical placement, some of whom were bemused or threatened by my frequent questions, and some were tolerant of my striving to do and know the right way to do things. As a junior staff nurse I was extremely fortunate to have experienced colleagues who forgave me my sometimes insensitive challenges of not only procedures and routines but also their clinical practice. During this time I frequently received critical, balanced feedback about my technical skills, my application of knowledge to clinical situations and developments in my own practice, much of which was helpful and constructive. Indeed it continued through further training which led to my becoming a Registered Nurse (Mental Health) and a staff nurse on a rehabilitation/challenging behaviour/continuing care unit for people with 'severe and enduring' mental health needs. But in all this time I had little guidance to help me examine, analyse, and explore the reasons as to why I did what I did, said what I said, behaved the way I behaved. It is reasonable to suggest that I gained insights through reflection upon and within my practice, by discussions with peers and colleagues, and from being exposed to praise, criticism and indifference by others. But I was frequently aware that there was something missing from the picture, although I didn't know what.

After nine months of working in the inpatient unit, I commenced a course in

'Understanding Therapeutic Relationships' which was run within the Trust by the Psychology Department. An integral part of the course was a module that involved clinical supervision by a psychologist with the aim of participants learning more of the processes that occur in their interpersonal therapeutic relationships with clients. Throughout the ten-week term we brought issues from our clinical practice on alternate weeks to the supervision group of a psychologist. We alternated the sessions between us, which generally lasted between an hour and ninety minutes. We had received teaching as to the purpose of the sessions, which were not specifically to address issues of technique or clinical knowledge but to gain an understanding about 'process'. This meant that our descriptions of interactions between us and our clients were less valuable than the exploration of what we thought was going on whilst the interaction or events occurred.

Formative group supervision sessions

The issues I brought to the group were to do with the difficulties I was experiencing in developing a therapeutic interpersonal relationship with a resident in the unit of which I was a staff member. I had been allocated as the key worker to a male resident, Dave, who had been an inpatient for several years in various mental health units within the Trust. The difficulty that I was experiencing was how to stop Dave from interrupting conversations with noisy demands for staff to listen to what he wanted to say about his voices. A nursing care plan had been in force which reflected the general perception of staff that Dave was behaving without reasonable consideration for accepted social norms as well as a clinical view which did not consider engagement in discussion about the content and meaning of auditory hallucinations as being therapeutic. Dave often became more insistent in his demand to be listened to, leading to mutual frustration, anger on his part and no successful resolution to his requests. My training had not equipped me with a conceptual therapeutic model with which to compare this oft-repeated scenario.

As I described what I thought was a reasonable therapeutic approach, i.e. to reinforce generally accepted social norms in line with the prevailing philosophy of the unit, my supervisor asked me to reflect on what was happening in the interpersonal dynamics between Dave and members of staff. She asked me directly how I felt whilst Dave was demanding attention from me. She asked me to speculate how Dave was feeling when he was told he couldn't talk about something he thought was very, very important. I realised we both felt powerless, angry, ignored, devalued.

I have never forgotten the impact of realising that for what had seemed good reasons I was colluding in a system that was resulting in anger and frustration for both Dave and members of staff. That supervision session I became aware that I had no conceptual justification for refusing to listen to Dave talk at me about his voices other than I did not know what to do to help him if I did. I also became aware of my emotional response to Dave which was interfering in the therapeutic interpersonal relationship that I was intending to be encouraging (Peplau, 1988). For example, in recognising and admitting to my own sense of irritation, indignation, or anger when Dave confronted me or colleagues I was able to ask myself whether my response was justified (in the context of being therapeutic). To my discomfort I was able to identify that some of my reaction was because I felt and thought that I, a staff nurse, should be shown more respect, perhaps more gratitude, from this rude, thoughtless, demanding man! I had become an authority figure who Dave was challenging as he had challenged his father since he was a child, although for years I would have espoused the idea that a nurse should work co-operatively with patients, promoting their sense of independence and challenging passivity and dependence.

It was through this I now understood how Dave's expectations of me (and others) were based on experience of previous relationships when he had taken a subordinate but rebellious role. I now had an experience of working with transference and counter-transference, as described by Brown and Pedder (1991). I had discovered what transference felt like, and once enlightened was able to respond to his behaviour in a way that did not confirm unhelpful thoughts and feelings that he had towards authority figures, a way that empowered him and affirmed him as an individual. I did this by failing to meet his unhelpful expectations of me. For example, when Dave did or threatened to do something which was potentially problematic, such as go to the pub to get drunk, he was no longer told he couldn't. Instead I discussed with him what his wants were, what the organisational requirements were and together a mutually beneficial solution was reached. What was avoided was an unhelpful reprise of an authoritarian father figure and a rebellious child (Harris, 1973). The outcome of this was that Dave reduced the number of assaults he made on staff for the next two years and felt able to arrange sessions when he and I would talk about his voices.

By bringing more examples of my interaction with Dave to supervision I was able to gain a deeper understanding of the nature and quality of the transactions that occurred between Dave and myself. More importantly I was able to change and adapt my own practice to the benefit of Dave. Instead of attempting to control Dave's demands for attention I began to actively seek opportunities for him to ventilate his frustrations and fears about the voices that caused him distress. It became possible to reject a view, which had not been challenged throughout my training, that voices were symptoms and not to be encouraged, and this led me to the new developments in cognitive behavioural therapy (Kingdon and Turkington, 1991; Alford and Beck, 1994; Birchwood and Tarrier, 1992) to 'treat' hallucinations and delusions. I was also able to appreciate that Dave's behaviour towards me might have had less to do with me and rather more to do with historical relationships.

My continuing experience of clinical supervision has been with my line manager. I agree with Bond and Holland (1998), Cutcliffe and Proctor (1998a,b) and Butterworth and Faugier (1992) that difficulties are likely to arise when line managers offer supervision, because the focus of the supervision can easily move from the needs of the supervisee to those of the manager and the employer. I could ignore the identity of my supervisors or pretend that my situation was the exception that proves the rule. The latter case has some validity as I have a strong character and robust personality and have by nature and inclination sought out people with the skills and insights to help me. I could even argue that in my case the supervisors were particularly skilled and were committed to offering supervision in the absence of formal requirement by our employers. The truth is that there were some issues I felt unable to take to my formal supervisor for different reasons. One was that in admitting to some thoughts and feelings I was concerned that this would prejudice my professional standing with my manager. This certainly illustrates some unresolved transference issues of my own but is also a reasonable concern. A second reason, closely related to the first, is that are some issues which practitioners are not comfortable about in exploring even with themselves, and to do so with someone in authority is even more problematic. In my own case this has included feelings of anger towards a patient who I was becoming frightened of. Fortunately I was able to take this issue (and others) to someone who I implicitly trusted and who did not feel obligated to inform my employer of our discussion. Because I had a place of safety I was able to express raw feelings, thoughts and emotions without fear of censure. In return I was relieved of the guilt and shame I had for merely experiencing human emotions, and was thereby empowered to change some of my own thoughts and beliefs, change my working practice and to develop strategies for managing the behaviour of the patient involved. If this proves anything it is that clinical supervision allows us to be human and professional. In my case it permitted me to continue working in a homely environment with people who had or were likely to assault or threaten me and to do so in a therapeutic way without resorting to authoritarian attitudes. I believe that this example also illustrates a danger of receiving supervision from a line manager, no matter how strong the professional or personal ties are. Regrettably, I could provide testimonies from dozens of colleagues whose 'clinical supervisors' consider supervision sessions to be about their own issues, about caseload management or about control. This is not clinical supervision and can only be detrimental to patient care and the professional development of the nurse being supervised.

Further development

The importance of this second phase in my experience of clinical supervision was that it occurred after I had spent eighteen months as a team member upon the unit, and it was during a period of considerable change within the ward. The needs of the residents meant that many of them had been in residential care for many years and new residents were likely to require high levels of support whilst resident within the unit or on discharge. A new ward manager brought a new sense of team identity, new expectations in the aims and objectives to be achieved by nursing interventions and new approaches to old difficulties or problems. I had also completed the course on which I first experienced supervision and now had an understanding of how to engage with clients and their needs and difficulties in a way that was more collaborative and more dynamic. But it was only because I had a forum for exploring the difficulties I experienced as a clinician and a team member that I retained such effectiveness as I had.

Whilst the supervision took place over several years there are specific examples that illustrate the effectiveness and value of the supervision I received. One example involved a resident who had recently been admitted to the unit after a period of time on an acute psychiatric admission ward which had followed a deterioration in his relationship with his parents. Jack was resentful of not being allowed to live with his parents because of his disturbed and aggressive behaviour. He expressed bizarre ideas about being influenced by aliens and the occult in the past and thought his real mum had been replaced by the present woman who looked like her and sounded like her but couldn't be her because his mum would have him to live at home. He was disturbed by some of these ideas and even more troubled by the sense of abandonment he felt. Jack was skilled in many activities of daily living although chose not to attend to his hygiene or grooming. He was also careless with personal possessions and became verbally aggressive when he had mislaid or used up his supply of tobacco. As his primary nurse, I had responsibility for developing a nursing care plan to address his various needs. As an individual I occasionally interpreted this as having a responsibility for Jack. Through several supervision sessions I was able to recognise that I was emotionally responding to Jack's explicit and implicit demands to be mothered, to be nurtured, to be rescued from the consequences of his own choices and actions. My supervisor facilitated this understanding by asking me how I felt or what I thought was being demanded from me by Jack, when he behaved in ways which were apparently careless or rebellious. It wasn't that I was thoroughly unaware of what Jack was doing, but by exploring the transference and counter transference I was able to respond with self-awareness. I was able to recognise the unhelpfulness of my own unconscious desire to help, to nurture, and to parent. Identifying the transference/counter-transference that was present meant that I was able to act in a way that was to eventually result in an increased sense of personal autonomy and responsibility for Jack. Because I resisted the urge to rescue him from distress and/or of feeling angry that he wasn't following a mutually negotiated and agreed care plan, because I gained a sense of empowerment through supervision, I felt increasingly able to empower Jack in having an expanding area of choice and responsibility. We were able to revisit parenting issues that he had experienced in ways that were more appropriate to our ages and abilities, and Jack was able to describe these issues as he gained an understanding of them.

Growth of self-awareness

It is not accurate to suppose that I brought such issues to supervision knowingly. Whilst I gave thought to what I wanted to talk about beforehand invariably I would incidentally describe with some emotion an event that had occurred, without immediately realising its significance. Thus when I talked of being confused or angry or sad it became apparent that Jack or whoever was experiencing similar or the same emotions. This became a powerful tool as I became more self-aware as I could then reflect back to a client that emotion, albeit in a tentative way, and encourage them to increasing awareness of their own mood states.

For example, this was particularly helpful in developing my therapeutic relationship with Dave, as he was not skilled in recognising and adapting to rising levels of anger or sadness. One evening Dave had become angry when a member of his family had made comments which Dave had difficulty in 'hearing', and he assaulted this family member. It was clear that further assaults were going to occur and that Dave was past the point at which he could be talked down. Nor did he respond to usually effective de-escalation techniques (Maier, 1996). He was informed of our next response, which would be to hold him until the threat of violence was withdrawn, as at that stage there was no likelihood that a further assault could be prevented due to the physical arrangement of the room. Dave was also reminded that we recognised that he would dislike this and we had no wish to harm him and would prefer for him not to have to endure that. The situation eventually required a physical intervention that within a minute resulted in Dave saying he was calm and that he would go to his room. (An interpretation of this rapid reduction in Dave's emotional arousal could be that there had been a resolution of the bind he was in. He had been angry but didn't have the skill to express this more effectively. Nor was he able to back down in that situation without losing face. Intervention by nursing staff conformed to past interventions he had experienced in previous establishments, including hospital environments, and so he was able to follow the part he had played on numerous occasions. Significantly there was a difference in the part played by the nursing staff, in that throughout the incident dialogue was maintained in a way that did not emphasise a need to control Dave but to manage the situation.)

It was as Dave returned to his room I felt an almost overwhelming sense of sadness and loss and instead of interpreting this as my own personal response to a violent incident I decide to check out with Dave how he felt. A few minutes later, with his permission, I was sat on his bedroom floor, drinking a cup of tea and describing how I felt to Dave, speculating that I was not the only one who felt sad. Instead of denying he felt bad and saying he was all right, a habitual shorthand way of avoiding any difficult discussion or realisation, Dave acknowledged sadness and we sat and cried together. He was able to own his emotion in that situation and showed some empathic understanding of others as well. He also was able to appreciate that his actions had resulted in unpleasant consequences for lots of people, and was able to accept responsibility for his part in the incident. A further benefit was that he did not get his revenge on anyone involved in the restraint procedure, which was also a departure from the norm.

Reflecting on critical incidents

I would argue that the effectiveness of critical incident analysis is also increased if carried out in the context of ongoing, skilful clinical supervision. That is to say, the process by which an incident can be analysed by gathering information to establish what happened, how it happened, why it happened and thereby gaining some insight into any lessons that could be learned from the incident is greatly enhanced if all participants can contribute freely to the process.

This was borne out by two violent incidents in which I was involved. The first involved my mishandling a situation but in the second even in hindsight there was nothing that could reasonably have been done that would have prevented the assault. The first occurred when I entered, with permission, a resident's bedroom, to discuss something that was causing him some distress and about which he was beginning to get agitated. Missing the danger signals I overstayed my welcome and had a shoe thrown at me. I was saved from further assault by the timely intervention of another member of staff. Team members provided a debriefing that shift but it was during a supervision session I was able to explore my reasons for staying in the bedroom when others would have made a tactical exit. I am certain that had it not been that I trusted my supervisor I would not have had the opportunity to examine the intrapersonal process I was going through in that bedroom. We were able to identify the technical mistakes I made: e.g. allowing an increasingly agitated patient get between me and the door, not leaving the room earlier and trying to sort a problem out rather than letting it subside with time. We could also discover how I felt at the time, why I did what I did and what I was hoping to achieve by acting the way I did. The supervision did not result in self-condemnation but in self-realisation and the opportunity to change my practice.

The second incident involved a resident who with no warning made an aggressive demand that something of his be given to him. Despite following an approach that was the optimum for de-escalating the situation. I was subjected to a bodily assault, which resulted in a period of sick leave. Critical incident analysis did not indicate any change in my actions at the time. It was supervision that enabled me to acknowledge my true thoughts and feelings to the assailant as I prepared to return to work. I had adopted an attitude which was admirable had it been true, that of understanding and forgiveness. My moral and ethical background is grounded in Christian notions of forgiveness and turning the other cheek. I also have strong ideas regarding justice and fairness. In addition to this I have been exposed to a great deal of nursing literature which uncritically exhorts nurses to have unconditional, positive regard for patients (Rogers, 1952). In truth I did bear feelings of anger, betrayal, sadness and fear. What I was able to do was own up to these feelings to my supervisor, secure in the knowledge that, barring confessions of illegality or gross professional misconduct, I could admit to perceived failure or weakness and not fear censure. Of course I had to work through the feelings, but I would not have done so on my own.

A need for caution

I am still surprised and saddened when I hear of colleagues who are suspicious about the introduction of clinical supervision to their normal working practice. I suppose it is with some justification that nurses are cautious or sceptical when they see a hastily developed policy implemented with no consultation and little thought given to the training of supervisors. I have heard many stories of how managers use supervision sessions as a management tool. I have read written policies on clinical supervision that have been based on sound principles described by Proctor (1986) applied by supervisors who have appointed themselves, who dictate the agenda of the supervision sessions, and who verbalise their belief it is all a waste of time anyway. I have worked with colleagues who are offended or frightened by the suggestion that they open their practice up to the gaze of anyone else. **But I have experienced how, when done adequately, clinical supervision is about growth and development not about censure. As importantly it has enabled me to improve my service to patients and they have directly benefited by changes in my clinical practice.** This was important when working in an inpatient environment but has an even greater importance in my present area of work – the community.

Towards clinical excellence

When I moved jobs to work as a GP attached CPN I experienced a culture shock. Whilst I was used to individual work with clients I was not fully prepared for the implications of having no one to take over at the end of a shift. The most pressing need is the requirement to carry out assessments as to the risk of suicide, significant self-harm or risk to others within a limited time period. Unlike a ward environment there is no one to complete the assessment over the next few hours. I was also faced with the different demands and opportunities presented by a different client group, and how to apply existing knowledge to different clinical problems. At my job interview I was assured that clinical supervision was considered to be part of normal working practice, and this has been the case, although this wasn't true at that time throughout the Trust. I was able to access informal supervision on an *ad hoc* basis, discussing difficulties and successes as we met coincidentally within the office. Formal supervision sessions were planned, noted in our diaries and given priority over other meetings and appointments. Because of the emphasis given to clinical supervision in the CPN team of which I am part a culture of support has developed that encourages a sharing of experiences. The team has acknowledged the importance of the opportunities to have colleagues listen to us ventilate feelings, help explore and resolve technical or practical difficulties and also be free to pass their own reflections upon issues raised. It is not a replacement for clinical supervision but is a helpful side effect. This also serves to give a group identity to practitioners who otherwise work independently for many hours each week.

The issues I have continued to bring to supervision continue to involve transference and counter-transference. It has been of considerable help to bring to supervision situations where clients have adopted roles which don't permit therapeutic nursing to occur (Peplau, 1988). For example, I have seen numerous clients who are referred not because they themselves want help but because a partner or parent has insisted they see a doctor. In the absence of a mental illness or disorder that poses significant risk to them or others nursing interventions are not helpful, effective or reasonable. However, whilst I can know this I don't always feel comfortable discharging a client when I believe there is real potential for change. Supervision gives me the opportunity to express this discomfort and in doing so I usually recognise that my feelings have to do with my agendas, to be seen as effective, to help people whether they want it or not. My supervisor can sometimes enable this process by allowing me to continue talking; sometimes it involves questioning.

Similar situations have also occurred when I have mistaken my agenda for the client's need. An example of this was whilst I was still seeing Bob. He had lost his job as an HGV driver two years previously due to arthritic changes in several joints, which continued to cause him physical discomfort despite prescription of strong painkillers. He had developed severe depression to the extent he paid no attention to personal hygiene and was at risk of severe neglect without the support of close family. He expressed a sense of hopelessness about the future and a belief there was nothing left to live for. My difficulty was that he wasn't interested in engaging in a process to challenge the thoughts that were exacerbating the hopelessness and depression. He was only bothered how I could help him get to an outpatient's appointment to see an orthopaedic consultant without him 'cracking up'. I brought my frustration to supervision. By being asked what it was that Bob wanted I was able to see my error. I agreed it wasn't wrong for him to have an agenda that was different from mine. He had to cross a hurdle before he could give attention to the problem he thought I had invented for him. My frustration evaporated as I decided to work with Bob instead of giving him nursing care. I subsequently discovered that when eventually our agendas coincided he quickly came to understand how changing his thinking would enable him to adapt to his changed circumstances. Within a short time he was free of both depression and pain.

Final thoughts and reflections

My assertion is that in receiving clinical supervision from skilful, knowledgeable, compassionate supervisors I was allowed to gain insights into

my own practice that had direct benefits to the clients I was working with. It could be argued that I, as a someone who habitually reflected upon his own practice, would have worked much of this out anyway. My point is that it was the few issues that got under my radar that I needed supervision for. I have found out that an outside view is frequently necessary. **The art and craft of nursing is such an all embracing human activity that it is too easy to be caught up in the doing and to lose sight temporarily of the processes that we are involved in.**

But I believe that supervision has an equally important benefit. I have been able to chart my development. I have had the opportunity for someone I trust to acknowledge the changes, the successes that have arisen out of my clinical development. I have had a regular opportunity not only to let off steam but also to act constructively as a result. And I remain as hungry to develop myself and clinical services to benefit patient care as ever after twelve years of nursing. I don't believe my experience is unique. There are many people who could write persuasive arguments to support the use of clinical supervision. The disappointing thing is that the nursing profession still seems to be deciding whether it is worth the effort. I hope my experience, outlined in this chapter, will help convince nurses that clinical supervision is worth the effort.

References

Alford, B A and Beck A T (1994) Cognitive therapy of delusional beliefs. *Behavioural Research and Therapy* 32, pp369–380.

Birchwood M and Tarrier N (eds) (1992) *Innovations in the Psychological Management of Schizophrenia*. Chichester, John Wiley and Sons.

Bond M and Holland S (1998) *Skills of Clinical Supervision for Nurses*. Buckingham: Open University Press.

Butterworth A and Faugier J (1992) *Clinical Supervision and Mentorship in Nursing*. London: Chapman and Hall.

Brown D and Pedder J (1991) *Introduction to Psychotherapy: An Outline of Psychodynamic Principles and Practice* (2nd edition). London: Tavistock/Routledge.

Cutcliffe J R and Proctor B (1998a) An alternative training approach in clinical supervision, Part One. *British Journal of Nursing* 7, 5, pp280–285.

Cutcliffe J R and Proctor B (1998b) An alternative training approach in clinical supervision, Part Two. *British Journal of Nursing* 7, 6, pp344–350.

Harris T A (1973) *I'm OK – You're OK*. New York: Harper and Row.

Kingdon D G and Turkington D (1991) The use of cognitive therapy with normalizing rationale in schizophrenia. *Journal of Nervous and Mental Disease* 197, pp207–211.

Maier G J (1996) Managing threatening behaviour. *Journal of Psychosocial Nursing* 34(6), pp25–30.

Peplau H E (1988) *Interpersonal Relationships in Nursing* (2nd edition). Basingstoke: Macmillan.

Proctor B (1986) Supervision: a co-operative exercise in accountability. In Marken M and Payne M (eds) *Enabling and Ensuring*. Leicester: National Youth Bureau for Education in Youth and Community Work.

Rogers C R (1952) *Client-Centred Therapy*. London: Constable.

12 Maintaining quality care in the independent sector

Clinical supervision: a key piece of the jigsaw?

Mike Nolan and Sue Smit

Editorial

This chapter focuses on the potential role of support systems, in particular clinical supervision, for nurses who work in the independent sector. It illustrates that current negative stereotypical views of nursing homes, whilst inaccurate, add to the already high stress levels experienced by these nurses. Despite an acknowledgement of the need for more formal support mechanisms, clinical supervision is not a widespread phenomenon within the independent sector. Furthermore, the chapter points out the need for a move towards a more person-centred approach to care, and with this evolution of practice comes an even greater need to receive regular, effective clinical supervision.

We believe that this chapter points out an important issue: the relationship between emotional labour and clinical supervision. Working in a more person-centred way is likely to produce an increase in emotional labour for the nurse and thus amplify the need for more support. Clinical supervision can provide the support and facility necessary to deal with these increased demands. Thus, we believe to increase the demand on the nurses in this sector, without simultaneously providing additional support, would only serve to further burden an already pressured nursing work force.

Introduction

The number of nurses working within the independent sector has grown significantly over recent years and currently companies such as BUPA employ the largest group of nurses outside the NHS. Moreover, in addition to those working within well structured organisations, increasingly many staff are also employed in small or single homes. While a number of these nurses are delivering acute care the vast majority are working with older people and providing continuing care in residential and nursing homes to an elderly population with high levels of physical and cognitive frailty.

The importance of work with such individuals cannot be underestimated, for despite an active policy of community care (Davies, 1995) the increasing numbers of older people, particularly over the age of 85, means that some form of alternative care provision will always be needed (Victor, 1997). Due to the vulnerability of the client group in these environments it is essential that the highest quality of care is maintained and that sufficient numbers of well qualified and motivated staff are recruited and retained. This is often difficult to achieve as despite the high levels of skills required to work in care homes (Buswell, 1999) the sector often has a poor image making it difficult to attract the quality of staff required (Nay and Closs, 1999). Moreover, nurses can often find themselves geographically and professionally isolated, a situation that exacerbates feelings of being undervalued and marginalised (*RCN News*, 1999). It is the purpose of this chapter to consider the potential role of support mechanisms, particularly clinical supervision, as a key component of an infrastructure necessary to maintain and promote care standards. We argue that for quality care to be achieved it is necessary to value both institutional alternatives and the staff working in them.

Creating a 'new face' for institutional care

The current negative image of nursing homes is due in no small measure to the ambiguous role of institutions in society. Over the last 30 years there has been a sustained critique of institutional care from both policy makers and academics, which has been reinforced by a largely negative media coverage (Jack, 1998). This has resulted in a public perception of admission to residential and nursing homes as the 'final sign of failure' (Victor, 1992). Furthermore current policy emphasis on community care is underpinned by the belief that older people would prefer to live in their own homes and that care in institutional environments cannot be stimulating or of a high quality (Meredith, 1995). While there is an intuitive appeal to the argument that older people would prefer to live at home this is not invariably the case nor is it necessarily true that care in the community is inherently superior (Baldwin *et al.*, 1993).

It is therefore important to overcome stereotypical views of nursing home care as, despite the promises of community care, some form of alternative will always be required (Jani-le-Bris, 1993; Victor, 1997; Jack, 1998). Therefore, although more frail older people may be cared for in community settings, significant numbers, especially of very frail individuals, are living in residential and nursing homes. For example, the Royal Commission on Long Term Care (1999) estimated that 600,000 older people receive formal care at home compared with 480,000 who are in some form of care home. These figures do not of course include the much greater numbers of people who receive care primarily or exclusively from their family but they nevertheless provide an indication of the relative balance in formal service provision.

Considered another way, although only about 1 per cent of the older population between the ages of 65 and 74 are in care, this figure increases to about 20 per cent at the age of 85 (Victor, 1997). Given that the fastest growing section of the older population is among those aged 80+ (Health Education Authority, 1998), the need to both maintain and value care home provision is inescapable. It is therefore no longer acceptable that institutional care is perceived as 'universally dysfunctional' (Higham, 1994) and there is a pressing need, as Salvage (1995) suggests, to create a 'new face' for institutional alternatives so that they are viewed as desirable and accessible. Such a 'new face' must comprise a vastly improved public perception of care homes with work in such environments being accorded status and value.

This presents a considerable challenge as work within institutional environments has never been accorded a particularly high status (Kayser-Jones, 1981; Diamond, 1986; Gilloran *et al.*, 1993; Lee-Treweek, 1994) and Glendenning (1997), drawing on the work of Pillemer and Bachman-Prehn (1991), concludes that well qualified staff do not choose to work in nursing homes. Glendenning (1997) summarises a number of reasons for this: work is physically demanding; financial rewards and status are low; there is a 'high risk' of physical and verbal abuse; and turnover and sickness rates are therefore high which compounds problems of low staffing.

Recent work (Baillon *et al.*, 1996) has suggested that despite positive attitudes towards working with older people, stress levels among staff are high, often due to the lack of support mechanisms and educational opportunities for staff. This was a point reiterated in a recent review of the literature on the importance of training in long-term care environments (Nolan and Keady, 1996).

It has been recognised for some time that the education and training of most professional groups, whether at basic or post-qualifying levels, provides an inadequate grounding for work with older people (Redfern, 1988; Kenny, 1988; Gill, 1988), a situation which is compounded by the unidisciplinary nature of most courses. As a consequence many practitioners are poorly prepared for the complexity of needs which older people present. This is particularly so in long-term care settings where, as noted above, the work lacks status and prestige. Nolan and Keady (1996) argue that a number of fundamental prerequisites need addressing before better qualified and trained staff can be recruited and retained in such environments. Therefore, in addition to adequate training in basic skills such as dealing with problem behaviour, wandering and aggression, a range of more therapeutic interventions should be introduced to staff. This provides an important conceptual distinction. For even though there is a need for training in techniques which deal with a particular problem, this alone is too reductionist and is likely to reinforce the perception that older people are basically problematic. To counter this a number of authors have stressed that training for work in long-term care (LTC) must include material on topics such as normal ageing, common pathologies of old age, communication skills, and working with families (Chartock *et al.*, 1988; Weber, 1991; Jones *et al.*, 1992; Kihlgren *et al.*, 1993; Blackmon, 1993; Baltes *et al.*, 1994) before attention is narrowed to particular difficulties. Such training should involve both qualified and unqualified staff and is particularly beneficial when it is multi-disciplinary in nature (Jones *et al.*, 1992; Nolan and Walker, 1993).

As Nolan and Keady (1996) argue, however, training must also be linked to a coherent staff development programme, as staff who have been empowered by training need to be exposed to a work environment that values and indeed promotes innovation and change. In its absence the likely consequence is raised but dashed expectations, resulting in increased frustration and disenchantment. Training, while important, is a necessary but not a sufficient condition for improved care (Nolan and Keady, 1996). Staff need to have an explicit and agreed philosophy of care (Alfredson and Annerstedt, 1994), with a set of operational parameters derived from that philosophy (Armentorp *et al.*, 1991; Murphy, 1992; Nolan and Walker, 1993). Many advocate the use of an individualised care planning programme for this purpose (Berg *et al.*, 1994; Nystrom and Segerston, 1994).

It is taken as an axiom here that staff cannot provide high quality care unless they themselves feel valued and supported. This is particularly so if they are to develop the close relationships with older people necessary to provide 'constructive' care. Therefore the formation of relationships between staff and individuals in LTC and the provision of stimulating activities must be seen as both a legitimate and a valued activity (Nolan *et al.*, 1995; Lawton *et al.*, 1995), and not viewed as 'skiving' (Gilloran *et al.*, 1995).

Recognising the importance of such 'people work' (Kitwood, 1993) also requires that support for staff is available on at least two levels. First there is a need for positive feedback on performance from peers and managers (Murphy, 1992; Kuremyr *et al.*, 1994; Nystrom and Segerston, 1994; Alfredson and Annerstedt, 1994; Gilloran *et al.*, 1995) in order to reinforce both the competence required to conduct such work and its basic worth. Second there must be explicit recognition of the emotional impact on staff that the forging of close relationships with people in their care engenders (Kuremyr *et al.*, 1994; Scott, 1995; Sumaya-Smith, 1995). Therefore the provision of good emotional support for staff is essential if they are not to exhaust their own emotional resources (Kuremyr *et al.*, 1994), especially when someone dies (Sumaya-Smith, 1995). It has been strongly suggested that the introduction of a system of clinical supervision provides the most effective means of providing such support (Kuremyr *et al.*, 1994; Alfredson and Annerstedt, 1994; Berg *et al.*, 1994).

Promoting clinical supervision

The stressful nature of work within the independent sector has been recognised for some time (Nazarko, 1996), particularly, but not exclusively, among mental health nurses (Dionne-Prolux and Pepin, 1993; Faugier, 1994; Everitt, 1994; Morris, 1995). Such stress is often exacerbated both by the high levels of physical and cognitive frailty among older people (Nazarko, 1996) and the relative isolation which qualified staff may experience (Dunn *et al.*, 1994; *RCN News*, 1999). Motivation and standards of care can therefore be difficult to maintain, especially when there is limited supervision and few opportunities for education and training (UKCC, 1994). However, as noted above, adequate support mechanisms are essential if staff are to feel valued. In other words, staff need to feel cared for themselves if they are to provide adequate care for older people (Nichols, 1992).

Clinical supervision is often promoted as one way of providing staff support (Tingle, 1995) and yet exactly what this means is far from clear, with the literature describing a range of different models (Johns, 1993; Fox, 1994). According to the UKCC (1995) the purpose of clinical supervision is to 'assist colleagues with the development of their clinical skills, knowledge and values in order to promote and maintain high standards and innovation in clinical practice.'

However, despite the benefits of clinical supervision being widely endorsed there is considerable misunderstanding as to what clinical supervision entails and what the actual outcomes of the process are (Malin, 2000). The result has been ambivalence amongst many nurses who are uncertain as to whether professional or managerial concerns are driving the agenda (Malin, 2000), the former being essentially designed to empower the supervisee while the latter focuses on ensuring accountability and responsibility. For example, in a recent study exploring the introduction of clinical supervision within community homes for people with learning disabilities, Malin (2000) describes the difficulties that were encountered. While there was tacit endorsement for the introduction of clinical supervision by management there was far less in the way of tangible resources and the process was not given a high priority. Moreover, staff tended to view clinical supervision primarily as a vehicle for achieving accountability rather than for empowering them. Therefore, although there were perceived benefits, particularly in terms of improved team-working, Malin (2000) argues that the notion of clinical supervision must be more actively 'sold' to staff if it is to be of optimum benefit. This will require education as to its potential benefits and a clearer understanding of its aims and purposes.

The above case example highlights many important lessons for the introduction of clinical supervision within the independent sector, an area that has received relatively little attention (Smit, 1998). A recent exploratory study by Smit (1998) suggested that if supervision occurs at all it is often on an *ad hoc* and informal basis, with relatively little structure. Although the benefits of informal support should not be underestimated (Kaberry, 1992) it is also important that more structured approaches are adopted (Wright *et al.*, 1997). A programme therefore needs careful planning and a systematic approach to its introduction if it is to be successful (Farrington, 1995), together, as noted by Malin (2000) with clarity as to its purpose. We would argue that its primary aim should be the empowerment of practitioners using a growth and support model (Faugier, 1994) rather than addressing a management agenda.

Of course any formal process is not resource neutral and it is essential to recognise the logistical and practical requirements of introducing a system of clinical supervision. This requires a commitment of both time and money (Johns, 1993) as well as the availability of sufficient supervisors. This is a particular challenge for the independent sector and the benefits of partnerships with local education providers and others need exploring (Devine, 1995). Staff release is also an issue and the implications of providing an adequate support infrastructure, of which clinical supervision forms an important component, should be factored into the equation for calculating the costs of nursing home care.

This will require continued investment in all staff working in residential and nursing home environments; without this, care is unlikely to improve. The central importance of this was noted over 30 years ago in the Report of the Williams Committee which considered the role of staff recruitment and training in local authority residential establishments in the UK. This concluded with a plea for greater investment in staff, thus:

> Unless this money is spent there is no hope of any significant improvement in the number and quality of the staff who enter and remain in residential work; and unless there is significant improvement in these respects it is not possible to provide the amount and quality of care that is needed. The happiness and welfare of the hundreds of thousands who must be cared for in residential homes depends on our willingness to spend this money. We do not consider the extra cost excessive in relation to the amount of human happiness involved.
>
> (Williams, 1967, pp191–92)

This is as true now as it was then. However, in addition to adequate staff support, standards are unlikely to improve unless there is greater clarity as to the values underpinning continuing care. As Kendy and Brooke (1999) note, practitioners are being constantly urged to confirm the 'personhood' of the people they care for while simultaneously managing a range of professional and organisational tensions. Achieving person-centred care is therefore unlikely unless the concept can be described more clearly.

Articulating person-centred care

Given the previously described largely negative perceptions of institutional care and the overt promotion of community care, such facilities occupy an increasingly denigrated and ambiguous niche in society. If, as is frequently the case, they are perceived as the environments of 'last resort' (Jani-le-Bris, 1993) and are utilised only when other care options have 'failed' (Victor, 1992), what function do they serve and how is it possible to create and sustain quality care and job satisfaction among staff? Indeed, what does 'quality care' mean in such a context?

One of the fundamental challenges is to conceptualise adequately the care needs of very frail older people. This process is particularly important as levels of frailty and dependence in care environments are rising and will continue to do so (Jani-le-Bris, 1993; Victor, 1997). Without a basic framework within which to consider key concepts, the quality of life of such individuals cannot be enhanced nor is it possible for an adequate discourse to begin about creating a meaningful and satisfying work environment for the individuals providing care. The unclear or 'taken for granted' manner in which the parameters of good care have been defined effectively inhibits achieving acceptable standards. For example, although benchmarks such as privacy, dignity, independence, choice, rights and fulfilment (DOH/SSI, 1989) are presented as the hallmarks of good care, what such ideas really mean and how they can be achieved in the context of very high levels of physical and mental frailty is far from clear. Gilloran *et al.* (1993) argue that it is simplistic and misleading to use 'buzzwords' such as autonomy and individuality without agreement as to their definition.

Moreover, even if consensus as to a definition can be reached, what value do concepts such as autonomy and individuality have for individuals who might be both physically and cognitively frail? To present benchmarks for quality which are either unrealistic, unachievable, or simply inappropriate does nothing to enhance quality of care, and indeed might even hinder it. This is not to argue that such values have no place but rather is a plea for more meaningful discussion about their applicability in all contexts. This is particularly important for staff who, if unrealistic or unobtainable goals are set, are likely to become increasingly disenchanted. For example, one of the basic failures in the nursing care of frail older people has been the lack of agreed outcomes for care. The application of a curative or rehabilitative model is often inappropriate (Reed and Bond, 1991) but in the absence of a viable alternative the result is often either 'good geriatric care' in which patients and the ward are kept clean (Reed and Bond, 1991) or 'aimless residual care' (Evers, 1991) where there is no discernible purpose. Such considerations apply equally in all environments which care for frail older people.

In the absence of agreed criteria for positive outcomes it is all too easy for older people to be viewed as commodities. Some years ago Diamond (1986) in the US vividly described the way in which people were treated as 'feeders' rather than individuals who needed assistance to meet their nutritional needs. Eight years later, and across the Altantic, Lee-Treweek (1994) portrayed a depressingly similar picture of life in a nursing home in the UK. She suggests that the motivation behind the activity of the unqualified care staff, who give the majority of 'hands on care', is to present the 'lounge standard patient'. This is an individual who is smartly attired and looks neat and tidy whilst on public display in the lounge. Within their work world the presentation of a 'well-ordered body' symbolises a job well done. In order to achieve this it was considered both necessary and legitimate to be ruthless in the delivery of care. Individuals who did not reach the required 'lounge standard' were confined to their own rooms, but in order to ensure that as many individuals as possible were presentable then 'mistreatment and being hard towards patients' became seen as an essential attribute of the good worker (Lee-Treweek, 1994).

While such practices are no doubt in the minority it is nevertheless of paramount importance that we are able to articulate clearly the aims of institutional care and accord them value and worth in the spectrum of care. Many would argue that maintaining the quality of life of residents is the key purpose (Denham, 1997; Twinning, 1997) but the challenges of identifying what constitutes a good quality of life for frail older people in any setting are well recognised (Stewart and King, 1994; Baltes, 1994; Twinning, 1997). Baltes (1994) suggests that 'ageing well and institutional living' are something of a paradox, hinting that the two concepts are incompatible. She argues that there is a need to achieve a delicate balance between overcompensating for deficits by doing too much for older people and optimising potential by placing too many unrealistic demands on them. This, as Baltes (1994) notes, represents the tension between security and autonomy.

Therefore although concepts such as privacy, dignity, choice and so on still have an important role to play, as has been reaffirmed in studies which confirm their importance in other cultures and contexts (Lowenstein and Brick, 1995), the challenge becomes how do we achieve these laudable aims at the more extreme ends of frailty where most care is carried out by another individual, and personal space is frequently invaded. It seems clear from most of the recent literature that the key to quality hinges largely on the nature of interpersonal relationships and the recognition that the older person, no matter how frail, has the status of a human being. It is therefore essential that older people are seen to have the potential for continued growth and development, something which is still conspicuous by its absence in many care settings (Koch *et al.*, 1995). Kadner (1994) suggests that intimacy is the essence of a therapeutic interaction and that to achieve this requires the self-disclosure of personal information. As Scott (1995) highlights, constructive care requires that staff perceive themselves as an instrument of care and that they have a personal investment in the people they are caring for. In other words caring has no meaning unless the recipient of care in some way 'matters'. Scott (1995) recognises that this role is a profoundly demanding one in terms of energy, imagination, time and emotion but as Kayser-Jones (1981) notes 'A personal relationship between staff and the elderly in long-term care institutions is desirable and essential' (p49). Developing and nurturing such relationships is not, however, simply a matter of intuition and being a 'good' person, for as Goodwin (1992) points out 'TLC and enthusiasm without proper knowledge and skills is, at best, ineffective and, at worst, disastrous' (Goodwin, 1992, p39).

Unfortunately caring has never been accorded particular value or status, whether provided in the home by families or by paid individuals (Davies, 1995). Davies (1995) argues that what she describes as 'care work', that is care provided by unqualified and often untrained staff on low wages, is largely invisible and is not seen to require particular skill. This, she believes, essentially devalues the therapeutic potential of the interpersonal dynamic between care workers and those in receipt of care. According to Davies (1995), even professional care delivered by well trained and relatively well paid personnel struggles to find recognition in a health service dominated by masculine values. Even within the 'New NHS', Davies believes that essentially masculine concepts such as independence and autonomy still predominate.

In relation to older people one increasingly worrying development is the current emphasis on 'successful ageing' (Kivnick and Murray, 1997) and its conflation, particularly in recent UK policy, with the promotion of independence (Handford *et al.*, 1999). Minkler (1996) argues that the uncritical acceptance of aims such as independence stigmatises and disempowers those who do not meet current criteria for 'success'. She believes that empowerment of older people should be the goal to aim for and that, particularly for frail older people, this will mean recognising the importance of interdependence rather than independence. This is particularly relevant in a continuing care environment and it is therefore important that the nature of the interdependencies between staff and older people are envisioned more clearly. One potentially useful framework is that outlined by Nolan (1997).

Nolan (1997) was concerned with the lack of a therapeutic rationale for work in long-term care settings with older people and identified six 'senses' which he believed might both provide direction for staff and improve the care older people received. The term 'sense' was selected deliberately to reflect the subjective and perceptual nature of the important determinants of care for both older people and staff. The 'senses' are briefly described in Table 12.1.

As yet the senses require further conceptual refinement and empirical testing but early work indicates that they are meaningful and robust within an acute care environment for older people (Davies *et al.*, 1999). Moreover, staff also identify with their properties and consider that they provide a useful framework within which to locate many of the dimensions of person-centred care.

Mulrooney (1997) argues that if standards of care for older people are to improve then three sets of conditions must be met. These are:

- valuing person-centred care;
- respecting interdependence;
- investing in caregiving as a choice.

The mutually reinforcing nature of these conditions are readily apparent as staff are unlikely actively to choose to work with frail older people unless there is a clear rationale for care and such care is valued appropriately. Person-centred care and interdependence are essential components in the care equation but we must have some notion of what both entail. The senses framework offers a set of parameters, albeit as yet incomplete, within which to locate both person-centredness and interdependence.

Person-centred care, clinical supervision and care for the older person in the independent sector

The authors of this chapter argue that the widespread introduction of clinical supervision into the independent sector is one way of addressing the two key

Table 12.1 The six senses

A sense of security

For older people: Attention to essential physiological and psychological needs, to feel safe and free from threat, harm, pain and discomfort.

For staff: To feel free from physical threat, rebuke or censure. To have secure conditions of employment. To have the emotional demand of work recognised and to work within a supportive culture.

A sense of continuity

For older people: Recognition and value of personal biography; skilful use of knowledge of the past to help contextualise present and future.

For staff: Positive experience of work with older people from an early stage of career, exposure to role models and good environments of care.

A sense of belonging

For older people: Opportunities to form meaningful relationships, to feel part of a community or group as desired.

For staff: To feel part of a team with a recognised contribution, to belong to a peer group, a community of gerontological practitioners.

A sense of purpose

For older people: Opportunities to engage in purposeful activity, the constructive passage of time, to be able to achieve goals and challenging pursuits.

For staff: To have a sense of therapeutic direction, a clear set of goals to aspire to.

A sense of fulfilment

For older people: Opportunities to meet meaningful and valued goals, to feel satisfied with one's efforts.

For staff: To be able to provide good care, to feel satisfied with one's efforts.

A sense of significance

For older people: To feel recognised and valued as a person of worth, that one's actions and existence is of importance, that you 'matter'.

For staff: To feel that gerontological practice is valued and important, that your work and efforts 'matter'.

(Based on Nolan, 1997)

points highlighted in this chapter. Those being: the need for a movement towards a more interpersonal, interdependent, person-centred approach to care, and the need for more formal support systems for the nurses who work in this sector.

Thus, it can be suggested that if a supervisee experiences person-centred clinical supervision, they may be better placed (or equipped) to provide person-centred care to their clients.

It is often argued that the dynamics and processes of practice can be mirrored in the clinical supervision session. What practitioners experience in the clinical supervision can, similarly, be transferred to the practice setting. Butterworth (1992) hypothesised that students who are trained in a learning environment which encourages active listening, empathy and support will develop into qualified nurses who will foster similar therapeutic exchanges between themselves and clients. Thus, it can be suggested that if a supervisee experiences person-centred clinical supervision, they may be better placed (or equipped) to provide person-centred care to their clients.

Whilst the arguments for moving towards person-centred caring practices are cogent, this development also appears to create a difficulty; that of the potential increase in the 'emotional labour' the nurses may have to experience. Several authors have alluded to the nature of the nurses' own 'reaction' to interpersonal work (for example Strauss *et al.*, 1982; James, 1989) and that this emotional labour is often viewed as less prestigious than technical work (Smith, 1991), even though such endeavour can be difficult, demanding and draining. This potential increased 'load' can be addressed, at least in part, by providing the nurses with clinical supervision. This argument was supported by Cutcliffe and Cassedy (1999) who reasoned that if nurses become more empathic towards their clients and thus move towards person-centred care:

> this is likely to increase the emotional labour of nursing and the nurses will therefore need the facility and support to be able to process these thoughts and feelings. This appears to be reinforcing the need for all nurses to receive and participate in clinical supervision, as this would be the ideal forum for obtaining the additional support they require.

Whilst acknowledging that informal support systems do exist in the independent sector, and the value of these should not be underestimated (Smit, 1998), this level of support may be insufficient to meet the current demands made on the nurses in this area. To increase the demands without simultaneously providing additional and importantly, more effective systems of support, would appear to be an ill advised development. Since support is central to the concept of clinical supervision, the authors argue that a more appropriate development would be for the widespread introduction of clinical supervision to run parallel with a move towards person-centred care.

Conclusion

The independent sector constitutes an essential element of the healthcare landscape and in respect of older people provides care to some of the most frail and vulnerable members of society. This is skilled and demanding work which rarely receives the recognition it is due.

Care is on the whole provided by dedicated staff but if standards are to be maintained and improved then there is a need for more adequate support mechanisms and a more clearly articulated rationale for the care given. Clinical supervision is likely to form a key component of any supportive infrastructure but for its potential to be realised there is a need for more work which clarifies its contribution to the overall development of quality in the independent sector. Crucially the resource implications of providing adequate staff support must also be recognised and included within any calculation of the costs of providing care of the highest quality to those in the later years of their life.

References

Alfredson B B and Annerstedt L (1994) Staff attitudes and job satisfaction in the care of demented elderly people: Group living compared to long term care. *Journal of Advanced Nursing* 20, pp964–74.

Armentorp N Gossett R D and Eucherpoe N (1991) *Quality Assurance for Long Term Care Providers*. Newbury Park: Sage.

Baldwin N Harris J and Kelly D (1993) Institutionalisation: Why blame the institution? *Ageing and Society* 13, pp69–81.

Baillon S Scothern G Neville P G and Bowle A (1996) Factors that contribute to stress in care staff in residential homes for the elderly. *International Journal of Geriatric Psychiatry* 11(3), pp219–26.

Baltes M M (1994) Aging well and institutional living: A paradox? In Abeles RP, Gift HC and Ory MG (eds) *Aging and Quality of Life*, pp185–201. New York: Springer.

Baltes M M Neumann E M and Zank S (1994) Maintenance and rehabilitation of independence in old age: An intervention programme for staff. *Psychology and Ageing* 9(2), pp179–88.

Berg A Hansson V W and Hallberg I R (1994) Nurses' creativity, tedium and burnout during one year clinical supervision and implementation of individuals planned nursing care: Comparison between a ward for severely demented patients and a similar control ward. *Journal of Advanced Nursing* 20, pp742–9.

Blackmon D J (1993) *Nursing Assistants in Nursing Homes: The Impact of Training on Attitudes, Knowledge and Job Satisfaction*. Unpublished PhD Thesis, University of Akron, USA.

Buswell C (1999) The value of care home nurses. *Elderly Care* 11(4), 25.

Butterworth T (1992) Clinical supervision as an emerging idea in nursing In Butterworth T and Faugier J (eds), *Clinical Supervision and Mentorship in Nursing*. London: Chapman and Hall.

Chartock P Nevin A and Rzatlelny H (1988) A mental health training programme in nursing homes. *Gerontologist* 28(4), pp503–7.

Cutcliffe J R and Cassedy P (1999) The Development of empathy in students on a short skills based counselling course: A pilot study. *Nurse Education Today* 19, pp250–257.

Davies B (1995) The reform of community and long term care of elderly persons: An international perspective. In Scharf F and Wenger GC (eds) *International Perspectives on Community Care for Older People*. Aldershot: Avebury.

Davies S Nolan M R Brown J and Wilson F (1999) *Dignity on the Ward: Promoting Excellence in Care*. London: Help the Aged.

Denham M J (1997) Quality issues for older people in continuing care accommodation. In Denham M J (eds) *Continuing care for older people*, pp3–16. London: Stanley Thornes.

Department of Health/Social Services Inspectorate (1989) *Homes Are For Living In*. London: HMSO.

Devine A (1995) Introducing clinical supervision: A guide. *Nursing Standard* 9(40), pp32–34.

Diamond T (1986) Social policy and everyday life in nursing homes: A critical ethnography. *Social Science and Medicine* 23(12), pp1287–95.

Dionne-Prolux J and Pepin R (1993) Stress management in the nursing profession. *Journal of Nursing Management* 1, pp75–81.

Dunn L A, Rout U Carson J and Ritter S (1994) Occupational stress amongst care staff working in nursing homes: An empirical investigation. *Journal of Clinical Nursing* 3, pp177–183.

Everitt J (1994) Stress and clinical supervision in mental health care. *Nursing Times* 92(10), pp34–35.

Evers H K (1991) Care of the elderly sick in the UK. In Redfern SJ (ed.) *Nursing Elderly People*. Edinburgh: Churchill Livingstone.

Farrington A (1995) Defining and setting the parameters of clinical supervision. *British Journal of Nursing* 4(15), pp874–875.

Faugier J (1994) Thin on the ground. *Nursing Times* 90(20), pp64–65.

Fox J (1994) Clinical supervision: A real aspiration. *British Journal of Nursing* 3(6), p805.

Gilloran A J McGlew T McKee K Robertson A and Wight D (1993) Measuring the quality of care on psychogeriatric wards. *Journal of Advanced Nursing* 18, pp269–75.

Gilloran A Robertson A and McGlew T (1995) Improving work satisfaction amongst nursing staff and quality of care for elderly patients with dementia: Some policy implications. *Ageing and Society*, 15: pp375–91.

Glendenning F (1997) The mistreatment and neglect of elderly people in residential centres: Research outcomes. In Decalmer P and Glendenning F (eds), *The Mistreatment of Elderly People* 2nd edition, pp151–62 London: Sage.

Goodwin S (1992) Freedom to Care. *Nursing Times* 88(34), pp38–9.

Handford L Easterbrook L and Stevenson J (1999) *Rehabilitation for Older People: The Emerging Policy Agenda*. London: King's Fund.

Health Education Authority (1998) *Older People in the Population*, Fact Sheet 1. London: HMSO.

Higham P (1994) *Individualising Residential Care for Older People*. Paper given at British Society of Gerontology Annual Conference, University of London, September 1994.

Jack R (1998) Institutions in community care. In Jack R (ed.) *Residential vs Community Care*, Basingstoke: Macmillan, pp10–40.

James N (1989) Emotional labour: skill and work in the social regulation of feelings. *Sociological Review* 37, pp15–42.

Jani-le-Bris H (1993) *Family Care of Dependent Older People in the European Community*. Luxembourg: EU Publishers.

Johns C (1993) Professional supervision. *Journal of Nursing Management* 1, 9–18.

Jones G M M, Ely S and Miesen B M L (1992) The need for an interdisciplinary care curriculum for professional working with dementia. In Jones G M M and Miesen B M L (eds), *Caregiving in Dementia: Research and Applications*. London: Routledge, pp437–53.

Kaberry S (1992) Supervision – support for nurses? *Senior Nurse* 12(5), pp38–40.

Kadner K (1994) Therapeutic intimacy in nursing. *Journal of Advanced Nursing* 19(2), pp215–18.

Kayser-Jones J S (1981) *Old and Alone, Care of the Aged in Scotland and the United States*. Berkeley: University of California Press.

Kendy H and Brooke C (1999) Social perspectives on community nursing. In Nay R and Garrat S (eds) *Nursing Older People: Issues and Innovations*, pp40–63. Sydney: Maclennan and Petty.

Kenny W T (1988) Services for the elderly by the Year 2000. Education and training issues. *Journal of Advanced Nursing* 13, pp419–21.

Kihlgren M Kuremeyr D and Norberg A (1993) Nurse-patient interaction after training in integrity promoting care in a long term ward: Analysis of video recorded morning care sessions. *International Journal of Nursing Studies* 30(i), pp1–13.

Kitwood T (1993) Person and process in dementia. *International Journal of Geriatric Psychiatry* 8, pp541–5.

Kivnick H Q and Murray S U (1997) Vital Involvement: An overlooked source of identity in frail elders. *Journal of Aging and Identity* 2(3), pp205–225.

Koch T Webb C and Williamson A M (1995) Listening to the voices of older patients: An existential-phenomenological approach to quality assurance. *Journal of Clinical Nursing* 4, pp185–93.

Kuremyr D, Kihlgren M and Norberg A (1994) Emotional experience, empathy and burnout among staff caring for patients at a collective living unit and nursing home. *Journal of Advanced Nursing* 19(4), pp670–9.

Lawton M P, Moss M and Duhamel L M (1995) The quality of life among elderly care receivers. *Journal of Applied Gerontology* 4(2), pp150–71.

Lee-Treweek G (1994) Bedroom abuse: The hidden work in a nursing home. *Generations Review* 4(2), pp2–4.

Lowenstein A and Brick Y (1995) *The Differential and Congruent Roles of Qualitative and Quantitative Methods to Evaluate Quality of Life in Residential Settings.* Israeli Gerontological Society, Israel.

Malin N A (2000) Evaluating clinical supervision in community homes and towards survey of adults with learning disabilities. *Journal of Advanced Nursing* 31(3), pp548–57.

Meredith B (1995) *The Community Care Handbook.* London: Age Concern.

Minkler M (1996) Critical perspectives on ageing: new challenges for gerontology. Ageing and Society 16(4), pp467–487.

Morris M (1995) The need to reduce stress amongst mental health nurses. *British Journal of Nursing* 4(10), pp572–573.

Mulrooney C P (1997) Competencies needed by frail caregivers to enhance elders' quality of life. In *16th World Congress of Gerontology*, Adelaide.

Murphy E (1992) Quality assurance in residential care (Editorial). *International Journal of Geriatric Psychiatry* 7, pp695–697.

Nay R and Closs B (1999) Staffing and quality in non-acute facilities. In Nay R and Garret S (eds) *Nursing Older People: Issues and Innovations*, pp172–190 Sydney: Maclennan and Petty.

Nazarko L (1996) Nursing homes' nurses need support to update skills. *Nursing Times* 92(42), pp38–40.

Nichols K (1992) Understanding support. *Nursing Times* 88(13), pp34–35.

Nolan M R (1997) *Health and Social Care, What the Future Holds for Nursing.* Keynote address at 3rd RCN Older Person European Conference and Exhibition: Harrogate.

Nolan M R and Keady J (1996) Training for long term care: The road to better quality. *Reviews in Clinical Gerontology* 6, pp333–42.

Nolan M R and Walker G (1993) *The Next Best Thing To My Own Home: An Evaluation of a Sheltered Tenant Housing Scheme in Clwyd*, Bangor: BASE Practice Research Unit, University of Wales.

Nolan M R Keady J and Grant G (1995) Developing a typology of family care: Implications for nurse and other service providers. *Journal of Advanced Nursing* 21, pp256–65.

Nystrom A M and Segerston K M (1994) On sources of powerlessness in nursing home life. *Journal of Advanced Nursing* 19(1), pp124–33.

Pillemer E J and Bachman-Prehn R (1991) Helping and hurting: Prediction of maltreatment of patients in nursing homes. *Research in Aging* 13(1), pp74–95.

RCN News (1999) Home at last. *Elderly Care* 11(5), pp124–133.

Redfern S (1988) Services for elderly people by the year 2000. Education and training issues. *Journal of Advanced Nursing* 13, pp418–19.

Reed J and Bond S (1991) Nurses' assessment of elderly patients in hospital. *International Journal of Nursing Studies* 28(1), pp55–64.

Royal Commission on Long Term Care (1999) *With Respect to Old Age*. London: Stationery Office.

Salvage A V (1995) *Who Will Care? Future Prospects for Family Care of Older People in the European Union*. Luxembourg: EU Publishers.

Scott P A (1995) Care, attention and imaginative identification in nursing practice. *Journal of Advanced Nursing* 21(6), pp1196–1200.

Smit S (1998) *A Qualitative Study of Four Mental Health Nurses Working in a Private Sector Nursing Home: Their Perceptions and Experiences of Support*. Unpublished BSc(Hons) Dissertation, Bradford University.

Smith P (1991) The nursing process: raising the profile of emotional care in nurse training. *Journal of Advanced Nursing* 16, pp74–81.

Stewart A L and King A C (1994) Conceptualising and measuring quality of life in older populations. In Abeles R P, Gift H C and Ory M G (eds) *Aging and Quality of Life*. New York: Springer.

Strauss A Fagerhaugh S Suczek B and Weiner R C (1982) Sentimental work in the technological hospital. *Sociology of Health and Illness* 4(3), pp254–277.

Sumaya-Smith I (1995) Caregiver-resident relationships: surrogate family bonds and surrogate grieving in a skilled facility. *Journal of Advanced Nursing*, 21(3): pp447–51.

Tingle J (1995) Clinical supervision is an effective risk management tool. *British Journal of Nursing* 4(14), pp794–795.

Twinning C (1997) Quality of life: Assessment and improvement In Denham M J (ed.) *Continuing Care for Older People*, pp107–30. London: Stanley Thornes.

UKCC (1994) *Professional Conduct – Occasional Report on Standards of Nursing in Nursing Homes*. London: UKCC.

UKCC (1995) *Position Statement on Clinical Supervision for Nurses and Health Visitors*. London: UKCC.

Victor C (1992) Do we need institutional care? In Laczko F and Victor C (eds), *Social Policy and Elderly People*. Aldershot: Gower.

Victor C (1997) *Community Care and Older People*. Cheltenham: Stanley Thornes.

Weber C (1991) Training staff to care for people with Alzheimer's disease. In O'Neill D (ed.) *Carers, Professional and Alzheimer's Disease. Proceedings of the 5th Alzheimer's Disease International Conference*. London: John Libbey.

Williams (Chairman) (1967) *Caring for People (The Williams Report)*. London: George Allen and Unwin.

Wright S G Elliot M and Schofield V (1997) A networking approach to clinical supervision. *Nursing Standard* 11(18), pp39–41.

13 Clinical supervision for nurse educationalists

Personal perspectives from a postgraduate mental health nursing course

Peter Goward, Joe Kellet and John Wren

Editorial

This chapter considers clinical supervision for nurse educationalists. It sets such practice within the context of a postgraduate mental health nursing course. It provides some background to the development of the course, identifies the nature of the supervision provided and goes on to discuss the value of supervision for nurse educationalists. The chapter also points out the differences in the organisational structure between universities and the NHS. As a result, the well documented problems that arise from a person having the dual roles of clinical supervisor and line manager may not be as significant an issue for university staff as they could be for NHS staff.

We believe that if practitioners are providing clinical supervision, then it would be prudent (if not necessary) for them to also receive clinical supervision. This position applies equally to clinicians and educationalists. Indeed, many nurses educationalists continue to practise as clinicians, which adds further weight to this argument. Clinical supervision, we believe, should be a career-long activity, and the authors of this chapter provide further evidence to support this position.

Introduction

During the latter part of the last decade local and national commissioning intentions have responded to the need to increase the number of qualified nurses who are capable of meeting the increasingly complex needs of mental health care provision. The move from a predominantly NHS-based setting into higher education institutions encouraged the deliverers of educational programmes to think more closely about the nature and level of such provision.

Our local analysis resulted in the development of the Pre-Registration Postgraduate Diploma in Health Care Studies with professional registration as a mental health nurse. This two-year programme is designed for those who hold a first level or higher degree in a health related subject such as psychology or sociology in accordance with Statutory Instrument 1456, Rule 14A(8)(c)(i).

Successful students are able to access an option to continue in pursuance of a master's degree. In keeping with most current thinking (Sainsbury Centre, 1997; Norman *et al.*, 1996) the course development team were very clear that the programme needed to be primarily skills based with the underlying theory clustered around practical interventions that would ensure previous knowledge could be contextualised within good mental health practice. For us this clearly indicated the need to include reflective practice and clinical supervision as central themes throughout the whole length of the course. In this chapter we will consider the wider context within which this initiative began, the influence of the curriculum, the nature of the supervision, the responses and experiences of those who acted as supervisors and a discussion of the role of supervisor in an educational context.

Supervision in context

Supervision has been present in some form amongst some mental health nurses for decades, with many nurses adopting the kinds of practices associated with other professions such as psychologists, counsellors and social workers (UKCC, 1996; Butterworth and Faugier, 1994). In the early 1990s, the document *Vision for the Future* (DoH, 1993) promoted the use of clinical supervision through identified policy targets. Within the profession itself, *Working in Partnership* (DoH, 1994), and *Pulling Together* (Sainsbury Centre, 1997) reinforced the notion of supervision within mental health nursing. Butterworth's and Faugier (1994) report on supervision qualified and quantified the development of supervision within mental health nursing and helped to clarify the models in use.

These developments have occurred at both a macro and micro level. At a macro level, policy initiatives dictate levels of excellence through processes and initiatives that are concerned with promoting quality, for example, clinical governance. At a micro level individual practitioners reflect on their practice through the use of PREP (UKCC, 1990) and supervision (UKCC, 1996). Nursing no longer utilises a fixed body of knowledge and procedures which is simply delivered to a patient who is a passive recipient of care. Nursing and nurses must constantly reflect on practice and learn from research, theory and new skills gained in practice itself, to develop their knowledge and practice in order to meet the demands of a continually changing healthcare system.

Part of this learning process is facilitated by supervision with the supervisor enabling the supervisees to reflect on their own practice and explore its knowledge and research rationale thus enabling reflection through insight (Cutcliffe and Burns, 1998). The authors believe that group supervision greatly enhances the opportunity for reflection and new learning to occur, it also provides opportunities for support, experiences of group cohesion and enhances opportunities for communication skills training (Markham and Turner, 1998). The supervisor facilitates the reflection of both the individual, and the whole group, and focuses this reflection on the clinical issues raised in a session. In addition the supervisor can facilitate examination of the dynamics of the group which may enlighten relationship issues between the supervisee and the client as a parallel of the client nurse relationship (Playle and Mullarkey, 1998).

Supervision of students

The clinical supervision sessions for students were located and sequenced so that the students had sufficient exposure to practice that could be used as a basis for discussions. It was noted in the groups that students often had previous experience of caring in a variety of ways, but mainly as support workers for people who had either a diagnosis of mental illness or learning disability, this proving to be a useful ingredient in addition to their other life experiences. Early sessions with the students were taken up with setting ground rules and checking out and confirming that we all had a clear understanding of what clinical supervision meant to us in the context of this group and relating this closely to the Butterworth and Faugier (1992) approach of seeing clinical supervision as the developing of skills through the medium of sharing and reflecting on experiences (from a work situation).

This approach to the implementation of clinical supervision reflected that of Twinn and Johnson (1998) in that the three stages of normative, formative and restorative practice were followed although each aspect also led into or feedback to one another, so that comfort or competence in one would provide a sound base to move on to the next one. This meant that as the course progressed the level of the sessions moved from focusing on what had happened in their practice to developing some of the aspects identified by Proctor (1986) in the formative part of her model, such as links with ethical and skill enhancement.

In the last six months of the course the students started to take on the lead facilitating role for the groups and the lecturer, as the original facilitator, moved to being a type of co-facilitator and providing feedback to the student who had led the session. This in itself was an extension of the clinical supervision, the supported movement from supervisee to supervisor. In undertaking this way of operating, the group members experienced a number of positive outcomes. From a content point of view they received opportunities where they could explore caring issues, with the outcome of considering alternative caring strategies, that members should receive opportunities to explore their attitudes in caring situations and that members should be exposed to the ideas and attitudes of others. From a process point of view the students could focus on and model the strategies used initially to enable exploration of caring issues in members, consider how issues were dealt with by the group and quantify the link between work in the group and the impact upon practice outside the group. It is important to note that in this respect the supervision sessions linked with one another as issues were not dealt with in isolation but were seen as ongoing from session to session.

As the sessions progressed the students identified a range of issues that they believed had helped and enhanced their learning within the supervision groups.

Establishing boundaries

Boundaries are essential to provide an environment where supervisees feel supported in disclosure. Broadcasting (having boundaries written down and distributed) and discussing them is an essential component to enabling work in the group to begin. The boundaries allowed for some initial prescription on the part of the supervisor with greater freedom to explore developing later in the session and through the development of the group. Haddock (1997) highlighted the feelings of anxiety evoked in groups where boundaries and structure were not evident and there was little cohesion or support experienced as a result. Supervisees were encouraged to explore and communicate their worries and suggest ways in which they could explore their practice but feel safe. It was not the intention to remove all risks, as risk taking would be part of developing as a nurse and an aid to disclosure in the group.

Confidentiality

Initially through the setting of ground rules confidentiality and the supervisor's role was explored. For a supervisor who is a registered nurse there were limits on confidentiality; for example, if a supervisee disclosed serious criminal abuse of clients then action by the supervisor would be inevitable. Generally issues raised in the group would remain in the group. If supervisees needed to raise an issue for themselves with their personal tutor then they would be supported in this; however, it would not be the supervisor's role to report anything of the group to a personal tutor.

Disclosure was also discussed and this was closely aligned to purpose. The purpose being to have a forum where supervisees could reflect on their practice. Disclosure of personal material relevant to practice would be the responsibility of the supervisee. For example, the supervisor may intuit from the supervisee that their caring might be inhibited by a similar experience in their own life which is inhibiting their caring. If this were acknowledged by the supervisee it would be up to him or her whether he or she wished to disclose and explore this issue. Supervisees were always given the option to opt out.

Keeping to focus

One of the problems for the supervisor was enabling the supervisees to focus on the purpose. Even though the purpose was highlighted in the boundaries, supervisees still drifted away from the purpose. As supervisor it was important to use communication skills to focus supervisees onto a self-reflective cycle rather than an other-reflective cycle. Supervisees tended to confuse reflecting on others' practice with their own, and programme theory or practice issues with their own assessments, judgements or rationales for their caring time. To aid focusing, written explanations as well as verbal examples were given of self reflection and Mezirow's (1981) critical reflectivity was used as a tool to aid reflection. Enabling supervisees to focus on what was their experience of caring rather than an observation of others, was a fundamental step in the development of supervisee skills.

Exploration of issues

Once supervisees began to bring their own practice issues to the group the supervisor's purpose was to enable as broad an exploration of each issue as possible. Once again Mezirow (1981) was used as a guide along with the Hawkins and Shohet (1989) process model (Figure 13.1). Actively listening to the supervisee (and encouraging other members to do the same) the supervisor would probe aspects of the issue raised as well as clarify with questions. For example, asking: what do you think about your judgements at the time? What decisions did you make? What was your rationale for your decision? How did the episode make you feel? All these questions enabled exploration of the issue for the supervisee, and in verbalising his or her thoughts enabled and developed within the supervisee some clarity about the situation. This enabled movement on to the next phase of the process model, exploration of the strategies and interventions used by the carer. The supervisee bringing the issue was encouraged to look at alternative strategies in the situation reflecting on theory and research and their own nursing philosophy. Alternative scenarios were considered and if necessary practice, or plans, initiated by the supervisee were made for practice outside the supervision session. In this respect outcomes were very important to each session, the supervision not being seen as an isolated bubble but a springboard for change in future practice. Thus work in the supervision group might produce changes in practice reflected in a learner's portfolio of learning or discussed as an issue in theory in one of the action learning groups. Links between supervision and other reflective processes in nursing are well

---

The focus of the supervision session
- Reflection on the content of the caring time
- Exploration of the strategies and interventions used by the carer
- Exploration of the caring process and relationship
- Focus on the carer's blocks to facilitating care

The focus of the supervisors session
- Focus on the here-and-now process as a mirror or parallel of the there-and-then process
- Focus on the supervisor's counter-transference

Figure 13.1 Process model of supervision

Based on Hawkins and Shohet (1989).

documented (Lowry, 1998). Feedback was often expected in the following or subsequent sessions. Lastly in the sessions exploration of the caring process and relationship as well as focus on the carer's blocks to facilitating care were explored. Was there anything within the supervisee that was hindering his or her progress with the client? Issues of gender, self-perception, race, discrimination, culture, previous negative experiences were all raised at this point and, if the supervisee agreed, gently explored.

Credibility

Throughout the sessions comment was often made comparing the supervisor's role to that of a university lecturer. In the initial sessions there seemed to be an acceptance that lecturers had clinical as well as educational credibility. As the sessions progressed and the students felt more able to challenge and confront it was enormously useful for lecturers as supervisors to be able to relate that they not only worked in the clinical arena for part of their time but also received supervision themselves. **That supervisors were also supervisees enabled them, in the views of the students, to play a major role in translating the curriculum into a functioning course at the point of delivery to learners.**

Supervision for supervisors

One of the major criticisms around supervision is that those who supervise are insufficiently equipped for the role of supervision (Fish and Twin, 1997). When setting up the clinical supervision for the students we had to consider the fact that we needed supervision in terms of the course in order to avoid the frequently levelled criticism of lecturers teaching theory without the related practice. In considering the process of setting up supervision for lecturers we had to address a number of issues which highlighted the similarities and differences between health oriented services and educational organisations and the perceived value for those concerned.

Occupational stress

Whilst recognising that all occupations have their own unique pressures, some activities are inherently more stressful than others and therefore it is incumbent on organisations to diligently seek out any measure that will ameliorate the damaging effects stress has on overall well-being. There is literature that identifies the caring professions including nursing as being particularly stressful (Parry-Jones *et al.*, 1998; Wing, 1999; Hardy, 1995) either because of the particularly turbulent climate caused by changes in social policy concerning the locus of care or through the primacy of the interpersonal aspects of the role and the essential therapeutic role of self (Peplau, 1988; Altschul, 1997; Barker, 1997; Gallop, 1997).

Nursing students, teachers and lecturers engaged in health focused programmes are also identified as being particularly stressful (Youseff and Goodrich, 1996; Sawatzky, 1998; Jones and Johnston, 1997; Hamill, 1995), possibly because the organisational turbulence and personal investment are not dissimilar (Humphreys, 1996). People involved in nurse education can therefore be seen to be doubly at risk as they are constantly exhorted to be active in the clinical as well as the educational domain (Hopton, 1996). If, as all the evidence – albeit partially anecdotally – suggests, supervision has a part to play in promoting a person's well-being, it is clearly something that should be available to nursing students and nursing lecturers. This may be increasingly important as recent moves into higher education have placed different, if not greater, imperatives on role performance (Rodriguez and Goorapah, 1998).

Choosing a supervisor

In seeking supervision the lecturers concerned elected to ask the head of department to act as their group supervisor, based on a number of considerations. Some writers emphasise when choosing a supervisor the primacy of the interpersonal skills of the person such as warmth, trust and understanding (Jones, 1996), the possession of relevant knowledge and skills (Sloan, 1999) and the ability to reflect and analyse (Fisher, 1996). Undoubtedly many within the university possess this laudable range of skills and attributes but this may not necessarily be sufficient to overcome the inherent dialectic created when heads of department are asked to become supervisors. **The tendency of those in senior roles to focus on performance and action rather than exploring the subtitles of process (Morris, 1995), the potential for material offered during supervision to be used in a disciplinary manner (Burrow, 1995; Wilkin *et al.*, 1997), the tendency to focus on management issues as the major agenda (Sloan, 1998) and the confusion caused by the duality of supervisory and managerial roles (Adcock, 1998) all contribute to the difficulties when such people undertake the role of supervisor.**

Despite these warnings the sessions appeared to go well and feedback from all participants indicated their worthwhileness. This clearly is not wholly congruent with some of the literature and therefore leads to a consideration as to why this may be. Underpinning the above writers' concerns appears at least in part to be the potential to misuse the power differential created by hierarchical involvement. Power differentials are created by the extent to which one person is dependent on another in terms of resources and outcomes (Brass and Burkhardt, 1992) and therefore is determined not only by the personal approaches of the participants but crucially by the nature and culture of the organisation by whom they are employed (Mullins, 1993).

The locus of most literature on clinical supervision is understandably within care delivery arenas. Because of its military origins, nursing and hospitals in general are often seen as the epitome of bureaucracy. Whilst this term has acquired pejorative overtones and has become synonymous with 'red tape' and 'officialdom', Hoyle (1986) paraphrases Max Weber in describing bureaucracies as organisations containing bureaucracy, specialisation, centralisation, procedural rules and a sense of order, security and predictability.

Many clinicians would look at their current practice and yearn for such order, symmetry and rationality but Hoyle suggests that whilst seldom seen in its pure form most organisations approximate it to some degree. The degree to which there is an observable and operational hierarchy within nursing is marked, this being supported by such things as clinical grading, differing levels of educational qualification, clerical specialists and the various tiers of management either general or clinical.

In contrast, higher education, in which most Schools of Nursing and Midwifery now belong, arose from a more monastic, discursive origin which is reflected in their culture and operations. Most positions of apparent authority are roles not posts and alternate between people over a set period of time, the main decision-making bodies are committees not individual officers and 'academic freedom' is acknowledged as a central facet of operational policy. It is suggested, therefore, that universities as organisations resonate more clearly with the organisational structure known as organised anarchies than with bureaucracies (Enderud, 1980). Whilst anarchy is not necessarily less pejorative then bureaucracy it points to organisational characteristics such as ambiguous goals, sub-unit autonomy, less positivistic means–end relationships and a variety of responses to external influences (Cameron, 1980), all of which are observable within our own university.

It would follow therefore that nurses working within a more hierarchical structure would have a greater concern about the potential abuse of power differentials and that would inform their views and actions regarding the choice of supervisor. **For lecturers working within a less overtly structured culture issues of power and potential coercion would not be as pervasive and therefore they may not see the hierarchical roles as antagonistic to supervisory roles.**

It is our view that the differences outlined create a milieu within university departments that is significantly different from the corresponding locus of activity within healthcare delivery. Therefore when 'managers' are involved in supervision it is significantly less problematic as the power difference is negligible and therefore does not compromise the internal dynamics and processes that are essential to effective supervision. This should not be misinterpreted as suggesting that nurses are more passive and reactive whereas nursing lecturers are in some way bolder and more proactive, but is more about the effects of organisational structures and cultures on the perceptions of equally valuable and worthwhile people.

In fact it could be argued that as newer care-oriented developments such as a greater involvement of users and carers, more multidisciplinary working, nurse consultancy, clinical governance, health action zones and primary care groups begin to take effect then current bureaucratic structures will, of necessity, become more anarchic. They will therefore become increasingly reliant on high quality non-power coercive clinical supervision from people with the appropriate skills irrespective of the position they hold.

The value of supervision for educationalists

The perceived benefits of supervision have been available to some of the caring professions i.e. midwifery and psychotherapists, for some time (Thomas and Reid, 1995; Farrington, 1995) and it is only relatively recently, under the guise of clinical supervision, that nurses have had access to these. Indeed, Fowler (1996) identified the use of supervision by others as being one of the reasons why nurses are now seeking access to such a helpful device. The benefits to nurses appears to outweigh the difficulties associated with supervision and are thought to include developing skills and knowledge that will equip practitioners to meet future healthcare needs (Barton-Wright, 1994), increased feelings of support, well-being, confidence and higher morale (Cutcliffe and Proctor, 1998), reduction in staff stress and burnout (Farrington, 1995), clarifying status thereby reducing uncertainty and confusion (Lowry, 1998)) and an increased confidence to tackle work related problems (Bowles and Young, 1999).

There is much less published work relating to how supervision can help educationalists; however, our own personal experiences would suggest that this is indeed the case. One of the first issues that arose during our sessions resonates with Lowry's (1998) notion that supervision aids role clarity. It very quickly became evident that the course leader felt that he had legitimate power in respect of this role and it was therefore questionable as to how much he had to listen to, consider or take on board the views of the other group participants. Clearly he needed to come to terms with the reality that this was not just an exercise to demonstrate that we practise what we preach but a meaningful attempt at increasing the feelings of support and well-being that Cutcliffe and Proctor (1998) suggested.

Addressing and ultimately resolving this issue arose during a session when one of the lectures in the group raised the question as to how decisions should be reached and agreed relating to course implementation. Fidelity to the previously agreed ground rules ensured that a reasoned and seemly debate ensued with everyone attempting to respect the views and feelings of their peers. By the end of the session a democratic system of reaching agreement through a majority viewpoint had been agreed, with the proviso that everyone then accepted and stuck to that decision.

In setting the initial ground rules, it was unanimously agreed that no written record of the meetings would be kept. This was partly to ensure congruency with the approach taken in the student groups but also to ensure total confidentiality within the group setting. Obviously the results of our discussions could be utilised to the benefit of the course as was the case when a better system of disseminating assignment information arose from discussions within the supervision group. Our approach to records did mean however that we were in danger of potentially going over the things time after time either through lapses in memory, the identification of further evidence or at times an effort to use prevarication and delaying tactics in order to gain personal advantage. In order to try to avoid an almost farcical situation arising it was decided to ask the supervisor to keep brief notes of the key headings, which were prompted and ratified by the supervisees. This constituted part of the facilitator's summarising function at the end of one session and his introduction at the beginning of the next.

The next challenge came when one supervisee wanted to raise an issue about what had happened in their supervision session with the students. This raised an ethical dilemma in that student supervision groups had an agreement not to raise any matter to others unless it fell into one of the areas where it had to be disclosed, e.g. illegal activities. Therefore it was felt not possible to discuss this issue in detail, but in an attempt to help it was decided to use hypothetical illustrations. At the end of this particular session there was an agreement that such a course of action had been of great use and had increased the individual's repertoire of skills for helping students in distress.

Perhaps the most meaningful indication that the supervision sessions were of value was the level of attendance. The rules of the sessions stipulated that all members had to be present in order to enhance ownership and commitment. Whilst fully recognising that this rule was incredibly ambitious and could have promoted pressure to attend and therefore resentment, in fact attendance was good with only a very small minority of sessions being cancelled, which was particularly noteworthy during a period of increased activity and annual leave.

Conclusion

It is often stated, especially in health arenas, that things appear to be essentially cyclical. Old activities could be seen to reinvent themselves as new and exciting initiatives, leading cynics to suggest that things are just the same as they have always been only with a new name. Within higher education it is possible to level this criticism at supervision for nurse lecturers and students. Students have personal tutors whose remit includes a pastoral element, course leaders who often address issues that may affect a student's progress, assessors and mentors during clinical placements who oversee skill development.

Lecturers have annual staff appraisal interviews, peer assessment of teaching and for those new to the organisation a 'probation' period for up to three years that includes regular supervision sessions. A question that arises therefore is that within this milieu, is there a niche for the type of supervision described in this chapter or is it merely repetition of other support mechanisms under a different guise? It is the firm belief of the authors that this is not the case and there is something significant and worthwhile about the process we have undertaken. Often other forms of support are task-oriented and focused on increasing the person's repertoire of knowledge or how to make something work within the given organisation.

The key thing that emerged from our supervision sessions was the felt sense of well-being and emotional support. These are outcomes that are difficult to empirically quantify and therefore could be questioned in a cost effective, financially driven arena. However, perhaps the challenge for those who advocate supervision in either clinical or educational settings is to establish appropriate ways of demonstrating its worth to those who have not experienced the warmth and power of the process.

References

Adcock L (1998) Clinical supervision in practice. *Journal of Community Nursing* 13(5), pp406.

Altschul A (1997) A personal view of psychiatric nursing. In Tilley S (ed.) *The Mental Health View: Views of Practice and Education* pp1–14, London: Blackwell Science.

Barker P (1997) Toward a meta theory of psychiatric nursing practice. *Mental Health Practice* 1(4), pp18–21.

Barton-Wright P (1994) Clinical supervision and primary nursing. *British Journal of Nursing* 3(1), pp23–29.

Bowles N and Young C (1999) An evaluative study of clinical supervision based on Proctor's three function interactive model. *Journal of Advanced Nursing* 30 (4), pp958–964.

Brass D J and Burkhardt M E (1992) Centrality and power in organisations. In Nohria N and Eccles R G (eds) *Networks and Organisations*. Boston: Harvard Business School Press.

Burrow S (1995) Supervision: Clinical development or management control. *British Journal of Nursing* 4(15), pp879–882.

Butterworth T and Faugier J (1992) *Clinical Supervision and Mentorship in Nursing*. London: Chapman and Hall.

Butterworth T and Faugier J (1994) Clinical supervision: a position paper. Manchester University School of Nursing Studies.

Butterworth T (1998) Clinical supervision and mentorship. In *Nursing*. Faugier J and Burnard P (2nd Edition) Cheltenham: Stanley Thornes.

Cameron K (1980) Critical questions in assessing organisational effectiveness. *Organisational Dynamics* (Autumn) American Management Association, pp66–78.

Cutcliffe J and Burns J (1998) Personal, professional and practice development: clinical supervision. *British Journal of Nursing* 7, 21.

Cutcliffe J and Proctor B (1998) An alternative training approach to clinical supervision I. *British Journal of Nursing* 7(5), pp280–285.

Department of Health (1993) *A Vision for the Future*. London: HMSO.

Department of Health (1994) *Working in Partnership: a Collaborative Approach to Care*. London: HMSO.

Enderud H (1980) Administrative leadership in organised anarchies. *International Journal of Institutional Management in Higher Education* 4(3), pp235–251.

Farrington A (1995) Models of clinical supervision. *British Journal of Nursing* 4(15), pp876–878.

Fish D and Twinn S (1997) *Quality Clinical Supervision in the Health Care Professions, Principled Approaches to Practice*. London: Butterworth Heinemann.

Fisher M (1996) Using reflective practice in clinical supervision. *Professional Nurse*, 11(7) pp443–444.

Fowler J (1996) The organisation of clinical supervision within the nursing profession: A review of the literature. *Journal of Advanced Nursing* 23, pp471–478.

Gallop R (1997) Caring about the client. The Mental Health Nurse; Views of Practice and Education (Tilley S ed.) pp28–42 London: Blackwell Science.

Haddock S (1997) Reflection in groups: contextual and theoretical considerations within nurse education and practice. *Nurse Education Today* 17, pp381–385.

Hamill C (1995) The phenomenon of stress as perceived by project 2000 student nurses: A case study. *Journal of Advanced Nursing* 21, pp528–536.

Hardy S (1995) Promoting a healthy workforce: A clinical case presentation. *British Journal of Nursing* 4(10), pp583–586.

Hawkins P and Shohet R (1989) *Supervision in the Helping Professions.* Milton Keynes: Open University Press.

Hopton J (1996) Reconceptualizing the theory–practice gap in mental health nursing. *Nurse Education Today* 16(3), pp227–232.

Hoyle E (1986) *The Politics of School Management.* London: Hodder & Stoughton.

Humphreys J (1996) Educational commissioning by consortia; some theoretical and practical issues relating to qualitative aspects of British nurse education. *Journal of Advanced Nursing* 24, pp1288–1299.

Jones A (1996) Clinical supervision; a framework for practice. *International Journal of Psychiatric Nursing Research* 3(1), pp290–299.

Jones M C and Johnston D W (1997) Distress, stress and coping in first year student nurses. *Journal of Advanced Nursing* 26, pp475–482.

Lowry M (1998) Clinical supervision for the development of nursing practice. *British Journal of Nursing* 4(10), pp583–586.

Markham V and Turner P (1998) Implementing a system of structured clinical supervision with a group of DipHE (Nursing) RMN students. *Nurse Education Today* 18, pp32–35.

Mezirow A (1981) A critical theory of adult learning and education. *Adult Education* 32, 1 pp3–24.

Morris M (1995) The role of clinical supervision in mental health practice. *British Journal of Nursing* 4(15), pp886–888.

Mullins L J (1993) *Management and Organisational Behaviour* (3rd edition). London: Pitman.

Norman I J, Redfern S J and Bodley et al. (1996) *The Changing Educational Needs of Mental Health and Learning Disability Nurses.* English National Board for Nursing, Midwifery and Health Visiting.

Parry-Jones B Grant G McGrath M Ramcharan P and Robinson C A (1998) Stress and job satisfaction among social workers, community nurses and community psychiatric nurses: implications for the care management model. *Health and Social Care in the Community* 6(4), pp271–285.

Peplau H E (1988) *Interpersonal Relations in Nursing.* London: Macmillan.

Playle J F and Mullarkey K (1998) Parallel process in clinical supervision: enhancing learning and providing support. *Nurse Education Today* 18, pp559–556.

Proctor B (1986) Supervision: A cooperative exercise in acountability. In Marken M and Payne M (eds) *Enabling and Ensuring.* Leicester: Youth Bureau and Training in Community Work.

Rodriguez P and Goorapah D (1998) Clinical supervision for nurse teachers: The pertinent issues. *British Journal of Nursing* 7, 11, pp663–669.

Rouy K (1999) Balancing act. *Occupational Health,* S1:9, pp19–22.

Sainsbury Centre (1997) *Pulling Together. The Future Roles and Training of Mental Health Staff.* The Sainbury Centre for Mental Health.

Sloan G (1998) Good characteristics of a clinical supervisor: A community mental health nurse perspective. *Journal of Advanced Nursing* 30(3), pp713–722.

Sloan G (1999) Understanding clinical supervision from a nursing perspective. *British Journal of Nursing* 8(8), pp524–528.

Swatzky J V (1998) Understanding nursing students stress: A proposed framework. *Nurse Education Today* 18, pp108–115.

Thomas B and Reid J (1995) Multidisciplinary clinical supervision. *British Journal of Nursing* 4, 15, pp883–885.

Twinn S and Johnson C (1998) The supervision of health visiting practice: a continuing agenda for debate. In Butterworth T Faugier J and Burnard P (eds), *Clinical Supervision and Mentorship in Nursing* (2nd edn). Chelterham: Stanley Thornes.

UKCC (1990) *Post Registration Education and Practice Project.* London: UKCC.

UKCC (1996) *Position Statement on Clinical Supervision for Nursing and Health Visiting* London: UKCC.

Wilkin P Bowers L and Monk J (1997) Clinical supervision: Managing the resistance. *Nursing Times* 93 (8), pp48–49.

Wing M (1999) Nursing makes you sick. *Nursing Times* 95, 7, pp24–25.

Youseff F A and Goodrich N (1996) Accelerated versus traditional nursing students: A comparison of stress, critical thinking ability and performance. *International Journal of Nursing Studies* 33, 1, pp76–82.

14 Providing cross discipline group supervision to new supervisors

Challenging some common apprehensions and myths

Paul Cassedy, Mike Epling, Liz Williamson and Gale Harvey

Editorial

This chapter is concerned with cross discipline group supervision. It describes how, at the request of their local NHS Trust, two mental health nursing tutors provided a series of group supervision sessions to registered general nurses who were about to take on the role of clinical supervisor for the first time. It shows how the groups were established, illustrates some of the experiences of being in this group, and identifies some of the issues that arose, mainly during the early stages. It draws attention to one particularly important issue, which is that some novice supervisees may be discouraged from participating in supervision if their supervisor is from a different discipline. However, exposure to and experience of supervision provides such novices with an awareness that the supervisor's skill in providing supportive, reflective and challenging supervision is more important than sharing the same discipline.

It is our experience that when first introduced to the practice of clinical supervision, many practitioners have perfectly reasonable concerns that only another practitioner from their discipline could understand the nuances of their world. As stated previously, we do not believe there is one correct way of operationalising clinical supervision, so for some, having a supervisor from the same discipline may work well. However, we would advocate that potential supervisees be mindful of the benefits in having a supervisor from a different discipline. Benefits not only described in this chapter, but also described by many of the supervisees we have trained over the years. Such mindfulness may help the supervisee to find supervisors with whom they can establish a relationship, work well with and thus develop as a practitioner and as a person.

Setting up the supervision groups

Back in 1997 clinical supervision was a new concept for the majority of the 1500 registered nurses in the large teaching hospital where two of the authors were employed. They had the task of implementing a pilot project to introduce supervision within the Trust. Volunteers were asked to be trained as supervisors and 18 registered nurses came forward. The supervisees were drawn from six areas which volunteered for the pilot project, but the supervisors came from all across the hospital.

Purposeful time had been spent by a working party to consider and provide a framework for implementation that would be carefully planned, covering as many aspects as possible to establish a culture and provide high quality clinical supervision. In keeping with the structures suggested in the relevant literature (Hawkins and Shohet, 1989; Butterworth, 1992; Bond and Holland 1998), and since this was to be a new experience, supervision for the supervisors was identified as essential within this framework, providing the much needed support.

Links had been established with the local education provider in particular through the supervision course that was offered to the Trust. As the facilitators of that course, the first two authors were therefore approached by the second two authors to facilitate group supervision to these new supervisors for the duration of the pilot study (six months). An arrangement was set up with a number of aims and valuable opportunities in mind. These aims are described in Table 14.1.

In addition to providing this learning experience, the group would be valuable for the new supervisors in providing an experience of what it feels like to be a supervisee. Participation in the group offered a unique means of learning, enabling empathic qualities to develop as more insight and respect can be gained as one begins to value the whole process of supervision.

The first two authors accepted this invitation with a mixture of enthusiasm and anxiety. Although both these authors have many years of experience facilitating groups in practice and educational settings, this was the first time they would be formally supervising general nurses in a setting and environment that is alien to our own. Both these authors have a background in mental health, human relations, counselling and training. Each of these subjects can be regarded as somewhat 'mystical' to those unfamiliar with the idiosyncrasies of the subject and as a result, may have caused a degree of caution in the potential group members. These anxieties existed on several levels. First, there

Table 14.1 Arrangement and aims of the group supervision

- An educative and supportive arena in which supervisors could explore and develop this new role
- To share their experiences with one another
- To increase confidence in carrying out their role as supervisor
- To experience group supervision
- To use the two facilitators as role models
- To provide the foundations for the groups to continue as peer supervision following the pilot study

was the initial anxiety of the supervision itself. The authors felt that they would be focusing on their role of supervisor rather than the role of general nurse, but concerns existed regarding the possibility that issues could arise about practice that was beyond our understanding and experience of the authors. Second, the authors had anxieties that mental health backgrounds might prove to be an issue in facilitating group supervision for general nurses.

Supervisors and supervisees sharing the same discipline

It is the authors' experience from running training courses in clinical supervision that when first embarking on the concept, the supervisee initially wants someone from the same discipline and background to supervise him or her. There is probably an element of safety here, in that potential supervisees don't want to feel vulnerable and exposed and they have always previously gone to a colleague for support. **However, as knowledge and experience is gained supervisees gradually realise there is a greater opportunity for development in choosing someone, irrespective of his or her background, who will stretch them and be more challenging.**

Bernard and Goodyear (1998) suggest that technical competence can be achieved when the supervisory dyad is of a different discipline even when an essential component is missing. This is the function of developing a sense of professional identity and helping the supervisee to socialise into that profession by serving as a role model. Socialisation in this sense means that it is pertaining to the overall welfare of the community or organisation. This is a strong argument for the supervisory dyad to be a member of the same profession particularly when working with a recently qualified practitioner. Although we were not from the same discipline we were from the same profession of nursing so some of these contentious issues could be explored.

The fact that the facilitators were from different backgrounds did not manifest itself as a significant issue for the group members. When the initial arrangements were being formulated and during the preliminary sessions, the new supervisors welcomed the opportunity of working with someone with more experience in supervision. The potential supervisors suggested that they were concerned with the skills the facilitators exhibited as supervisors rather than their clinical backgrounds. **It's the authors' belief that it is more important for the supervisor to be competent in and understand the process of supervision, than it is to share the same clinical background as the supervisee.**

The new supervisors were divided into three groups of six members in each; there was a considerable range of specialities and grades within each group. Only two had received supervision before and there was an even mix of those who knew one another and those who did not. There was apprehension about taking part in group supervision alongside the anxiety of taking on the role of supervisor for the first time. Page and Wosket (1994) allude to the notion that becoming a supervisor is rather like learning to swim. Although the new supervisors would be getting their feet wet by going in at the shallow end there was also the opportunity of taking lessons and learning along side a more experienced swimmer. The facilitators felt qualified to take on the role of group supervisor as Carroll (1996) and Scanlon (1980) suggest, having previous supervision experience and the transferable skills of teaching and facilitating, so this was about to be put to the test.

The group experience

There were no pre-conceived ideas or guidelines about how to use the sessions, only that these supervisors would need considerable support as this new role was in its infancy. As in any new role or setting the nurse may find herself in, there needs to be a period of mentorship and nurturing. To help safeguard this new journey, it was considered important to create a contract for the supervision group to enable some degree of control over the experience. A good starting point for encouraging empowerment and ownership is to discuss the very issues that may cause concern to the individuals involved (Hawkins and Shohet, 1989; Bond and Holland, 1998). Airing these anxieties provided a forum to share and explore a range of issues which are not only important to the supervisor in the group, but may also parallel the very same concerns of the supervisee in the work setting.

The group decided that the time allowed for each member would be divided equally but urgent matters would take precedence. As status within the group was diverse, it was considered to be important to address this and the group wanted to ensure that it was put to one side to create an egalitarian approach. The facilitator would be mindful of this and challenge the use of a status position or pulling rank as a means of authority. The authors attempted to create a 'level playing field' to provide supportive challenge that would avoid competitiveness and encourage reflection, exploration and sharing. Each member agreed to be prepared for supervision, and the group would decide the agenda on the day.

Confidentiality was discussed; the decisions reached were analogous to the agreements that were stated between supervisors and supervisees. Revisiting the UKCC guidelines for professional practice (1992) proved to be a good starting point. A breach of this code, a breach of law or serious exploitation or endangerment to others would normally be occasions to disclose information to another source (Morton-Cooper and Palmer, 2000).

Concerns of disclosure, which would involve reporting serious malpractice and how these could be dealt with in the supervisory alliance, were aired, but also 'what if' scenarios were brought to the fore (see Cutcliffe *et al.*, 1998a,b). Many issues are not easily answered; reminding the group that they were also in a supportive relationship and would not be left isolated can calm anxiety about the possibility of serious disclosure. An issue that was related to confidentiality emerged in one group and had an effect on both the attendance and dynamics. Feltham and Dryden (1994) point out that group supervision does have its drawbacks; notably the group dynamics can be a complicating factor.

Blurring of relationship boundaries

A member of the group had a close friendship with another group member's supervisee. This was not disclosed or picked up by the facilitator at first, but there was some absenteeism and when all were present some hesitance and holding back of material. A group member finally revealed this in a group evaluation round. Although the names of the supervisees were not used in the group, identities in this small world can be recognised so anonymity cannot be maintained, only the conditions of confidentiality can be provided. This was explored and discussed with the group with the conclusion that it would be more therapeutic to be open and honest about such matters and that we as a group needed to establish strategies to overcome such issues. Many staff, even within large hospitals, are going to have some awareness or acknowledgement of one another. Even if not, certain persons still may be able to be identified from the material the supervisor is working on. The issue here for the group and subsequent supervision arrangements is to maintain the boundaries and responsibilities of clinical supervision. Some group members will know one another and their supervisees; a group member may have a different role over another member's supervisee, which could cause a blurring of boundaries or conflict of roles.

Power (1999) argues that a supervisor should not agree to supervise anyone that he or she has a close relationship with. Bond and Holland (1998) state that it is the responsibility of the supervisor to hold tight boundaries and keep any other role outside the supervision sessions. Perhaps both of these views can be substantiated, but when a supervision group finds itself with such issues practical measures may be needed. One such method would be for group members to disclose a supervisee's first name and then perhaps his or her area of work. If any group member recognises the supervisee as someone well known to him or her, he or she should acknowledge this and leave the room whilst this supervision work is being presented. Another method would be, following negotiation with the group, to have the last ten minutes of the session for an individual to work alone with the supervisor if his or her supervisee was well known to another in the group. By making every effort to respect confidentiality, this would help maintain objectivity and avoid the potential damages of avoidance or collusion.

The early stages: finding our feet

Attendance of one group was spasmodic in the early stages, which could have had a number of contributing factors. Some will always drop out for unplanned unexpected reasons, e.g. leaving the area. There is also the notion that in the initial stages of implementing supervision anxiety levels of staff will be raised, in particular if it is to be group supervision (Hawkins and Shohet, 1989). This could result in absenteeism either from the supervision sessions or from work itself, as staff are apprehensive and uncertain of attending. It is well documented that receiving supervision can reduce stress levels in the supervisee (Butterworth *et al.*, 1997). However, undertaking the role of supervisor for the first time can have the opposite effect and increase the supervisor's level of stress.

This, in some small way, seemed to be the case here. In the pilot evaluation supervisors did admit to some anxiety about the size of the group and they felt uncomfortable with self-disclosure, which affected levels of reflection. A few supervisors found the whole process too much and opted out while for some others the group size created some reticence. One supervisor during the evaluation stated that 'it wasn't until my group reduced to three supervisors that I really felt comfortable and was really able to reflect on my performance.' Another mentioned that 'it wasn't that I didn't trust all the group members, although I did feel some concern about the makeup of the group and possible impact on outside working relationships. The group felt too big and a little intimidating.' Then went on to add, 'I never felt sufficiently at ease to want to address important issues, especially due to the fragmented nature of the group in the early sessions.'

A delicate balance is needed here, as Charleton (1996) points out that supervision is approached with a mixture of anxiety and relief: anxiety at the thought of exposing their clinical practice and relief that there is someone to who will really listen and provide support. It can be a problem to maintain attendance and keep commitment and motivation high, in particular in the early stages of the group when only meeting once a month in what can be a disquieting experience. Support and encouragement is certainly needed but what also needs to be built in is a professional approach to value the whole process of supervision, and a responsibility to make and keep that commitment. If we do not take that personal responsibility, then we are not only letting ourselves and our profession down, but arguably our patients or clients as well.

The supervision sessions themselves were also fragmented at the start of the pilot in the work setting. Some found it hard to meet regularly, there were cancelled appointments and when some meetings did occur there were perceived to be no major issues to discuss or explore. So for some new supervisors the relationship with the supervisee was difficult to get going and the alliance slow to develop. This meant that those supervisors who hadn't met with their supervisees felt inhibited or even embarrassed about attending the group sessions. Further exploration with the group revealed that some form of parallel process might have been occurring. Although this is a very complex phenomenon a simple definition would be that at times the dynamics of the relationship between client and nurse become paralleled or mirrored in the relationship between nurse and supervisor. Carroll (1996) gives a comprehensive overview of this phenomenon from a psychoanalytical and counselling perspective, while Power (1999) goes into some detail from a nursing perspective. Therapeutic relationships do take time to grow and develop, even more so when the meeting is only for one hour a month. So the rather fragmented start to the supervision process for some in the work setting appeared to mirror that of one of the supervision groups in the pilot project. Perseverance, commitment and enthusiasm were needed by all those concerned in the process as well as the full backing and co-operation of those on the periphery. The supervision group needed to become aware of this so that we could address the issue and work on our own group co-operation.

An advantage of group supervision over individual supervision is that participants can share their abilities and resources for a common purpose. Listening to other group members presenting their supervision work can help others in the group to identify and express issues in their work setting. This is particularly valuable, as new supervisors may well experience similar difficulties (Bond and Holland, 1998). There are developmental opportunities as each member can be a co-supervisor for one another, enabling reflection and supervision skills to develop. Creativity has an opportunity to be rediscovered and developed for the task in hand. The authors needed to remind themselves to take risks and were eventually rewarded with a greater richness of learning and experience. Tuckman's model (Tuckman, 1965) of group development suggests there will be confusion and conflict in the early stages but if successfully managed it will lead to a successful performance of the task.

Themes arising from the group

There were common themes of material that emerged from the group supervision sessions. Rather than the supervisee focusing on his or her clinical practice it tended to be relationships with other members of staff or his or her own personal development issues. It seemed that at least initially most supervisees needed to focus on the formative and restorative aspects of supervision rather than on the normative function. There could be several reasons for this; it would seem that there is little already available in terms of support systems to focus on personal issues related to team working and professional development. **Such issues may therefore have been stored away or built up over a period of time leading to a backlog of concerns or issues needing to be addressed before the supervisees could move on to examining their own practice in more depth.** This is not to suggest that there is no need for supervision in the normative function for general nurses.

Bond and Holland (1998) propose that the focus of supervision leads from the restorative to the formative and finally to the normative when safety in the relationship and process has been established. The experiences the group reported in the nature of the material brought to supervision can therefore be viewed as following such a pattern and process, which needs to be worked through in the development of the supervisory relationship. Progressing onto exploring issues relating to practice would be the next phase of the process.

It's possible that initially the supervisees need to feel fully supported to reflect more in depth on their care and relationships with patients. There is a misconception that it is only when nurses are working with patients intensively over a long period that there is need to reflect on that work and the relationship. Nurses working in areas with a rapid turnover of patients often underestimate the significance of their relationship with patients and families for the patients and themselves. Even brief relationships may leave unresolved issues for the nurse, which could be explored in supervision.

The supervisors new to their role may have allowed some supervisees to keep their focus on 'familiar' issues as this gave them an opportunity to build up their own confidence in their role before having to face more demanding situations that may raise anxiety, e.g. dealing with uncertainty.

A common theme also emerged in how the supervisors tackled these issues and the types of interventions they used. Perhaps because the supervisors were apprehensive of this new role and of being viewed in a position of responsibility, they tended to be rather prescriptive and solution focused in their interventions. This tendency to focus on the actions and activities of the supervisee with problem solving in mind was seen to be a measure of success. There was also the misconception on the supervisors' part that solutions to problems identified in supervision could be written up for the evaluation in order to demonstrate its value to the organisation. Indeed, following the pilot and evaluation a number of supervisors reflected that this was primarily a symptom of their lack of experience with supervision and that it fitted more comfortably with their more familiar nursing role.

What emerged from the group sessions and proved to be valuable learning were the ways the new supervisors perceived their authority and how comfortable they felt with it. Pickvance (1997) states that new supervisors will bring to the role their own feelings and experiences regarding authority. The facilitators felt that it was paramount that the supervisors did not over-identify with an authoritarian role by being too prescriptive and being seen to have all the answers. Conversely there should not be denial of the role by an avoidance of challenging supervisees and leaving sessions without clarity or focus. Both these characteristics appeared in the supervision sessions as some supervisors found it easier to stay purely supportive while others wanted to focus intently on outcomes. This will have the effect of undermining the supervisee and the whole purpose and process of supervision. What needed to be established in the supervision relationship was a genuine space for reflection, thinking and development, not only for the supervisee but also the supervisor.

Seeing the big picture

This ability did develop during group supervision and the supervisors were able to work with their supervisees in a different style from any previously experienced. This was not only to be more facilitative in their approach but also to have a wider vision. Hawkins and Shohet (1989) refer to this as helicopter vision, which is the ability of the worker to switch perspectives at various times. The purpose is to help the supervisor to take a broader perspective on the supervisee. This is to not only focus on their practice and work setting but also to consider their (the supervisors') own behaviour and experience and the reasons for acting as they do. There is a matrix of relationships and possible issues to be explored and reflected upon.

One supervisor presented a case where the supervisee felt left out and not part of the ward team. What they both initially began to explore was to find a solution to the problem and how to resolve it. This was in part due to the supervisor's desire to problem solve as this was her usual way of working. During group supervision this was processed and other possible interventions and ideas reflected upon. Following this exploration the supervisor felt more able and thus competent to utilise facilitation skills and help the supervisee to reflect more deeply. When the case was next presented in supervision, it surfaced that the supervisee felt more isolated with herself rather than with others and a broader picture emerged. She worked part time, was caring for an elderly relative and had just returned to practice following maternity leave. She now lacked confidence in herself and questioned her ability in a changing ward environment.

The supervisor had helped the supervisee to focus more on how to build up her self-esteem and confidence, what she actually wanted for herself and how to develop more supportive relationships in her team. Eventually there was more insight and understanding and the supervisee felt more able to disclose her feelings to others. She began to update herself with practice issues which enabled her once again to feel involved. Hawkins and Shohet (1989) point out the skill of seeing things in a wider context is difficult at first and can only fully be developed during the actual supervision process. This was also our experience as the skills began to emerge and then develop during the life of the group.

Moving towards supervisee centred skills

Perhaps also due to a lack of skill or experience, there was some initial anxiety of utilising more the catalytic or facilitative type of intervention and its links to helping in a counselling type of role. Supervision is not counselling, although many of the skills and certainly the qualities that make the working alliance are transferable. The overall intention and purpose of each is different: counselling is focused solely on the person being counselled while the focus of supervision is primarily on issues that ultimately affect the supervisee's practice. However, this should not discount the need for support for the supervisee as a person and in his or her emotional and psychological development. As Bond and Holland (1998) argue, support is open-ended. Good supervisors need to develop their use of counselling skills as well as feeling confident and comfortable with that process. There needs to be an ability to be aware of their appropriate and inappropriate use as well as to recognise when they may need to refer elsewhere. The supervisor needs at least to be able to contain any emotional material the supervisee brings to supervision and have at least some understanding of the psychological processes that may be occurring. A fear that new supervisors may often have is saying the wrong thing or not wanting to put their foot in it. However, if they truly are actively listening and communicating their empathic understanding there needs to be no such fear. Communication skills such as paraphrasing and reflecting back key words or feelings are very powerful in enabling the supervisee to be really heard and understood. But what the new supervisor will need is to feel supported in this different way of working and have a forum, such as their own supervision, to explore any issues that may arise.

The essential ingredients of good communication, learning and supervision are Rogers' core conditions of warmth, genuineness and empathy (Rogers, 1962). It is important for us all to re-establish this at times, in particular when the relationship is difficult or demanding and when rapport is hard to establish. We endeavoured to create these conditions in the group to create a climate and culture to serve as a good model for relationships.

Final reflections

Overall, the involvement in group supervision for the new supervisors was a positive experience. Although it took some time for trust to develop with the facilitators we all felt the benefits by the end of the pilot project. The facilitators have learned that there is a fine balance of support and challenge needed at the start of a group, alongside being able to keep the balance of commitment, enthusiasm and responsibility to the task. Perhaps the facilitators did not successfully juggle all the aspects together at the beginning. The facilitators have also gained a wider experience in group facilitation and felt it is successful to supervise others of a different discipline in this capacity. We are also indebted to the various group members for providing us with material and valuable learning that we can take back into our educational setting and the supervision course.

The group members report that they will take away the experience of being supervised, in that levels of self-awareness regarding the role of supervisor have increased significantly. The development of facilitation skills and the ability to view the supervisees' work in a wider perspective have also been fostered. The supervisors reported that it was important that they were supported and nurtured through this beginning process of being a guardian to another (their supervisees). The analogy of parent and grandparent that Page and Wosket (1994) refer to is a useful one to use here. If the supervisor is acting as a 'parent type figure' to the supervisee then the supervisor of the supervisor is similar to a 'grandparent figure'. The supervisor who is new to the role will need fostering for some time while he or she becomes more effective and competent in that role. This analogy also addresses the question of where the continuous line of supervision ceases. The supervisor of the supervisor (grandparent) can eventually withdraw as they place more trust in their supervisors. However, they can be a reassuring figure in the background for welcome support when needed or at times of emergency. Grandparents will occasionally seek out help and support from other adults or peers in a similar role; the facilitators certainly did this at times, with certain colleagues and ourselves. They would share some of our ideas or findings or check out with one another some small detail.

Through their development and learning most group members felt they had now reached a stage where they could function more autonomously as a supervisor. Some have arranged to meet in small peer groups while others can utilise their own clinical supervision at times to reflect on their supervision role. The arrangements for providing support for the supervisors will inevitably vary. This will depend on the overall amount of supervision work the nurse is undertaking, but will need to be monitored. All the supervisors will however, continue with their own clinical supervision. As the UKCC (1996) position statement proposes, this will assist life long learning, as indeed, some will eventually step into the role of 'grandparent' and become a supervisor of supervisors themselves.

References

Bernard J and Goodyear R (1998) *Fundamentals of Clinical Supervision* (2nd edition). Boston: Allyn and Bacon.

Bond M and Holland S (1998) *Skills of Clinical Supervision for Nurses*. Buckingham: Open University Press.

Butterworth T (1992) Clinical supervision as an emerging idea in nursing. In Butterworth T and Faugier J (eds) *Clinical Supervision and Mentorship in Nursing*. London: Chapman and Hall.

Butterworth T Carson J White E Jeacock J Clements A and Bishop V (1997) It is good to talk. Clinical supervision and mentorship. An evaluation study in England and Scotland. University of Manchester: The School of Nursing, Midwifery and Health Visiting.

Carroll M (1996) *Counselling Supervision, Theory, Skills and Practice*. London: Cassell.

Charleton M (1996) *Self-Directed Learning in Counsellor Training*. London: Cassell.

Cutcliffe J Epling M Cassedy P McGregor J Plant N and Butterworth T (1998a) Ethical dilemmas in clinical supervision, part 1 – need for guidelines. *British Journal of Nursing* 7 (15), pp920–923.

Cutcliffe J Epling M Cassedy P McGregor J Plant N and Butterworth T (1998b) Ethical dilemmas in clinical supervision, part 2 – need for guidelines. *British Journal of Nursing* 7 (16), pp978–982.

Feltham C and Dryden W (1994) *Developing Counselling Supervision*. London: Sage.

Hawkins P Shohet R (1989) *Supervision in the Helping Professions*. Milton Keynes: Open University Press.

Morton-Cooper A and Palmer A (2000) *Mentoring, Preceptorship and Clinical Supervision* (2nd edition). Oxford: Blackwell Science.

Page S and Wosket V (1994) *Supervising the Counsellor*. London: Routledge.

Pickvance D (1997) *Becoming a Supervisor* In *Supervision of Psychotherapy and Counselling*. Shipton G (ed.) Buckingham: Open University Press.

Power S (1999) *Nursing Supervision, a Guide for Clinical Practice*. London: Sage.

Rogers C (1962) *On Becoming A Person.* London. Constable.

Scanlon C (1980) Towards effective training of clinical supervisors. In V Bishop (ed.) *Clinical Supervision in Practice.* London: Macmillan.

Tuckman B W (1965) Developmental sequences in small groups. *Psychological Bulletin* 63 (6).

United Kingdom Central Council (1992) *Code of Professional Conduct* (3rd edition). London: UKCC.

United Kingdom Central Council (1996) *Position Statement on Clinical Supervision for Nursing and Health Visting.* London: UKCC.

15 Developing methods for evaluating clinical supervision

Julie Winstanley

Editorial

This chapter focuses on evaluating the effects of receiving clinical supervision, and indicates that some progress has been made in this area. It reviews current methods that have been suggested as a means to conduct this evaluation and discusses the various techniques used by nursing researchers, in relation to their usefulness and validity (see Winstanley, 1999). The chapter also reviews the results and assessment instruments which were used to evaluate clinical supervision in the largest study to date of this kind (Butterworth *et al.*, 1997). Following a new study by the same research team, this chapter then reports on the progress made with the development of an evaluation scale, specifically for evaluating clinical supervision (Winstanley, 2000). In addition, the chapter also includes key findings from this study.

We believe that this chapter shows two important developments in the substantive area of clinical supervision. First, that notable progress has been made in the development of validated and sufficiently sophisticated instruments used to evaluate the effects of receiving clinical supervision. Second, that the frequency and duration of sessions (in addition to the quality of training) appears to have significant influence on the supervisee's experience of supervision. This may not be entirely surprising. Since clinical supervision involves a relationship between the supervisee and supervisor, it is quite possible that these relationships need time to develop the sense of trust, safety and commitment necessary for effective clinical supervision to occur. Hence, the greater the frequency and duration of sessions, the sooner the supervision can become effective.

Introduction: Why the need for evaluation?

The importance of clinical supervision for nurses has been reiterated and emphasised with the introduction of clinical governance in 1999. The report entitled *The New NHS – Modern and Dependable* (DoH, 1998), stated that trusts should encourage a

self-evaluative and responsive culture amongst district nurses that will allow clinical practice to evolve and reflect emerging evidence of effectiveness.

Consequently, the combined effects impetus of evidence based practice, value for money and the introduction of clinical governance, has re-affirmed the need for the evaluation of clinical supervision.

A substantial link has been established between the good practice of clinical supervision and the responsibilities necessary for effective clinical governance, and a briefing paper by Butterworth and Woods (1999) has stated that:

Participating in clinical supervision is a clear demonstration of individuals exercising their responsibility under clinical governance. Organisations have a responsibility to ensure that individual clinicians have access to appropriate supervision and support in the exercise of their joint and individual responsibilities.

Now that clinical supervision has an established role to play in the working practices of the nursing workforce, effective evaluation of clinical supervision is one of the important challenges which currently face nursing. Most of the evaluation methods that have been used to date have been developed locally, and have tended to be qualitative in nature. This diversity has been largely due to the lack of a national standard protocol. A number of data collection methods have been employed: for example, audit forms, self-completion questionnaires, focus groups, personal interviews and feedback techniques.

Setting standards for evaluating clinical supervision

It has been suggested (Cutcliffe, 1997) that if one could establish a minimum standard of quality of supervision, future research studies and evaluations of clinical supervision could use this as selection criteria for participants. However, the quality of clinical supervision is dependent on so many factors that it may be beyond the control of either the supervisee or the supervisor. Cutcliffe emphasised that clinical supervision was not a skill that could be learnt fully in a couple of days and that should a nurse receive inadequate or insufficient training, then the quality of his or her supervision would be affected. In addition, there are several models to choose from, and a range of different ways of integrating clinical supervision sessions into the working environment. Proctor's (1991) model, which identified areas that the process of clinical supervision sought to address, has been widely accepted by the profession. These areas are the normative component (issues related to quality control and organisational responsibility), the formative (development of knowledge and skills) and the restorative (supporting personal well-being). Clearly an effective evaluation system would need to include elements which address all three components of Proctor's model and have the capacity to function in a variety of settings with proven validity.

Clinical supervision in practice

In practice, we know that clinical supervision takes place in a variety of ways. Once an NHS trust has decided to implement clinical supervision and has invested in the training of staff for the supervisory role, actual implementation is a lengthy process. It usually becomes established in 'pocket' areas of each trust to begin with, perhaps even within one speciality: evidence of these variations can be seen in the chapters in the 'Introduction' section. Variations in the structure and process of clinical supervision occur as a result of a variety of reasons, including:

- local policy and managerial decisions made within each Trust as to how to integrate the supervision process into working practice;
- the particular understanding or philosophical bent of those leading the implementation.

For example, the manner in which clinical supervision has been implemented into the working practice of community nurses varies considerably from that of hospital based nurses.

Why do we need a validated evaluation scale for clinical supervision?

The literature has largely considered clinical supervision to be a 'good thing' and there is an explicit assumption that it will assist in the application of nursing theory to practice. The main benefit of clinical supervision is the potential improvement in client care but, to date, the published research has been limited to reports of the efficacy of clinical supervision, in terms of increased satisfaction with the working environment (Begat *et al.*, 1997), or decreased levels of strain in nurses (Hallberg and Norberg, 1993). This has been due, in part, to the lack of a validated assessment scale specifically to measure clinical supervision. It has been suggested that the use of existing instruments to measure the effectiveness of clinical supervision has not been entirely successful (Butterworth *et al.*, 1997) and that more research is needed to devise new evaluation tools. Clearly prompt access to a validated instrument for measuring the efficacy of clinical supervision would serve to enhance opportunities for more quantitative research in this area.

Present systems for evaluation of clinical supervision

Qualitative

Focus group interviews

Focus group interviews have been used increasingly in nursing research (Macleod Clark *et al.*, 1996) and are said to be particularly suited to the study of attitudes and experiences (Kitzinger, 1994). Sessions are labour intensive but produce a vast amount of data of a qualitative nature. However, in this data collection method, the unit of analysis is the group and therefore this would not be a suitable method to evaluate the supervisee's or supervisor's individual experience of the clinical supervision process, if required. Thematic content analysis of data from focus groups has enabled a clearer definition of what makes a good supervisor (e.g. Sloan, 1998), but has not enabled measurement of the attributes associated directly with the effectiveness of the supervision given.

Semi-structured interviews

A sub-sample of individual supervisees and supervisors can be selected for interview, either randomly or purposively and these data may be transcribed for analysis. White *et al.* (1998) reported on the 'lived experience' of clinical supervision in findings from 34 in-depth interviews, conducted with a sample of nurses engaged in clinical supervision. Reaction was generally positive and valuable outcomes were reported in the areas of peer support, encouragement of openness and honesty, self esteem, staff morale and stronger relationships with colleagues. A different study which investigated mental health nurses perceptions and experiences of clinical supervision (Scanlon and Weir, 1997) also produced rich data using this method, but neither of these studies set out to explore the effectiveness of the supervision the supervisees received.

Self-completion questionnaires

Questionnaires for self-completion, which contain open-ended questions, can be developed to suit the local information needs required at the time of evaluation. Written responses from these instruments lend themselves to being thematically analysed and categorised. Although the time required to complete this type of questionnaire, compared with a personal interview, is often brief, the analysis of data can be time-consuming and may sometimes require some computational expertise. The Experience of Clinical Supervision Questionnaire (ESQ), for example, has been developed by Nicklin (1997) and consists of twenty items designed to elicit the perceived effectiveness of the supervision experience. This instrument has demonstrable reliability and is currently being used in several centres on a trial basis (Nicklin, personal communication 1999). Several other studies have reported on the development and use of simple self-completion questionnaires, sometimes referred to as audit forms or recording sheets. For example, an evaluation questionnaire developed for use in a nursing development unit (Mahood *et al.*, 1998) comprised several quantitative items, in a format for the measurement of some aspects of efficacy. Supervisees were asked to indicate the percentage of time spent during a supervision session in the areas of education, support, personal development and practice. This style of questionnaire, if carefully constructed, can yield a valuable mixture of qualitative and quantitative data.

Quantitative

Self-completion questionnaires

These instruments usually contain statements which require the respondent to indicate his or her level of agreement or preference using a Likert scale. For example, a Likert scale for agreement might range from 1 to 5; 1=strongly disagree, 2=disagree, 3=no opinion, 4=agree, 5=strongly agree. The responses can be analysed numerically, summarised using descriptive statistics and compared using standard non-parametric statistical tests (Siegel, 1956).

Several researchers have reported on the development of their own assessment scales for use in evaluation. For example, twenty-six qualified nurses took part in a pilot study conducted by Severinsson and Hallberg (1996a), aimed at evaluating the nurses' experiences of the effect of clinical supervision on psychiatric healthcare by questionnaire. The nurses completed a sixty-two-item questionnaire, of which twenty-four questions were designed to describe the respondents' views of the effects of supervision. Analysis identified three factors: improved communication skills, improved sensibility to patient needs and personal growth. Although this was a pilot study and had the limitations of small sample size, this study demonstrated the technique of using factor analysis to identify underlying concepts associated with effectiveness of clinical supervision. The same methods have been used in a different study, by the same research team, to investigate nurse supervisors' views of their supervisory roles (Severinsson and Hallberg, 1996b). The questions on a ten-item questionnaire were answered on a four-point Likert scale and results identified the supervisors' personal qualities and views of their leadership role.

Existing assessment instruments

The Clinical Supervision Evaluation Project (CSEP) (Butterworth *et al*, 1997) reported difficulties in the use of existing research instruments to measure the process of clinical supervision. This project was conducted over twenty-three sites in NHS Trusts from England and Wales, and looked at the effects of the implementation and evaluation of clinical supervision on the nursing workforce. To date, this study has generated the largest database from nurses engaged in the process of giving and receiving clinical supervision. The research team screened existing instruments available at the time, which were likely to evaluate the core components of clinical supervision, as defined by Proctor (1991). Five instruments (shown in Figure 15.1) were deemed likely to be sensitive to changes in at least two of the three components of clinical supervision. The third component, formative, relates to the process of developing knowledge and skills, and evaluation of this component was thought to be possible using educational audit and individual performance review.

Results from the completion of the five selected instruments accumulated a vast data set on levels of stress, coping skills, job satisfaction and psychological status from 586 nurses engaged in the process of clinical super-

Component	Instrument	Description
Normative	Minnesota Job Satisfaction Scale (Weiss, 1967)	20 items, rated from 1 to 5
Restorative	Maslach Burnout Inventory (Maslach and Jackson, 1986)	28 items, rated from 0 to 3
	General Health Questionnaire (Goldberg and Willaims, 1988)	30 items, rated from 1 to 5
	The Nurse Stress Index (Harris, 1989)	28 items, rated from 1 to 6
	Cooper Coping Skills (Cooper *et al.*, 1988)	22 items, rated from 0 to 6

Figure 15.1 Instruments used in the clinical supervision evaluation project

vision. These data have shown that occupational stress levels in nursing have risen in recent years (Butterworth *et al.*, 1999) and that (say) working in the community is more stressful than working in hospital settings. There was also evidence that grades of staff were affected differently by stressors and that proposed interventions for stress management should be tailored accordingly.

Although there was a wealth of positive feedback and evidence of the beneficial impact on staff (White *et al.*, 1998; Butterworth *et al.*, 1997), the quantitative data using the chosen existing assessment questionnaires showed only two instruments were sensitive to changes with respect to the clinical supervision process. As a result, recommendations were made in the final report that only the Minnesota Job Satisfaction Scale and the Maslach Burnout Inventory would be of value in future evaluation studies.

Significant findings using existing instruments

The Minnesota Job Satisfaction Scale

The study by Butterworth *et al.* (1997) reported that when supervision was withdrawn from supervisees during the second phase of the national project there was a significant decrease in levels of job satisfaction. The opposite effect was seen for the participants who had previously not been in receipt of supervision; that is, those who, in phase one of the study, had formed the control group. This group and the supervisors group showed a decrease in levels of satisfaction whilst not in receipt of clinical supervision and a stabilisation once supervision was introduced.

The Maslach Burnout Inventory

Levels of emotional exhaustion and depersonalisation showed an increase for nurses on the evaluation study who had not been receiving clinical supervision. Once clinical supervision had been introduced the instrument also showed that levels had stabilised, and in some cases decreased. A Swedish study (Palsson *et al.*, 1996) also analysed levels of burnout amongst groups of district nurses before and after systematic clinical supervision using a burnout measure developed by Schaufeli and Enzmann (1993). In contrast, they reported no significant change over time, within or between groups.

Development of the Manchester Clinical Supervision Scale

Nursing researchers from the Manchester School of Nursing have completed a further study, evaluating clinical supervision in a variety of nursing settings in the UK. The main aim of the study has been to develop and validate a quantitative instrument to effectively evaluate clinical supervision from the supervisee's perspective.

Source of items for the questionnaire

The first stage in developing the new scale was to search for potential items for inclusion in the first pilot questionnaire. Qualitative data was drawn from two rich data sources readily available to the research team: the Clinical Supervision Evaluation Project (CSEP) and the findings from a set of in-depth site interviews conducted by Professors White, Butterworth and Bishop. Following a comprehensive review of the literature, these data sources were thought to be the most suitable for developing appropriate and relevant items to be used in the construction of a new scale for measuring the effectiveness of clinical supervision. Both sets of qualitative data were collated and the comments made by the respondents were transformed into a set of statements. These formed the framework for the new questionnaire.

Piloting

Initially, a 59-item scale was developed and piloted at five centres in England and Scotland, representing a range of nursing specialities. Respondents were asked to score statements related to the clinical supervision they received, based on a five-point scale from 'strongly disagree' to 'strongly agree'. Responses from 467 completed scales were analysed. Exploratory factor analysis was used to identify significant factors associated with the process of clinical supervision and reduce the number of items on the scale to those of statistical value.

Field testing

Following the pilot stage, the scale was reduced to 45 items and field tested at a further three centres in the UK. A full replication study has been completed, using both pilot and field datasets, and a scale of 36 'common' items comprising seven factors has been established which can be replicated using different samples of nurses.

Factor	Related to:	Number of items	Content
Trust/rapport	Normative/ restorative	7	Level of trust/rapport with the supervisor during the session/ability to discuss sensitive/confidential issues
Supervisor advice/support	Restorative	6	Extent to which the supervisee feels supported by the supervisor and a measure of level of advice and guidance received
Improved care/ skills	Formative	7	Extent to which the supervisee feels that clinical supervision has affected their delivery of care and improvement in skills
Importance value of clinical supervision	Normative	6	A measure of the importance of receiving clinical supervision and whether the clinical supervision process is valued or necessary to improve quality of care
Finding time	Normative/ restorative	4	A measure of the ease of finding time for clinical supervision sessions
Personal issues	Restorative	3	A measure of how supported the supervisee feels with issues of a personal nature
Reflection	Formative	3	A measure of how supported the supervisee feels with reflecting on complex clinical experiences.

Figure 15.2 Components of the Manchester Clinical Supervision Scale

Calculation of sub-scales

The 36 items (statements) on the questionnaire identified seven factors, which when labelled, included elements of all three components of Proctor's model of clinical supervision, the model most widely used by the nursing profession. The seven factors of the Manchester Clinical Supervision Scale are shown in Figure 15.2. The calculation of sub-scale scores is achieved by simply adding together the scores (from 1–5) on each item within each factor.

Reliability issues

Cronbach's alpha coefficients were calculated to establish the internal consistency of the items within each sub-scale and between each of the sub-scales;

these values were all consistently high, above 0.8 (Cronbach, 1951). The intraclass correlation coefficients (Bland and Altman, 1996) for test–retest reliability on the sub-scales and total evaluation scores were all above 0.9.

Major findings from the study

The database from the study contains completed measures from 1027 nursing staff, comprised of two fairly equal groups of community and hospital based nurses. Analysis of the demographic characteristics of these two major staff groups showed striking differences. **Hospital based staff were more likely to have chosen their own supervisors and had supervision on a one-to-one basis. Their sessions were more likely to have been held within the normal workplace rather than away, were shorter and less frequent than those experienced by community based staff.** The results of these analyses, using the MCSS, have given new insight into how the various implementation strategies of clinical supervision work in practice.

Length and frequency of sessions

The protocol for the CSEP stated that the length of sessions for the participants of the project had to conform to certain characteristics, namely, that the supervisees should have received clincial supervision for 'not less than 45 minutes every four weeks' (Butterworth *et al.*, 1997). Based on their experiences in implementing clincial supervision at that time, this was an informed decision made by the researchers on the study. This criterion has also been used by other clinicians as a guide to best practice in relation to the delivery of clincial supervision (Nicklin, 1997).

Results of analyses, using the MCSS, support the recommendations that sessions should be of significant length to be effective. However, the results showed the outcome for the two staff groups were different. For hospital staff the greatest increase in the evaluation scores occurred when the length of session increased to between 46–60 minutes, whereas for community staff, the evaluation scores increased most when the session length increased to over one hour (see Figure 15.3). For hospital staff, these results indicate that clincial supervision sessions should be a maximum of one hour; for community based staff, there may still be some benefit from extending clincial supervision sessions to last longer than one hour.

For hospital staff, the benefits from receiving clincial supervision reduced significantly if the sessions were more than three months apart. In contrast, for community staff, scores associated with Improve care/ skills and Importance/value of clincial supervision reduced significantly if the sessions were less frequently than monthly (see Figure 15.4). These results support the hypothesis that supervisees benefit from more frequent clincial supervision sessions: supervisees in monthly or bimonthly sessions achieved the highest evaluation scores.

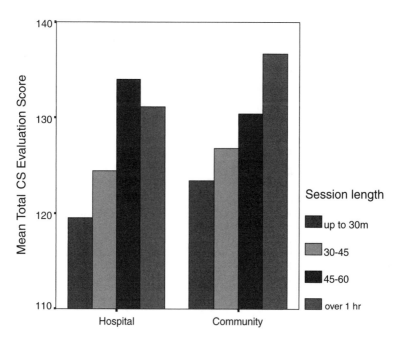

Figure 15.3 Mean total community supervision session length by community/hospital

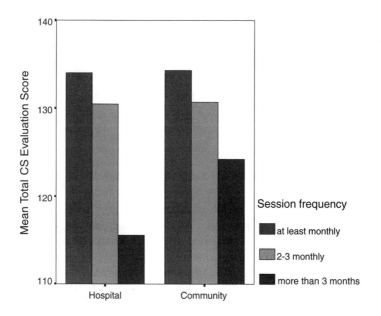

Figure 15.4 Mean total clinical supervision session frequency by community/hospital

Choice of supervisor

Much has been written about the quality of the supervisory relationship and what makes a good supervisor. Faugier and Butterworth (1994) stated for example, when describing aspects of the supervisory relationship, that 'without trust there is no relationship'. Wilkin (1992) suggested that 'the important factors for selecting a selecting a supervision partner seem to be mutual trust, respect for each other and feeling comfortable in each other's presence'. Nicklin (1997) included in his protocol for clinical supervision that 'where possible each nurse will be able to choose his/her own supervisor'. Using the MCSS, changes in the sub-scale scores indicated an increased readiness to

Factor	Hospital staff	Community staff
Length of sessions	Trust/rapport Supervisor advice/support Improve care/skills Importance/value of clinical supervision Personal issues Reflection Total CS evaluation score highest for sessions of one hour	All sub-scales and total clinical supervision evaluation scores higher as time increased
Frequency of sessions	All sub-scales and total clinical supervision evaluation scores reduced if more than three months apart	Improve care/skills Importance/value of clinical supervision Reflection Finding time Total clinical supervision evaluation score higher for sessions held at least monthly
Supervisor allocated or chosen	Trust/rapport higher if chosen Finding time higher if allocated	Trust/rapport Reflection higher if chosen
Within or away from the workplace	Not analysed, because most nurses were supervised within the workplace	Trust/rapport Improve care/skills Importance/value of clinical supervision Finding time Personal issues Reflection Total clinical supervision evaluation score higher if away from the workplace
One-to-one or group	Not analysed, because only ten per cent of staff in group sessions	Supervisor advice/support Finding time higher in group sessions

Figure 15.5 Summary of significant findings using the MCSS

learn from someone whom they had chosen as their supervisor, suggesting a more effective engagement between supervisor and supervisee was necessary for trust, rapport and challenge to develop (see Figure 15.5). For hospital staff only, there was also a difference associated with finding time for the sessions. As was reasonably expected, the score for finding time was found to be higher for the supervisees who had a supervisor allocated to them.

Sessions within or away from the workplace

White *et al.* (1998) reported that clinical supervision sessions had been 'intentionally held in quiet and comfortable, neutral places, away from the work areas of the participants' in the CSEP study. Supervision should take place in a designated room which is always available, free from disturbance and interruption (Wilkin, 1992). However, in practice, as shown in this study, many sessions were conducted within the workplace. These data have shown, for community based staff, that six sub-scales and the total score were higher if the sessions were held away from the workplace (see Figure 15.5).

One-to-one or group sessions

Evidence in the literature suggested that whether the session is held on a one-to-one basis with a supervisor or in a group situation was important. White *et al.* (1998) reported that the most common arrangement was a one-to-one basis, but amongst the list of other potential modes to use, based on definitions by Houston (1990), was group supervision within one's own discipline, peer group supervision or network supervision. The choice as to which mode to use may be influenced by staff resources available for clinical supervision, but one-to-one supervision has been viewed as the most effective method (Nicklin, 1997; Butterworth *et al.,* 1997).

These findings indicated that the supervisees in group sessions felt that the advice and support given by the supervisor was more effective than those receiving clinical supervision in a one-to-one situation. However, supervisees commented that other members of the supervision group also offered collective advice and support with any problems discussed at the session. These results have indicated that there may be some gain in using the technique of shared responsibility of supervision in some work settings. The difference associated with finding time was interpretable; group sessions can be pre-arranged and allow more staff to receive clinical supervision at one time, therefore there is less demand on staff to interrupt their work schedule for individual sessions. This result was not shown for the hospital staff.

Correlation with job satisfaction and burnout

Two Scandinavian research studies have reported that clinical supervision may have the potential to influence job satisfaction (Begat *et al.,* 1997;

Hallberg *et al.*, 1994). These findings had been established for a small sample of specialist nursing staff, but had not been confirmed for a more diverse sample of nursing staff from both community and hospital based settings. In this study, significant correlations were reported between the seven sub-scales and the Minnesota job satisfaction score, although, they were not of sufficient strength to be considered as an alternative to using the evaluation scale.

Hallberg (1994) reported no significant relationship between burnout and clinical supervision but, in contrast, the CSEP reported some significant changes in levels of burnout for nurses who were in receipt of clincial supervision. It could be speculated that high scores on the new scale may be associated with lower levels of burnout. Some elements of the Maslach Burnout Inventory were correlated with components of the new evaluation scale. In particular, for community staff, personal accomplishment was correlated with four of the components of the scale: trust/rapport, supervisor advice/support, improve care/skills and reflection. It was also noted that the factor associated with finding time was negatively correlated with emotional exhaustion and depersonalisation sub-scores on the Maslach Burnout Scale for both hospital and community staff. These findings have shown some associations between the scores on the new scale and levels of burnout, which can be interpreted. For instance, for hospital staff, finding time for the sessions in a busy work schedule may lead to increased levels of burnout for emotional exhaustion and depersonalisation. In addition, for hospital staff, depersonalisation was negatively correlated with trust/rapport, reflection and total score as would be expected. However, the correlation coefficients were small, although statistically significant, because of the large sample size.

Summary

Clinical supervision focuses on matters of central importance in the provision of safe and accountable practice. **Trials of the Manchester Clinical Supervision Scale have shown that clinical supervision is addressing improvement in skills, encourages reflective practice and attends to personal development. These can inform and be part of the systems of clinical governance which have been established since April 1999.**

The Manchester Clinical Supervision Scale (MCSS, Winstanley, 2000) is the first validated assessment instrument designed specifically to measure the effects of clinical supervision. This scale may now provide researchers with the capability to link the process of clinical supervision directly to patient outcomes. There are several assessment tools designed for measuring patient satisfaction and quality of care indicators, which could now be used for further controlled trials of clinical supervision, using the new scale. This is an opportune time to expand the programme of research into clinical supervision and its influence on the delivery of quality care. The availability of this new scale has opened fresh possibilities for new, high quality research into the effects of clinical supervision on the nursing workforce. Qualitative research into this substantive area is perhaps already more prolific, but the new scale will enable quantitative methodology to play an increasing and complementary role in the future.

References

Begat I Severinsson E and Berggren I (1997) Implementation of clinical supervision in a medical department: nurses' views of the effects. *Journal of Clinical Nursing* 6(5), pp389–94.

Bland M and Altman D (1996) Measurement error and correlation coefficients. *British Medical Journal* 313, pp41-42.

Butterworth T and Woods D (1999) *Clinical Governance and Clinical Supervision; Working Together to Ensure Safe and Accountable Practice*. University of Manchester.

Butterworth T Bishop V and Carson J (1996) First steps towards evaluating clinical supervision in nursing and health visiting. I. Theory, policy and practice development. A review. *Journal of Clinical Nursing* 5(2), pp127–32.

Butterworth T Carson J White E Jeacock J Clements A and Bishop V (1997) *It is Good To Talk. An Evaluation Study in England and Scotland*. University of Manchester.

Butterworth T Carson J Jeacock J White E and Clements A (1999) Stress, coping, burnout and job satisfaction in British nurses: Findings from the Clinical Supervision Evaluation project. *Stress Medicine* 15, pp27–33.

Cooper C Sloan J and Williams S (1988) *Occupation Stress Indicator Management Guide*. Windsor: NFER-Nelson.

Cronbach L (1951) Coefficient alpha and the internal structure of tests. *Psychometrika* 16, pp297–334.

Cutcliffe J (1997) Evaluating the success of clinical supervision. *British Journal of Nursing* 10–23 6(13), p725.

Department of Health (1998) *The New NHS – Modern and Dependable*.

Faugier J and Butterworth T (1994) *Clinical Supervision – A Position Paper*. Manchester: Manchester University Press.

Goldberg D and Williams P (1988) *Users Guide to the General Health Questionnaire*. Windsor: NFER-Nelson.

Hallberg I (1994) Systematic clinical supervision in a child psychiatric ward: satisfaction with nursing care, tedium and burnout and the nurses own report on the effects of it. *Archives of Psychiatric Nursing* 8, 1, pp 44–52.

Hallberg I and Norberg A (1993) Strain among nurses and their emotional reactions during one year of systematic clinical supervision with the implementation of individualised care in dementia nursing. *Journal of Advanced Nursing* 18(12), pp1860–75.

Hallberg I Hansson U and Axelsson K (1994) Satisfaction with nursing care and work during a year of clinical supervision and individualised care. Comparison between two wards for the care of severely demented patients. *Journal of Nursing Management* 1, pp296–307.

Harris P (1989) The Nurse Stress Index. *Work and Stress* 3(4), pp335–336.

Houston G (1990) *Supervision and Counselling*. London: The Rochester Foundation.

Kitzinger J (1994) The methodology of focus group interviews: The importance of interaction between research participants. *Sociology of Health and Illness* 16, 1, pp103–121.

Macleod Clark J, Maben J and Jones K (1996) The use of focus group interviews in nursing research: Issues and challenges. *NT Research* 1, 2, pp143–153.

Mahood N McFadden K Colgan L and Gadd P (1998) Clinical supervision: the Cartmel NDU experience. *Nursing Standard* 18–24 12(26) pp44–7.

Maslach C and Jackson S (1986) *The Maslach Burnout Inventory.* Palo Alto, CA: Consulting Psychologists Press.

Nicklin P (1997) Clinical supervision – efficient and effective? In *Final Report to the Research Steering Group* – Hexham General Hospital.

Palsson M Hallberg I Norberg A and Bjorvell H (1996) Burnout, empathy and sense of coherence among Swedish district nurses before and after systematic clinical supervision. *Scandinavian Journal of Caring Sciences* 10(1), pp19–26.

Proctor B (1991) Supervision: a co-operative exercise in accountability. In Marken M. and Payne M (eds), *Enabling and Ensuring: Supervision in Practice* Leicester: National Youth Bureau and Council for Education and Training in Youth and Communitiy Work, pp21–23.

Scanlon C and Weir W (1997) Learning from practice? Mental health nurses' perceptions and experiences of clinical supervision. *Journal of Advanced Nursing* 26(2), pp295–303.

Schaufeli W and Enzmann D (1993) The measurement of burnout: A review. In: Shaufeli W B, Maslach, C and Marek, T (eds), *Professional Burnout: Recent developments in Theory and Research*, pp199–205 New York: Hemisphere.

Severinsson E and Hallberg I (1996a) Clinical supervisors' views of their leadership role in the clinical supervision process within nursing care. *Journal of Advanced Nursing* 24(1), pp151–6.

Severinsson E and Hallberg I (1996b) Systematic clinical supervision, working milieu and influence over duties: the psychiatric nurse's viewpoint – a pilot study. *International Journal of Nursing Studies.* 33(4), pp394–406.

Siegel S (1956) *Non-parametric Statistics for the Behavioural Sciences.* New York: McGraw-Hill.

Sloan G (1998) Focus group interviews: defining clinical supervision. *Nursing Standard*, 12(42), pp40–3.

Weiss D J (1967) *Manual for the Minnesota Satisfaction Questionnaire.* Minneapolis, MN: Industrial Relations Center, University of Minnesota.

White E Butterworth T Bishop V Carson J Jeacock J and Clements A (1998) Clinical Supervision: insider reports of a private world. *Journal of Advanced Nursing* 28, 1, pp85–192.

Wilkin P (1992) Clinical supervision in psychiatric nursing. In Butterworth T and Faugier J (eds) *Clinical Supervision and Mentorship in Nursing.* London: Chapman and Hall.

Winstanley J (1999) *Methods for Evaluating the Efficacy of Clinical Supervision.* Clinical Monograph. London: Nursing Times Books.

Winstanley J (2000) Manchester Clinical Supervision Scale. *Nursing Standard* 14, 19, pp31–32.

16 Personal, professional and practice development

Case studies from clinical supervision practice in mental health nursing

John R. Cutcliffe

Editorial

This chapter focuses on current research concerns in relation to clinical supervision as the basis for suggesting the use of case studies as a means of evaluation. It highlights the argument for having both qualitative and quantitative data in order to illustrate the alleged link between receiving clinical supervision and improved client care. Three case studies from mental health nursing are presented and then submitted to a phenomenological, hermeneutic analysis, which enabled the author to induce a theory. This theory represents the key themes of how the clinical practice of psychiatric/mental health nurses appears to be influenced by their experience of receiving clinical supervision. These three themes are described as: personal development, professional development and practice development.

In addition to the much needed quantitative data (see previous chapter) we would argue that there is also a need for qualitative data, and case studies can provide this. Furthermore, it is important to note that these case studies highlight the value and centrality of support within clinical supervision. Supervision conducted without support ceases to be enabling and starts to become disabling and restrictive. While the insights and evidence gained from these case studies cannot be generalised and applied to all nursing situations, we believe there may be scenarios, behaviours and attitudes that all nurses can relate to their practice. We would also add that there is a need for more case studies of this nature, which could help produce a more thorough understanding of the process and experience of receiving clinical supervision.

Introduction

The need for healthcare practitioners to receive clinical supervision has been highlighted by several authors including NHS ME (1993), UKCC (1995), Bond and Holland (1998) and Cutcliffe and Proctor (1998b). Whilst the arguments made by these authors appear to have merit and validity, nurses face growing pressure to engage in the systematic examination of nursing practice and increasingly, need to demonstrate clinical outcomes to their practice. According to McKenna *et al*. (2000), no credible healthcare professional would deny that sound evidence should be an integral part of clinical decision making. Consequently, that healthcare practitioners should continue to receive clinical supervision without making any attempt to link supervision with improved outcomes is an untenable position. In response to the need to provide this evidence, scholars and researchers are seeking ways to discover these alleged links. This chapter therefore focuses on one such way of obtaining that evidence: the use of case studies from mental health nursing.

Methods of evaluating clinical supervision

Literature review

Several authors including Wright (1989) and Beardshaw and Robinson (1990) have posited that while the shift in psychiatric/mental health nursing away from ritualistic and custodial care towards evidence based care has resulted in benefits for clients, it has also created problems. This difficulty is not limited to psychiatric/mental health nursing. Correspondingly, general (or adult) nursing care that is founded in ritualistic practice (Walsh and Ford, 1988) creates similar problems for practitioners. For example, new practices need to be supported by evidence (Chambers, 1998), validated through research (Haines and Jones, 1994) and, in a climate that is increasingly concerned with 'value for money', shown to be cost effective. Given that its widespread introduction within nursing is a relatively recent phenomenon, it is logical, therefore, to examine the position of clinical supervision in terms of these three issues. According to Butterworth *et al.* (1996) initial attempts to evaluate clinical supervision centred on the three components of clinical supervision suggested by Proctor (1986): normative (personal organisation, personal ethics and personal quality/standards); restorative (support for staff); and formative (education and development). The variables examined in each of these components are described in more detail in Table 16.1.

Limitations of the evaluations

The merits of these initial attempts at evaluation should be recognised but accordingly, the limitations need to be acknowledged. One criticism that has been levelled is that these methods do not produce any empirical data that illustrates a direct link or causal relationship between receiving clinical supervision and improved client care. Indeed, the majority of the data produced is concerned with practitioner, not client, outcomes. Even the data produced in the research of the formative component may have limited validity due to the influence of the Hawthorne effect (Polit and Hungler, 1993).

In a climate where the consideration of economics has an ever increasing importance, and where the pressure to articulate and demonstrate the 'clinical outcome' of interventions is growing, NHS trust boards often require empirical

Table 16.1 Initial evaluation of clinical supervision using Proctor's (1986) three components

• Normative	Concerned with rates of staff sickness/absence, patients' complaints, and staff satisfaction (Butterworth *et al.*, 1996). It may also be worthwhile examining staff turnover and attrition rates.
• Restorative	Centred on measurements of staff stress levels, coping level questionnaires and burnout inventories (a measurement of the frequency of feeling 'burn out' (Butterworth *et al.*, 1996)
• Formative	Focuses on evaluating observed performance, possibly in the form of audiotaped recordings, videotape recordings, or observations of clinical practice (Butterworth *et al.*, 1996). This method of evaluation has already been used on 'Thorn' training courses (Gamble, 1995).

evidence to support new (and established) practices. Therefore, research needs to be carried out that identifies links between receiving clinical supervision and certain clinical outcomes (Butterworth *et al.*, 1996). At this point in time it is recognised that there are no empirical data to link receiving clinical supervision with improved client care, and furthermore, to establish such a link by means of research would be a methodological minefield. Some of the principal methodological problems that would be encountered in such a research study are listed in Table 16.2.

With the advancement of the research focused on supervision, some of these problems will be overcome. For example, the Manchester evaluation tool (MCSS; see previous chapter) now is sensitive and advanced enough to measure some of the phenomena. However, the principal methodological problem remains. Even if improved outcomes are detected in the clients who receive care from nurses who receive supervision and not in the group of clients who don't, how do we know that it is receiving clinical supervision that has made this difference and not some other variable?

Butterworth (1996) stressed that as clinical supervision is bound up with both the practice environment and the person's emotional state, any attempt at evaluation is fraught with difficulty. Furthermore, some current evaluation is limited in that it fails to include service-user evaluation of clinical supervision. Barker (1992) submitted that nurses need to embrace the clients' view of the care they

Table 16.2 Methodological problems of research into establishing a link between clinical supervision and improved client care

- Isolating the independent variable
- Establishing a control group
- Establishing a representative sample
- Ethical issues around providing supervision to some clinicians and not others
- Producing matched groups
- Absence of advanced or sufficiently sensitive measuring tools

receive and their views of their carer. If nursing really is concerned with forming and maintaining therapeutic relationships, then the views of the clients have to be taken into account. If a new variable is introduced into this relationship, as in this case, the new variable being clinical supervision, then the clients' views of how this affects the relationship need to be considered. This would be particularly important when trying to obtain data that indicate a direct link between receiving clinical supervision and improved client care.

Qualitative and quantitative data

Attempts to evaluate the effect of clinical supervision on client outcomes must include both qualitative and quantitative data (Bishop, 1994; Fowler, 1995; Severinnsson, 1995; Butterworth, 1996). Each research paradigm provides particular types of knowledge and can thus answer certain research questions. Quantitative methods provide 'know that' knowledge, where as qualitative methods provide 'know how' knowledge. Therefore, with regard to the evaluation of clinical supervision on client outcomes, qualitative methods would provide answers to such questions as: How does receiving supervision affect the care provided by the supervisee? How does receiving supervision affect the emotional state of the supervisee? How does the emotional state of the practitioner affect the care he or she subsequently provides? Quantitative methods would provide answers to such questions as: How many nurses experience the identified benefits of receiving supervision? How many clients experience improvements in the care provided by nurses who receive supervision? What are the differences, as experienced by clients, of care provided by nurses who receive supervision and nurses who don't?

It has been suggested that a simple equation exists which could be used as a hypothesis for preliminary research in clinical supervision and client outcomes. This equation suggests; a happy nurse is a healthy nurse, and a healthy nurse is an effective nurse. Thus, if it can be shown that receiving clinical supervision makes nurses feel 'happier' and healthier, then one can begin to see the relationship between receiving supervision and improved client outcomes. As pointed out previously, there is a current paucity of evidence that links clinical supervision with improvements in client care. Despite having only limited empirical data, some authors have produced qualitative data which suggests the link between clinical supervision and improved practice does exist (Hawkins and Shohet, 1989; Paunonen, 1991; Booth, 1992; Timpson, 1996; Butterworth et al., 1997). However, it is reasonable to say that many gaps still exist in the knowledge and that there are many unanswered questions, some of which appear to require qualitative methods.

Justification for case studies

Considering the need for qualitative research, the author suggests that one method of addressing this issue is the case of case studies. Yin (1989, p23) defined a case study as an empirical inquiry that 'investigates a contemporary phenomenon within its real-life context'.

Janesick (1994) added to this definition suggesting that case studies allow the writer/researcher to focus on the naturalistic, holistic, cultural and phenomenological (e.g. the lived experiences) elements of a given situation. They enable readers to juxtapose their own practice and experiences with those described in the studies, creating parallels between the case and their own actual experiences. Stake (1994) highlighted how case studies serve an epistemological function, allowing the reader to learn from actual 'real' cases. Furthermore, case studies provide detailed insight into these real situations, and enable understanding of how theoretical constructs have been applied within them. Therefore, case studies of clinical supervision provided to practitioners offer insights into the dynamics and processes involved in the world of the supervisor, supervisee and the clients they care for. They enable readers to ask, 'how is clinical supervision making a difference to the practice of the supervisee?', 'how is the practice of the supervisee changing as a result of the supervision they receive?', and 'how is the care the client receives altered by this changed practice?' While each isolated case cannot be taken to represent the nationwide picture, and it would be unwise to attempt to generalise from such finite investigation, case studies do reveal interesting patterns and commonalities, particularly, how receiving supervision can influence the ways practitioners think, feel and behave and thus how the subsequent care they deliver to the clients is different, and hopefully improved.

According to Mariano (1993), in order to have clarity and rigour, a researcher using a case study method should consider the following: the boundaries of the inquiry, the purpose/question, what unit of analysis is to be used, the design, the method of data collection, and what method of analysis is to be used. Therefore, each of these issues is addressed in turn.

The boundaries of the inquiry

In accordance with Stake's (1994) guidelines, the case needed to be a bounded unit. Consequently, the boundaries of the inquiry corresponded with the boundaries of the supervision sessions. Whatever the supervisee introduced into the session would thus also constitute legitimate data for inclusion in the case study analysis.

The purpose/question

The purpose of the case studies was to investigate the lived experiences of psychiatric/mental health nurses as they encounter clinical supervision. Therefore, the research question posed was: what influence or effect does receiving clinical supervision have on the practice of psychiatric/mental health nurses?

The unit of analysis

The unit of analysis was the clinical supervision session. In this instance each session needed to be conducted on a one-to-one basis, to last for at least one hour, and to be facilitated by a supervisor who had a minimum experience of two years as a clinical supervisor.

The design

Yin (1989) identifies two basic types of design: the single case design and the multiple case design. Since single case designs are suggested when the case represents a typical case, a critical case, an extreme or unique case or a revelatory case, and given the current depth of understanding of the nature of what would constitute a 'typical' or 'critical' supervision session, it would be prudent and appropriate to use a multiple case design.

The method of data collection

Data was collected by tape recording the accounts of the supervisors, each of whom described a recent clinical supervision session. In order to respect and maintain confidentiality, no client's or supervisee's real name was used.

The method of analysis

According to Yin (1989) there are two basic strategies for analysing case study data:

- developing a case description;
- employing the theoretical propositions on which the study is based to explain the case.

Consequently, since the author was concerned with obtaining an understanding of the lived experiences of psychiatric/mental health nurses and how these experiences appear to influence their practice, a phenomenological, hermeneutic analysis was undertaken. This would enable the author to undertake a thematic analysis and therefore induce a theory of the key themes that represents how the clinical practice of psychiatric/mental health nurses appears to be influenced by their experience of receiving clinical supervision.

Case study 1

Terry was a 42-year-old man with anxiety related problems. During his one-to-one counselling sessions he would often bring up his concerns and worries. Whenever any move to address these concerns was initiated Terry would be silent for a while and then move on to another of his concerns. This pattern was repeated over several sessions with Terry often bringing up the same problems again and again. This pattern was raised in clinical supervision and the supervisor and supervisee focused on the process of communication rather than the content.

The supervisor encouraged the supervisee to take a step back and attempt to view the whole of the situation (taking a more global view), rather than focusing on the dynamics or issues of one session. Even though Terry asked for help and information, he did not appear to be willing to accept it when offered. Therefore, the supervisor and supervisee explored the possibility that perhaps airing these concerns was therapeutic in itself, and that erudite answers and clever solutions were not necessary at this particular time. Perhaps the most important issue for Terry was that he needed to feel someone was listening to him.

A brief strategy was negotiated and agreed upon, that in the next session with Terry, the supervisee would be more concerned with listening and hearing rather than talking. The supervisor summed up this issue by suggesting that: 'Sometimes the hardest thing to do is nothing.'

In the next session the supervisee did not attempt to provide any solutions to Terry's problems but concerned himself with communicating his interest and empathy non-verbally. Again, Terry spoke of the issues that were bothering him and his feelings and exasperation became evident. The supervisee did not say a great deal but assured Terry that he was there for him and encouraged Terry to ventilate his frustrations. At the end of the session Terry looked visibly calmer, displayed far less evidence of agitation and said: 'Thanks for listening. I've been having an angry day and sometimes you just need to know that someone is hearing you.'

Case study 2

Sid was a staff nurse working on a challenging behaviour unit, a feature of which was the potentially violent clinical situations that he encountered. Sid had been involved recently in a particular stressful, violent incident where property had been damaged and the client had needed to be physically restrained. Following this incident, Sid raised the matter in clinical supervision as he was concerned about the anger he felt towards the client. He felt he would have to disengage from his role as the client's primary nurse. Sid said he could no longer work with this individual given the way he now felt about him.

The supervisor encouraged Sid to talk openly about the feelings he experienced during, and subsequent to, the incident. Sid spoke of a wide range of emotions including fear, anger, disappointment and guilt. The supervisor first offered Sid some support and reminded him that such a response to a violent situation is completely reasonable. Such intense violent situations often produce a response in the nurse that makes close interpersonal work with the client more difficult. Whittington and Wykes (1994) argued that, following such incidents, it is not unusual for the nurse to feel the need to withdraw. The supervisor felt that Sid needed to give himself permission to experience these feelings and that it was OK to express them.

The supervisor and Sid then explored the value of having a formal debriefing process in place in order to allow ventilation of the feelings provoked by such incidents. This would also allow practitioners to view each such incident as an opportunity for learning, both for themselves and for the client (Conlon *et al.*, 1995). Sid said he would talk to the ward staff about debriefing on his return. Importantly, as his feelings had been expressed and accepted, Sid said he felt less stressed. As his reaction had been validated as a reasonable response, not a response that should provoke feelings of guilt, he was able to avoid distancing himself or erecting barriers, and could once more engage the client. The consequences of this, according to Whittington and Wykes (1994), would be to lessen the likelihood of further violent incidents.

Case study 3

Nancy was a 31-year-old woman with low self-esteem who had recently separated from her long-term boyfriend. This event had a debilitating effect on her, eroding her self-confidence and further challenging her already compromised hope levels. The supervisee had chosen to adopt a humanistic approach when working with Nancy. At the same time he was keen to help Nancy move through her own process of bereavement. To this end, the supervisee was concerned with creating a safe, comfortable environment in which Nancy would be more likely to feel able to express any painful emotions.

In the early sessions very little progress was made, with Nancy expressing predominantly negative self-expressions of hopelessness. The absence of any evidence of or sense of progression caused the supervisee to become doubtful and question whether or not he was using the appropriate approach. This was discussed in the supervision session. The supervisor encouraged the supervisee to explore and explain his rationale for choosing this particular approach over an alternative approach. Consequently, as Powell (1989) suggests, such exploration ushered the supervisee into a process of reflection. Without feeling threatened, the supervisee could consider the philosophical and theoretical constructs that were guiding his practice.

The supervisee believed that Nancy would begin to move through her own process of bereavement in her own time and that such a process could not be forced or coerced. The self-development and personal growth of the client was mirrored in the supervision by the supervisor creating the appropriate environment e.g. warmth, empathy and unconditional positive regard (Rogers, 1952; Heron, 1990; Duck, 1992) necessary for the supervisee's personal and professional development.

The supervisee subsequently found his own answers and moved through his own phases of development, just as he believed, given the appropriate environment, that Nancy would do. Further sessions with Nancy thus took a similar approach, being non-directive, supportive and client-centred. When she began to feel safe enough, Nancy began to take her first steps towards resolving her bereavement, challenging some of her negative self-assumptions and adopted a more hopeful outlook.

Findings

The analysis and description of the data produced three key themes which form an emerging theory of the effect of receiving clinical supervision on the practice of mental health nurses. This theory is represented in diagrammatic form by figure one. Each of these key themes is then discussed in more detail.

Personal development

The essence of this key theme is the development of the practitioner as a person. It identifies that engaging in clinical supervision appears to have helped the practitioner develop and refine certain qualities. Support for the supervisee underpins all the other processes and dynamics in supervision. This is particularly highlighted by case study 2. Just as Heron (1990) writes that his six categories of intervention need to be carried out with a supportive underpinning and that the client's well-being is paramount, this is also the case with supervision. Supervision conducted without support ceases to be enabling and starts to become disabling and restrictive. Self-awareness is a prerequisite for mental health nursing (Peplau, 1988; Cutcliffe, 1997), and thus it can be argued that any activity that enhances the development of self-awareness in mental health nurses, has the potential to enhance the nurses practice. Case study 2 also demonstrates the growth of self-awareness in the supervisee. In this case, as a result of engaging in supervision, the supervisee realises that it is entirely understandable and reasonable to have reactions to clients and their behaviour. It is how one processes these feelings, what one actually does with them that is key. According to Cutcliffe (2000):

> To admit that one finds things difficult, or that one's feelings are provoked, essentially, that one is human, is no crime or case for misconduct. Quite the opposite, it is only when such feelings and issues are brought 'into the light' that they can be explored, understood and learned from.

Professional development

The essence of this key theme is the development of the practitioner as a professional. It identifies that engaging in clinical supervision appears to have helped the practitioner examine, reflect on and address professional issues. The case studies illustrate a dynamic which is described by Hawkins and Shohet (1989) as mirroring. This is where processes occurring in the supervision 'mirror' those processes that occur in the interaction with clients. Supervisors act as a role model in demonstrating ways that the supervisee can develop as a professional. For example, the case studies illustrate that the supervisors model the use of challenging skills (Cutcliffe and Epling, 1997), demonstrating the therapeutic potential of such interventions and simultaneously encouraging the supervisee to challenge aspects of his or her own thoughts, feelings and behaviours. The cases also indicate that the supervisee may wish to draw upon the supervisor's experience in order to consider professional issues. That is not to suggest that the supervisor provides answers to each of the supervisee's concerns about professional issues. Rather, it is a resource which the supervisee can draw upon. As Benner (1984) pointed out, this expertise is a rich source of knowledge and if the supervisee finds this appropriate, it can be used to assist him or her.

Practice development

The essence of this key theme is the development of the practitioner's practice. It identifies that engaging in clinical supervision appears to have helped the practitioner focus on particular practice problems (and successes). It is concerned with the process of reflection practice (Hawkins and Shohet, 1989). Indeed, Schön (1984) argues that without reflection, growth cannot occur. Without growth there is stagnation and this can only hinder the development of practice. It identifies how supervisees are encouraged to explore the possible reasons why approaches or interventions work and others not, and sometimes why they don't. This theme is also concerned with how within supervision attempts were made to strengthen the links between theory and practice. The case studies show that having reached an impasse, the process of supervision highlighted other options. Consequently, the problem was addressed, less time was spent searching for solutions, the practitioners had sound rationale for their interventions and the client consequently received a better service. Without the aid of supervision the practitioners would have been left floundering, since they would have no way of checking the validity or soundness of their judgement and decisions.

Discussion

Each of these case studies provides an example of how clinical practice can be influenced by the application of clinical supervision. They do not generate a wealth of quantitative data, but they do offer insight into, and evidence of, specific areas of growth and development. They indicate how the supervisee (and supervisor) can change as a direct result of supervision and how real clinical problems were overcome.

It is possible that other variables may have affected the outcome of the care. The clients could have received effective help from another source or experienced more support from their significant others. Alternatively, additional changes of the practice of the supervisee not brought about by the clinical supervision may have had an influence. Nevertheless, the case studies provide further qualitative evidence that supports the argument that receiving clinical

PERSONAL, PROFESSIONAL AND
PRACTICE DEVELOPMENT

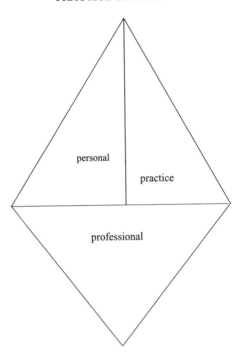

personal

practice

professional

Figure 16.1 The effect of receiving clinical supervision on the practice of mental health nurses.

supervision can affect the care provided by the nurses, and thus the clients can receive a better service.

If a nurse is developing as a person, as a professional and as a practitioner, her range or 'tool box' of skills, attitudes and interventions is increased. The nurse is better able to engage with people, and better able to deal with her emotional reaction provoked by engaging with the client. Additionally the nurse has an increased ability to monitor the effect she is having on the client. Therefore, given all these changes and developments, it is not unreasonable to argue that the client is going to receive a better service from a nurse who has experienced these developments when compared to a nurse who hasn't.

As stated previously, evaluating the effectiveness of supervision requires both qualitative and quantitative data, and the use of case studies represents one way of obtaining the qualitative data. Morse (1991) suggests that case studies allow an understanding of the meanings people ascribe to their particular experience and situations. Schultz (1967) states that phenomenological enquiry brings explicit clarity to the structures of the client's world; consequently, it is this clarity and understanding enabled by the case studies that highlights some of the processes of clinical supervision. Any argument used to convince sceptical trust boards of the benefits of clinical supervision would be more cogent if they included not only evidence that demonstrates that clinical supervision improves clinical practice, but in addition, evidence that explains how clinical supervision makes a difference to practice. Before quantifying how many supervisors and supervisees experience development and growth as a result of receiving supervision, one first needs to establish what the nature of this growth is, and furthermore, how this growth and development actually occurs.

Dickoff and James' (1968) work on theory generation suggests that there are four levels of theory: factor isolating; factor relating; situation relating and situation producing. Situation producing theory is described as the highest level of theory because the preceding levels of theory exist in part to enable higher level theory to be produced. Dickoff and James (1968) posit that situation producing theory can be described using the equation:

Variable A, causes variable B in the presence of variable C.

The current level of theory, induced from the case studies, appears to be factor relating theory, in that the factors, clinical supervision, clinical practice and client outcomes appear to relate. Having induced this level of theory, the next logical step would be to test out the theory, and hopefully obtain quantitative evidence that would then validate the relationships between these variables. Thus moving the theory to the level of situation producing theory. Thus, nursing intervention (variable A) in the presence of clinical supervision (variable C) causes improved client outcome (variable B).

The qualitative data produced from each case study, when compiled, illustrates that the benefits to mental health nurse practice (and consequently benefits to clients), as a result of receiving clinical supervision do not occur in isolation. Rather, enhanced practice arising out of engaging in clinical supervision appears to be a widespread phenomenon. Additionally, the qualitative data paves the way for quantitative study to examine and determine how many practitioners and clients have experienced these benefits in practice. Also, each case study that can illustrate an improvement in practice adds to the accumulating qualitative data that indicates a link between clinical supervision and improved client care. Thus these case studies add credence to the argument that receiving clinical supervision positively affects mental health nurses' practice and improves client care.

Conclusions

Case studies clearly add to the accumulating qualitative evidence that supports the widespread introduction of clinical supervision. They provide unique insights into the dynamics which occur, deepen the understanding of the processes and provide some tentative evidence of improved client care. While one cannot generalise from such findings, Denzin and Lincoln (1994) state, 'every instance of a case or process bears the general class or phenomena it belongs to. However, any given instance is likely to be particular and unique.'

Therefore, while the insights and evidence gained from these case studies cannot be generalised and applied to other nursing situations, there may well be scenarios, behaviours and attitudes that all nurses can relate to their practice. The author suggests that there is a need for more case studies of this nature, which could produce a wealth of information about clinical supervision. Such information and data would strengthen the links between receiving clinical supervision and improved client outcomes. Furthermore, each case study could then be included on a database, such as the database at the Network for Psychiatric Nursing Research (NPNR) based at the Royal College of Nursing Institute at Oxford. This information could then be made known to trust boards and purchasers of health care, in order to incorporate clinical supervision into future business plans.

This chapter is based on a paper that was originally published as 'Personal professional, and practice development: clinical supervision' in the *British Journal of Nursing*, 1998, Vol.7, No.21, pp 1319–1322.

References

Barker P (1992) Psychiatric nursing. In Butterworth T and Faugier J (eds) *Clinical Supervision and Mentorship in Nursing*, pp65–79 London: Chapman and Hall.

Beardshaw R and Robinson J (1990) Omissions in nursing research: Another look. *International Nursing Review* 35, pp165–8.

Benner P (1984) *From Novice to Expert: Excellence and Power in Clinical Nursing*. California: Addison-Wesley.

Bond M and Holland S (1998) *Skills of Clinical Supervision for Nurses*. Oxford: Oxford University Press.

Bishop V (1994) Clinical supervision for an accountable profession. *Nursing Times* 90, pp35–7.

Booth K (1992) Providing support and reducing stress: a review of the literature. In Butterworth T and Faugier J (eds) *Clinical Supervision and Mentorship in Nursing*, pp50–60. London: Chapman and Hall.

Butterworth T (1996) Primary attempts at research based evaluation of clinical supervision. *Nursing Times Research* 1(2), pp96–101.

Butterworth T Bishop V and Carson J (1996) First steps towards evaluating clinical supervision in nursing and health visiting: 1. Theory, policy and practice development. A review *Journal of Clinical Nursing* 5, pp127–132.

Butterworth T Carson J White E *et al.* (1997) *It is Good to Talk: An Evaluation Study in England and Scotland*. Manchester: Manchester University Press.

Chambers M (1998) Mental health nursing: the challenge of evidence based practice. *Mental Health Practice* 1(8), pp18–22.

Conlon L Gage A and Hillis T (1995) Managerial and nursing perspectives on the response to inpatient violence. In Crichton J (ed.) *Psychiatric Patient Violence: Risk and Response*, pp81–95. London: Duckworth.

Cutcliffe J R (1997) The nature of expert psychiatric nursing practice: A grounded theory study. *Journal of Clinical Nursing* 6, pp325–332.

238   *John R. Cutcliffe*

Cutcliffe J R (2000) To record or not to record: documentation in clinical supervision. *British Journal of Nursing* 19(6), pp350–355.

Cutcliffe J R and Epling M (1997) An exploration of John Heron's confronting interventions within supervision: Case studies from practice. *Psychiatric Care* 4, pp174–180.

Cutcliffe J R and Proctor B (1998a) An alternative training approach to clinical supervision: Part One. *British Journal of Nursing* 7(5), pp280–285.

Cutcliffe J R and Proctor B (1998b) An alternative training approach to clinical supervision: Part Two. *British Journal of Nursing* 7(6), pp344–350.

Denzin N K and Lincoln Y S (1994) Part Three: Strategies of inquiry. In Denzin N and Lincoln Y S (eds) *Handbook of qualitative research*, pp199–208. London: Sage.

Dickoff J and James P (1968) A theory of theories: A position paper. *Nursing Research* 17, 197-203.

Duck S (1992) *Human Relationships*. London: Sage.

Dudley M and Butterworth T (1994) The costs and some benefits of clinical supervision: An initial exploration. *International Journal of Psychiatric Nursing Research* 1, pp34–40.

Farrington A (1995) Models of clinical supervision. *British Journal of Nursing* 4(15), pp876–878.

Faugier J (1992) The supervisory relationship. In Butterworth T and Faugier J (eds), *Clinical Supervision and Mentorship in nursing.* pp65–79. London: Chapman and Hall.

Faugier J and Butterworth T (1994) *Clinical Supervision: A Position Paper.* University of Manchester.

Fowler J (1995) Nurses' perspectives of the elements of good supervision. *Nursing Times* 91, pp33–37.

Gamble C (1995) The Thorn Nursing Initiative. *Nursing Standard* 4(9), pp31–4.

Haines A and Jones R (1994) Implementing findings of research. *British Medical Journal* 308, pp1488–1492.

Halberg I R and Norberg A (1993) Strain among nurses and their emotional reactions during one year of systematic clinical supervision combined with the implementation on individualised care on dementia nursing. *Journal of Advanced Nursing* 18, pp1800–1875.

Hawkins P and Shohet R (1989) *Supervision in the Helping Relationships.* Milton Keynes: Open University Press.

Heron J (1990) *Helping the Client: A Creative Practical Guide.* London: Sage.

Janesick V J (1994) The Dance of qualitative research design: Metaphor, methodolatry and meaning. In Denzin N and Lincoln Y S (eds) *Handbook of Qualitative Research*, pp209–219. London: Sage.

King's Fund (1995) *Clinical Supervision: An Executive Summary.* London: King's Fund.

Mariano C (1993) Case study: the method. In Munhall P L and Boyd C O (eds), *Nursing Research: A Qualitative Perspective.* New York: National League for Nursing Press, pp311–337.

McKenna H Cutcliffe J R and McKenna P (2000) Evidence-based practice: demolishing some myths. *Nursing Standard* 14(16), pp39–42.

Morris M (1995) The role of clinical supervision in mental health practice. *British Journal of Nursing* 4(15), pp886–888.

Morse JM (1991) Strategies for climbing. In Morse J M (ed) *Qualitative Nursing Research: A Contemporary Dialogue* (2nd edition) pp127–145. London: Sage.

NHS ME (1993) *A Vision for the Future.* London: HMSO.

Paunonen N (1991) Changes initiated by a nursing supervision programme: An analysis based on log linear models. *Journal of Advanced Nursing* 16, pp982–986.

Peplau H (1988) *Interpersonal Relations in Nursing* (2nd edition). New York: GP Putnam.

Polit D E and Hungler B P (1993) *Essentials of Nursing Research: Methods, Appraisal, and Utilisation* (3rd edition). Philadelphia: Lippincott.

Powell J H (1989) The reflective practitioner in nursing. *Journal of Advanced Nursing* 14, pp824–832.

Proctor B (1986) Supervision: A cooperative exercise in accountability In Marken M and Payne M (eds) *Enabling and Ensuring*. Leicester: National Youth Bureau and Council for Education and Training in Youth and Community Work.

Rogers C (1952) *Client Centred Therapy: Its Current Practice, Implications and Theory*. London: Constable.

Schön D (1984) *The Reflective Practitioner*. New York: Basic Books.

Schultz A (1967) *The Phenomenology of the Social World*. Chicago: Northwestern University Press.

Severinsson E (1995) The phenomenon of clinical supervision in psychiatric health care. *Journal of Psychiatric and Mental Health Nursing* 2, pp301–309.

Stake R E (1994) Case studies. In Denzin N and Lincoln Y S (eds) *Handbook of Qualitative Research*, pp236–247. London: Sage.

Timpson J (1996) Clinical Supervision: A plea for 'pit head' time. *European Journal of Cancer Care* 5, pp43–52.

UKCC (1995) *Proposed Position Statement on Clinical Supervision for Nursing and Health Visiting*. London: UKCC.

Walsh M and Ford P (1989) *Nursing Rituals: Research and Rational Actions*. Oxford: Butterworth-Heinemann.

Whittington R and Wykes T (1994) An observational study of associations between nurse behaviour and violence in psychiatric hospitals. *Journal of Psychiatric and Mental Health Nursing* 1, pp85–92.

Wright S (1989) *Changing Nursing Practice*. London: Edward Arnold.

Yin R K (1989) *Case Study research: Design and methods*. Newbury Park: Sage.

17 Clinical supervision in multidisciplinary groups

Qualitative evaluation of clinical supervision using a focus group technique

John Fowler and James Dooher

Editorial

This chapter reports on the findings from a qualitative study that used multi-disciplinary focus groups to evaluate the experience of receiving clinical supervision. It provides findings from each of the multi-disciplinary groups who participated in the research and it contains a summary of the actions, outputs, and outcomes of clinical supervision. It concludes with a summary of the key findings and draws a very insightful analogy of clinical supervision as a campfire.

It is interesting to note that the findings in this study lend support to our position that there is no one 'best way' of conducting clinical supervision. Models and formats of supervision, that fitted within the parameters identified in Chapter 1, were developed to meet the needs of the different situations and individual members. As a consequence, practitioners gained a sense of ownership of the supervision and were thus perhaps more committed to ensuring it worked for them. It is also worth noting that across the wide variety of healthcare disciplines who participated in this research, the benefits of clinical supervision was unanimously recognised.

Clinical supervision and its evaluation

Traditional evaluation of healthcare practice has relied largely on professional judgement and the subjective experience of those either directly involved, or in positions of authority. The relatively recent demand for 'evidence-based practice' has stimulated managers and researchers to review this customary approach to evaluation. The factors that have triggered this move towards more rigorous evaluation are, according to Jenkinson (1997), twofold. First there is the fear that many healthcare procedures are of no benefit and may even be harmful, second is the acknowledgement that healthcare resources are finite, and that provision must be effective in terms of both cost and health gain. Thus the providers of healthcare look to research and other forms of enquiry to provide evidence of successful practices, and the resources they consume.

The often stated 'gold standard' of evaluative research is the randomised controlled study (RCT) (McGee and Notter, 1995; Greene and D'Oliveira, 1998). This method is frequently used for evaluating specific physical and chemical treatments and, if applied with scientific rigour, can allow the researcher to make statements regarding the effectiveness of a particular treatment. Arguably the strength of RCT lies in the ability of the researcher to identify and isolate a single variable and measure its effect against a control group. This requires three things: first the isolation of the variable, second a tool which can accurately measure its effect, and third two groups which are the same in every respect, one to be the experimental group and the other to be the control. Whilst these criteria can be met in laboratory conditions there are many healthcare practices which cannot be isolated into single variables, accurately measured or manipulated onto an experimental group.

Caring aspects of nursing practice and the interpersonal interactions associated with clinical supervision are difficult to isolate. This may lead to the false assumption that this lack of measurability indicates that they are of no use. Conversely the blind acceptance of practices that are somehow on a higher intellectual or aesthetic plane, because they are difficult to isolate or measure, is equally misplaced.

Where does this leave evaluation of clinical supervision? Although it is unlikely that clinical supervision will do harm, it does have the potential to consume and divert both human and financial resources from direct clinical contact. Although there are some published examples of evaluative studies (Dudley and Butterworth, 1994; Edberg *et al.*, 1996; Butterworth *et al.*, 1997; Fowler and Chevannes, 1998) they form the minority of published work regarding clinical supervision. If we accept that we should evaluate clinical supervision the next question must be what we going to evaluate? And how should we do it? Jenkinson (1997) postulates that evaluative research should be as critical and objective as possible and may use a variety of research methods to achieve this. In the evaluation of clinical supervision the strength and weaknesses of different research methods need to be examined against the problems to be investigated, and the questions of which answers are sought. In this regard, no one method should be assumed to be appropriate to every investigation but rather considered in relation to the identified problem or efficacy of the intervention.

Introduction to the study

In 1997 a community healthcare NHS Trust in Leicestershire developed a strategy regarding clinical supervision. Some areas and clinical teams within the Trust had previously established a form of clinical supervision, others underwent a training day to prepare them for its introduction. This study represents the independent evaluation of ten pilot sites, capturing the feelings and experience from real people. The aim of the study was to evaluate from the staff's perspective:

- the general structure of clinical supervision;
- the outcomes of clinical supervision for staff;
- the outcomes of clinical supervision for patient/client care.

Method

The Trust commissioning the study had already implemented clinical supervision making any form of pre- and post-evaluation (Bowling, 1997) difficult. Following discussions with the Trust managers it was clear that the objective at this stage was to have an objective evaluation based upon reflective discussions with staff who had been involved with clinical supervision.

A written questionnaire was considered, but it was felt that the lack of clear nationally accepted outcomes, and the different ways in which clinical supervision had been implemented within this Trust, would result in relatively superficial data. As the majority of the pilot groups had implemented clinical supervision using a group format, the possibility of an adapted focus group (Robinson, 1999; Clarke, 1999) was examined. Evaluation using focus groups would allow open questions to be posed to approximately seventy people. The groups would be evaluated in the style that they had implemented and operated clinical supervision. The disadvantages of this method were explored in that some staff might not be able to express dissatisfactions with other group members present, and more vocal members might dominate the discussions. To overcome these potential disadvantages it was planned that the group members would be given the opportunity to talk to the researchers on an individual basis either following the focus group or at a suitable time. A structured interview based upon the Trust's original objectives was developed. Notes were taken during the focus group evaluation and an audiotape of the session was made. The analysis was carried out thematically based upon the objectives set by the Trust but including any emerging themes.

Procedure

The facilitators of the ten pilot sites were written to informing them of the evaluation study. They were then contacted by phone and a convenient date, time and venue arranged for the focus group meeting. The evaluation meetings usually commenced with informal 'chat' and a cup of coffee, followed by the formal focus group which took approximately sixty minutes. All ten pilot sites were visited as part of the evaluation and out of a potential seventy-eight staff listed in the official membership list, sixty-one (seventy-eight per cent) were present during the various focus group evaluations.

Set questions were posed to eight of the ten groups and formed the focus of the evaluation study. In two groups it became apparent that these questions were not appropriate as the group's clinical supervision sessions had either never really started off or had been discontinued after only one or two sessions. For these groups the evaluation was focused on the reason for the groups not developing.

Ethical issues

An application was submitted to the local Ethical Committee and permission to proceed was granted. All facilitators of the groups were written to informing them of the nature of the evaluation and that it would be the researchers' wish to audio tape the focus groups, discussions.

Summary of ten pilot sites

Group 1. Health visitors

This group consisted of seven health visitors meeting for ninety minutes every two months. They appreciated the clinical supervision meetings as a time when they could mix with their peers in a way that other professional meetings did not allow. The health visitors felt that the clinical supervision sessions provided an arena where they could spend a little time discussing difficult clients with another health visitor, brainstorming ideas and gaining support from their peers. The group felt that clinical supervision had been useful. Initially the first three meetings had been about setting up the group, discussing ground rules and generally getting to know one another. The subsequent last three meetings were seen to be very useful although some members found the setting aside of time for the meeting and then protecting it, a stressful process.

Comment: This system allowed staff to review difficult clinical situations and discuss issues of professional concern. It served as a valuable professional support forum and had the potential to become even more supportive as the group continued to meet and relationships developed.

Group 2. Physiotherapists

This was a group of community physiotherapists and was the only group to structure clinical supervision on a purely individual basis.

JUNIOR PHYSIOTHERAPISTS

Junior physiotherapists on a rotational placement to the community met up once a week individually with a senior physiotherapist. The main focus of this meeting was to review the junior physio's caseload. Each patient was reviewed with any immediate problems identified and discussed. The junior physio's felt that these clinical supervision meetings were a useful and supportive system. Being new to community work they appreciated the opportunity to have a regular meeting with an experienced supportive senior physiotherapist.

SENIOR PHYSIOTHERAPISTS

The senior physiotherapists met approximately monthly for an hour and the meeting's focus was to review the workload and the organisation of the department. The content of the meeting tended to be rather *ad hoc* with the demands of the department dictating the discussions.

Comment: This was a system that supported and monitored the work of junior staff working in a new and very different environment. It allowed individual patient treatments to be reviewed and unusual conditions, treatments or family relationships to be discussed in detail. The supervision meetings for the senior staff were useful but with a little more structure and focus, and have greater potential than was currently being realised.

Group 3. Community hospital nursing staff

This was the only ward-based hospital group to be part of the clinical supervision pilot study. It was set up with the ward manager and five staff nurses. However, after the first couple of meetings that focused on discussing the ground rules, the ward manager and one of the staff nurses left the hospital for alternative jobs. This posed two main problems for the remaining members of the group. First, the ward manager who was the leader and key motivator of the clinical supervision group left and none of the remaining group took on that motivating role. Second, neither the staff nurse nor the ward manager was immediately replaced, leading to the remaining staff covering the shifts on the ward. After the ward manager left, the group no longer met. They admitted that their morale was low and that they 'just couldn't raise themselves any more'. They said that it would have been 'really nice if the group had advanced enough so that we stayed as a peer group'.

Comment: The system of group clinical supervision initially planned did not happen due to the resignation of the key motivator and lack of managerial interest. Paradoxically the area where the benefits of clinical supervision would be extremely valuable was the area least able to implement it. It was felt that this group would need resources and expert support to engender motivation and the basic ability to develop a useful system.

Group 4. Community nurses

This consisted of two groups, qualified nursing staff and health care assistants (HCA). The structure of both groups was planned to accommodate both group and individual supervision. A group meeting was held once a month for two months and then on the third month individual clinical supervision was introduced. The person taking on the supervisor role was decided upon by the manager of the department, but the manager did not participate in either of the groups. The HCA group continued for a further two or three meetings, but the qualified group never really started. The reasons why clinical supervision was not adopted were complex. The department was relatively new and as such was developing its role, function and structure. At the time that clinical supervision was introduced the lines of professional and personal management appeared unclear to the staff within this team. There appeared to be no formal or informal leader responsible for the direction of the team, indeed the concept of 'team' did not appear to be a dominant feature of these workers. Into this structure a number of the group felt that clinical supervision was 'thrown in by the management' and in their own way they 'threw it out'. Choice of supervisors was said to have been imposed on both supervisors and supervisees. Both groups expressed feelings that demonstrated that they felt no ownership of the process of clinical supervision. 'The way it was done put your back up,' said one member. In discussion as to why clinical supervision did not take off with either group the following factors were identified by the group:

Qualified group
- role of supervisor imposed upon us;
- didn't know what to expect from either the study day or clinical supervision and the training did not help;
- meetings took on the same format as others;
- senior managers did not appear motivated;
- no one was clear about roles and which hat to put on;
- there was a lack of enthusiasm;
- we weren't getting anything out of it;
- covering 24 hours of patient care makes meetings difficult.

HCA group
- the supervisor was from the team, someone from outside would have been better – not the facilitator herself but just someone from outside the team;
- they would be able to ventilate more;
- how can a manager who bullies you one minute, be your friendly supervisor the next?
- covering 24 hours of patient care made meetings difficult.

Comment: A lack of managerial commitment, team restructuring and the interpersonal difficulties caused by role ambiguity, created a dysfunctional group of workers who made a conscious decision to abdicate from clinical supervision. They felt that the role of supervisor should be less formal and should be developed according to the team structure rather than false hierarchical registered / HCA divide.

Group 5. Community nursing staff

There were twelve people at the focus group evaluation for this group. All staff were community nurses and included health care assistants and qualified nurses of various grades. The groups met for approximately 60–90 minutes every four to six weeks. The groups identified a number of examples in which clinical supervision had impacted upon their clinical practice. These included diabetic care, management of incontinence, certain accountability issues, development of critical thinking, and feeling happier at work.

Comment: Clinical supervision was a useful and professionally supportive system. It provided a forum in which staff could discuss professional issues, clinical conditions and explore difficult areas of communication or relationships. Staff felt supported and valued by being part of the groups.

Group 6. Health visitors and school nurses

This group consisted of six health visitors and three school nurses. They meet together for one hour every month during their lunch hour; during the meeting they eat their lunch and have a coffee. They decided that they did not want a 'chatty group or poor me', it should be focused on clinical situations. Clinical supervision sessions tended to focus on clinical situations looking at: 'what happened' or 'could it have gone better.'

This group felt that it was not appropriate for their sessions to be used for 'burdening others with personal stress' although issues of professional concern were discussed. The opportunity to discuss difficult client scenarios with peers was seen to be extremely valuable in that it gave reassurance that what was being proposed was appropriate, and this increased clinical confidence, and 'it gave power to move forward having discussed it with other professionals'. This reduced the potential stress of professional practice.

They felt that clinical supervision was a very positive experience for them and they 'got a lot out of it' but the group commented that they were fed up with yet more lunchtime meetings, and felt clinical supervision survives because staff donate their own lunchtimes.

Comment: This was a motivated and assertive group. It focused on professional work but in a way that was outside the standard management structure, and utilised a reflective cycle to review incidents. 'I wouldn't have attended if it was more management type meetings.'

Group 7. School nurses

This group consisted of six school nurses who met for one hour a month. They tended to meet for a sandwich lunch for thirty minutes then spent five to ten minutes in general chat, then spending the remaining fifty minutes on the 'business'. All the group were experienced school nurses and as such said that they tended not to talk about 'hands on clinical issues' but concentrated on issues of policy, time management, or general management situations. All the staff worked in isolation and talked about the benefits of clinical supervision as being one of mutual support and the opportunity to discuss issues with colleagues.

Sometimes clinical supervision sessions were used to discuss difficult situations such as when a headteacher was rude to one of the members, 'it was good to share it and gain support, we are all in the same boat.' Another session focused on behavioural approaches to management of some children.

Comment: This system provided a valuable time for staff to meet together and discuss issues that were pertinent to their speciality. It allowed difficult or unusual clinical situations to be discussed with peers working in similar situations.

Group 8. Occupational therapists

The staff present at this focus group represented two separate clinical supervision groups of occupational therapy staff. Initial allocation to either of the groups appears fairly random. Both groups met for two hours once a month during an afternoon. The department's work was either adjusted or covered by the remaining staff of the department. The groups developed differently.

1st group. This group gelled immediately and began focusing on clinical issues via presentations of patient studies. All participants found the group a 'pleasure to be a part of' and saw it a valuable time out. Discussions used a reflective format with a patient case study being presented for general discussion. A number of specific clinical issues were discussed usually via a case study presentation.

2nd group. Initially the group did not gel and for the first six months they seemed to be working through a number of role and personality issues. Attendance tended to be poor, 50–60 per cent attending each group and about five groups being cancelled in the first twelve months. Following a six month review the group began to progress, attendance was improved and people began to share clinical situations and clinical problems. At the time of the evaluation, trust and respect were beginning to develop and staff were beginning to work together.

Comment: Both groups contained a mixture of occupational therapists specialising in physical and mental health; this proved to be very beneficial particularly in the exchange of experience regarding dealing with patients with disruptive behaviour and mental health problems. Staff commented that their confidence in dealing with clinical situations had increased resulting from the reassurance they had received regarding their actions in dealing with certain clinical situations.

Group 9. Health visitors

This group consisted of eight health visitors meeting every two months for ninety minutes over a lunch time period. The meetings covered areas such as topics of interest, cases of interest and the possibility of guest speakers. An agenda was set for each meeting.

Although this group felt able to discuss difficult clients it had currently not done so. The sorts of areas covered were UKCC policies, hormone replacement therapy, measurement of head circumference, dealing with the police. This has led to a general questioning of some traditional health visiting practices. There was a general feeling that these were more than just professional discussions: 'at other meetings I tend not to be listened to or no action is taken, but here we can do something.'

Comment: Staff were using the clinical supervision sessions to discuss issues of professional interest and concern. They felt that their contributions were valued and that they were able to act upon some of the issues discussed. The group was considering meeting monthly as they felt that this would enhance continuity and enable more reflective reviews of specific clients.

Group 10. Clinic staff

This group consisted of four nurses and a consultant doctor. The group met once a month for one hour over lunch time and had been meeting for approximately fifteen months. Sociological and ethical issues relating to their speciality were discussed and the boundaries and extent of their role debated. The group felt that they had gained a lot of reassurance from finding out that they all faced similar anxieties and had explored different ways of dealing and coping with the professional problems raised. This had resulted in increased confidence in themselves, their clinical abilities and recognition of the nature and limitations of their role.

Comment: This was the only group to contain a consultant doctor and nurses. The mixing of disciplines proved useful and served to build relationships and helped both disciplines appreciate each other's role and routine functions. Specific clinical situations were discussed and support was gained regarding a number of difficult areas. Despite being experienced staff the group felt that clinical supervision had increased their clinical confidence.

An overview of the pilot site responses

In eight of the ten pilot sites clinical supervision could be said to be up and running. In the other two groups clinical supervision had either never commenced or floundered after two meetings. The reasons why clinical supervision did not take off in these two groups were complex but tended to focus on organisational and staffing issues.

Boxes 17.1–17.4 contain a selection of comments presented under the headings of questions posed to the eight groups that had implemented clinical supervision:

- Can you identify an event in which clinical supervision has had an impact on clinical practice?
- In what ways has clinical supervision supported you through difficult or stressful events?
- In what ways has clinical supervision helped you identify areas of weakness or inexperience?
- Has your clinical supervision been worthwhile?

As a general observation it appeared that the more frequently a group met the more likely it was to discuss and reflect upon specific patient / client care. Groups that met on average once a month tended to review one client in depth for part of the meeting and then discuss pertinent issues during

---

Box 17.1: Responses to the question; can you identify an event in which clinical supervision has had an impact on clinical practice?

We go through the notes and discuss patients, he (supervisor) says have you thought about this? Makes you think wider, broader, bouncing ideas off each other. – Physio

We spent one session discussing breast feeding; following that, I had a mother who had a lot of problems with breast feeding and I was able to put quite a lot of that into practice. – Health Visitor

I talked about one patient with this particular problem and it (clinical supervision) gave you alternatives and more effective ways of dealing with the situation. – School Nurse

I had a family that had several problems and I was getting bogged down; I presented the case and got several useful suggestions, it helped me see it with fresh eyes. I was able to put several of the ideas into practice and it gave me confidence to take the case forward. – Health Visitor

It makes you reflect not only on the person you're discussing but other clients that you have not talked about. – District Nurse

We talked about how to manage the paperwork of the job and how to manage time. – School Nurse

One person presented a patient who had mental health problems and some quite disruptive behaviour; some ideas were wanted on how to handle the situation better. We all learnt a lot from that session and it led to a specific training session on dealing with disruptive behaviour. – Occupational Therapist

Discussing aspects of measuring children, we found that we were measuring slightly different ways. We went away and reviewed our practice. – Health Visitor

Sometimes it is difficult in our work to know where the boundaries lie between ethical, professional, moral issues, where to let go. That's difficult to manage on your own. – Family Planning Nurse

---

Box 17.2: Responses to the question; in what ways has clinical supervision supported you through difficult or stressful events?

Coming from the hospital to this job in the community it was a time to check, gain some reassurance and not feel abandoned. – Physiotherapist

I had a family that I was dealing with, the relatives were quite obstructive to the treatment, it was reassuring to take this to supervision and feel supported that I was handling it OK. – District Nurse

I feel better knowing someone knows. – District Nurse

The fact that you know it's a confidential platform for discussing problems within the team or with colleagues. – School Nurse

When I gained promotion I talked through a lot of issues, it was very supporting. – District Nurse

We tend not to talk about personal issues, it doesn't seem right to burden others with your stress. – Health Visitor

It's reassuring, when you present a difficult case and know what we're doing as individuals is OK, this gives you confidence and power to move forward, that we have discussed it with other professionals. – Health Visitor

It's a kind of luxury when you work on your own, being given permission once a month to share with others about how they deal with certain situations. – Health Visitor

It's the permission to discuss and the time to explore those things that would normally be snatched over coffee or in the corridor. – District Nurse

Some of the ethical type issues are difficult to deal with on your own. – Family Planning Nurse

---

the rest of the meeting. It could be concluded from this that if a group wishes to focus in greater detail on individual patients / clients they will need to meet quite frequently.

The general view was that clinical supervision was a genuinely supportive system in terms of dealing with difficult or new clinical situations. Reassurance, confidence building and empowering were three terms that were frequently mentioned. Those staff that worked predominantly on their own or were the only member of their speciality working in a team felt that simply meeting with and discussing 'specialist' issues was very supporting. In a number of the groups there was a very definite, yet difficult to quantify, 'warmth of atmosphere'.

The majority of the people we interviewed were experienced staff who were professionally confident in the routine of their daily work. Areas that they tended to identify as 'weak or inexperienced' were those which tended to be unusual for their situation: for example, a person with learning disabilities for a health visitor, or patients with mental health problems but being 'treated' for a physical disorder. There were also some examples of general relationship and communication issues where people acknowledged that their way of dealing with the situation just wasn't working and they were seeking alternatives. What was evident in the majority of groups was the willingness to discuss such issues in a positive and problem solving way.

Box 17.3: Responses to the question: in what ways has clinical supervision helped you identify areas of weakness or inexperience?

IPR identifies formal needs, clinical supervision is more subtle, stops you getting complacent. I think I'd better find out what this medication is for, Peters (supervisor) is bound to ask me that. – Physiotherapist

One member knew a lot about asthma and led a session, I found that very useful as I was quite weak in that area. – School Nurse

Some of the new drugs and inhalers I didn't know about. – Health Visitor

I didn't really have much idea about how to communicate with a 15-year-old boy; that was very useful. – Health Visitor

Yes, diabetic foot ulcers, that was an identified need. We talked through it at supervision then I went to the leg ulcer clinic to gain some clinical knowledge. – District Nurse

I feel comfortable in the group being able to say, what do I do here? – Occupational Therapist

Trying to do too much myself, how to organise myself. – School Nurse

Tend to keep myself isolated, you get used to coping on your own, I need to share more. – Health Visitor

Communicating with patients with mental health problems. – District Nurse

---

Box 17.4: Responses to the question: has your clinical supervision been worthwhile?

Yes, both as a manager and as staff. – Physiotherapist

Yes, definitely. It's improving as well. The first three months it was plodding a bit but as we got to know one another it feels as though we are getting a lot more out of it. – Health Visitor

We were sceptical at first but can now see the scope of what we can get out of it. – School Nurse

Yes, support for one another, for new staff and those retiring. Reduced stress levels and sickness. – District Nurse

Work was impacting on private lives before, but now work related problems tend to be contained largely at work. – Health Visitor

Yes, coming together and protected time, we are all up against the same difficulties.

It brings people together, makes them think – Occupational Therapist.

Yes, definitely. – District Nurse

I missed one and felt quite distant from it all. – Health Visitor

Yes, empowering, stress relieving, you almost get a buzz from it. – Health Visitor

A summary of the actions, outputs and outcomes of clinical supervision

This summary focuses on the structure, process and outcomes of clinical supervision.

Structure of the sessions

- Most of the sites had implemented group clinical supervision, with only two examples of individual supervision. Both models were effective in the situations in which they were introduced.
- Group supervision was particularly useful for staff who worked predominantly on their own.
- Some sites had staff of mixed grades and disciplines. Others were segregated according to grade and discipline. As a general finding it appeared that a mixture of disciplines and grades was very useful in giving staff insight and understanding of other people's ways of working. At times however these groups would be restricted in the focus in terms of professional interest and potential depth of their discussions.
- Clinical supervision needs time for a relationship of mutual trust and respect to be developed between the staff. Depending on the frequency of the meetings this seems to take between three and six months. The 'productivity' or qualitative outcomes of clinical supervision sessions seems to be significantly greater once the relationships have gelled.
- Clinical supervision sessions ranged from weekly meetings to those occurring once every two months. Sessions lasted between sixty and ninety minutes. Where clinical supervision was used to review patient caseload then weekly clinical supervision is appropriate. Where clinical supervision is used to review longer-term patient situations and general professional issues then monthly meetings seem to be appropriate. Groups that met every two months found it harder to focus on specific clinical issues and discuss individual problems.
- Staff who cover twenty-four hour patient care by working shifts have considerable difficulty in organising and safeguarding a set time for a clinical supervision meeting.
- Staff who are in charge of their own 'diary' and are experienced in managing their own time were most effective in organising and safeguarding clinical supervision sessions.

Process of clinical supervision

- Different clinical supervision groups developed different focuses, functions and 'personalities'.
- Those groups where all members feel that they have ownership and control of clinical supervision appear to be the most productive.
- Those sites where clinical supervision became established and productive had mature leadership. The style of leadership varies within each site and there does not seem to be one style that is more favourable than another. With experienced staff groups a 'low key' leader who encouraged equality and joint responsibility between all members seemed particularly effective. With groups that had less experienced staff a slightly more

dominant leader who took responsibility for direction and focus appeared productive. There is a delicate balance between leadership that encourages, organises, motivates and empowers without appearing to dominate and take over.

- Mutual trust and comfortable working relationships appeared to be a feature of groups that met regularly and formed the basis for a number of beneficial outcomes.

Outcomes of clinical supervision

The following outcomes are based upon a general summary of the eight groups where clinical supervision had become established.

- Feedback to individuals that clinical actions and professional practices undertaken were appropriate and reassurance that these actions were 'good / best practice'.
- Discussion of alternative ways of dealing with unusual clinical problems and identification of creative solutions.
- Acted as stimulus to reflect upon one's own practice and helped prevent complacency developing.
- The safeguard and sanction of time to focus in depth on a specific client problem.
- Support from clinically knowledgeable peers regarding difficult relationships concerned with clients, relatives or colleagues.
- A formalised, structured system for staff to seek advice and gain support relating to professional work situations.
- A valuable support system for all staff but particularly effective for new staff and those changing roles.
- Provision of a platform from which individuals felt able to influence their practice and at times the organisation policy and practices.
- Provides a safe environment where one's areas of weakness could be disclosed, reviewed and positively managed.

Conclusions

- No single model of clinical supervision emerged as better than any of the others. Each developed to meet the needs of different situations and individual members.
- Sufficient autonomy should be given to each group to allow them to develop and tailor a model that is seen to be useful to themselves.
- When new groups are being established they should be encouraged to explore different approaches and established good practices but given the authority to develop and build upon these models so that they can develop a system specific to their needs.
- Implementation of clinical supervision required the support, permission

and encouragement of the organisation and immediate managers but it is essential that the ownership should be taken and maintained by the individual practitioners.

- Where the working environment is in a state of considerable organisational change, or staffing levels are significantly below the norm, then the introduction of clinical supervision is probably not appropriate at that time.

- Clinical supervision has to be seen as a long-term investment from both the organisational and practitioners' perspective. The benefits appear to be related to the cumulative effect of regular, planned meetings and the building up of trust and friendship between the healthcare practitioners.

- The actual and potential benefit of clinical supervision to staff was unanimously recognised and praised as a legitimate and professionally acceptable process by all participants. The wholly positive perception of benefits was illustrated by a range of clinical examples and anecdotal accounts, citing improved performance, increased confidence, a reduction in the use of both professional and personal support mechanisms, and a greater understanding of colleagues' clinical work.

- The benefits to clients were less tangible, with secondary gains being acquired from new knowledge of contemporary treatment methods, previously shared during clinical supervision. The professional's increased self-assurance in their own practice was said to have been projected onto clients, who were on the whole more confident and relaxed about the care they received.

- Where clinical supervision had been successfully established, the benefits to the organisation seemed to have their basis in an increased level of job satisfaction and morale. Staff felt clinical supervision had created an opportunity to consider the method and style of their clinical interventions which in turn made them more effective professionals.

The final picture – clinical supervision as a campfire!

All the groups where clinical supervision was up and running felt that the sessions had been worthwhile. People tended to feel that individually and professionally they gained from clinical supervision. For all staff it meant committing the time to attending, being prepared to talk honestly and having genuine respect for others. In both areas where clinical supervision did not take off staff were noticeably demotivated, lacked energy and appeared to have no professional leadership. These individuals did not feel in control of their daily working environment and poor staffing seemed to be a significant factor in one of the areas. Both areas were undergoing considerable organisational change, which appeared to be poorly planned and poorly implemented. **The introduction of clinical supervision appeared to be something else that was being imposed upon them and in which they had little say. Somewhat ironically, the support and direction that clinical supervision**

has the potential to offer was exactly what these two areas needed. However, the motivation and leadership required to introduce and develop such a system was not there.

An analogy of clinical supervision could be that of a group of people sitting around a campfire. If a group had dry wood they could with relative ease get a fire going and enjoy its warmth. Once the fire was established it would be relatively easy to keep it going. Even if it began to rain and their wood got damp the fire would keep going because the warmth of the existing fire would dry out the damp wood. However, another group is already wet and their wood is damp. They are sitting in a field where it is raining and the wood they bring to the fire is damp. This group will find it very difficult to get a fire started. People who are particularly skilled may be able to start the fire, but it will probably require some outside input, such as a carefully controlled dose of petrol.

In this analogy the wood is likened to people's motivation and energy: those who have an excess of energy, enthusiasm and motivation can throw it into the fire where it generates warmth, support and encouragement for others in that group. Once the group is established and positive relationships forged, then they will be able to 'keep the fire going' even when people are going through a hard, demotivating time. Those groups in which people do not have any spare motivation or energy – and this can occur for a variety of reasons – will not be able to get the fire going. Ironically it is these 'damp' groups that need the warmth and support of the 'fire'.

The moral of this analogy is to establish clinical supervision when the team is strong. When the team is weak, outside motivation will need to be injected and maintained until the group is established and self-supporting.

References

Bowling A (1999) *Research Methods in Health*. Buckingham: Open University Press.

Butterworth T Carson J White E Jeacock J Clements A and Bishop V (1997) *It is Good to Talk. An Evaluation Study in England and Scotland*. University of Manchester.

Clarke A (1999) Focus group interviews in health care research. *Professional Nurse* 14, 6, pp395–397.

Dudley M and Butterworth T (1994) The cost and some benefits of clinical supervision. *International Journal of Psychiatric Nursing Research* 1, 2, pp34–40.

Edberg A Hallberg I and Gustafson L (1996) Effects of clinical supervision on nurse patient cooperation quality. A controlled study in dementia care. *Clinical Nursing Research* 5, 2, pp127–149.

Fowler J and Chevannes M (1998) Evaluating the efficacy of reflective practice within the context of clinical supervision. *Journal of Advanced Nursing* 27, 279–382.

Greene J and D'Oliveira M (1998). *Learning To Use Statistical Tests in Psychology*. Milton Keynes: Open University Press.

Jenkinson C (1997) *Assessment and Evaluation of Health and Medical Care*. London: Open University Press.

McGee P and Notter J (1995) *Research Appreciation*. Wilts: Mark Allen Publishing.

Robinson N (1999) The use of focus group methodology – with selected examples from sexual health research. *Journal of Advanced Nursing* 29, (4), pp905–913.

Part IV

18 An Australian perspective on clinical supervision

Tania Yegdich

Editorial

This chapter focuses on the Australian perspectives of clinical supervision. It draws attention to the practice of clinical supervision in teaching and, as a result of this association, it highlights the current difficulty in conceptualising clinical supervision as an independent entity in Australia. The chapter then examines the extent of clinical supervision practice and discusses the current barriers and resisters to supervision. One such resister is the clinicians' confusion that arises by amalgamating clinical supervision with managerial supervision, and the resulting resistance to engage in supervision whilst it remains coupled in this way.

We believe that when considering the theory and practice of clinical supervision, the chapter illustrates how Australian nurses appear to have followed the lead provided by some British nurses. If this is the case, then perhaps it follows that the methods and means that have been used to address the resistance to clinical supervision in Britain may have some worth and application in Australia. Whilst recognising that variations in the culture, politics and practice would have to be considered, the commonality in experience should not be ignored.

Introduction

Some decades ago, the British psychoanalyst Donald Winnicott was described by his editors as that kind of creative genius who neglected to acknowledge his sources. Winnicott recognised that in much of his clinical theorising others before him had made similar revelations, nevertheless, he believed it important to discover those insights for himself. This now familiar reference to experiential learning, of making one's own discoveries, lies at the heart of meaningful knowledge, and best encapsulates the hopes for the formal introduction of clinical supervision clinical supervision into nursing, both in the Australian context and elsewhere.

While clinical supervision has become an important concept internationally, and particularly in the United Kingdom (Butterworth and Faugier, 1992), it is presently underdeveloped in Australia. Although all nurses would not hesitate to acknowledge supervision of some kind, the newer emerging concept of clinical supervision is not familiar in Australian nursing, apart from isolated developments in mental health nursing. Certainly the notion of self-directed discovery by critically thinking reflective practitioners has permeated Australia's nursing education system (Taylor, 1997; Gray and Pratt, 1991) as in other English-speaking countries worldwide. This philosophical shift in education methods has occurred across all professions in health, industry and education which, despite their fundamental differences in language, discourse and setting, broadly share similar strategies concerning training, supervision and outcome monitoring (Caldwell and Carter, 1993). Nevertheless, the Australian nursing imagination has been slow to engage the idea of clinical supervision for exploring and enhancing therapeutic interventions, notwithstanding local rhetoric on grounding the essence of nursing in the nurse–patient relationship (Sutton and Smith, 1995).

In parallel with changes in education are the changes in management philosophy. Where previously organisational supervision was characterised by a language pervaded by power and control (Saville and Higgins, 1990), contemporary trends within a broad spectrum of industry, including health and nursing, emphasise collaboration to inspire shared vision (Commonwealth of Australia [Karpin Report] 1995). According to Karpin, the supervisor of the 1970s became a coach for the 1980s and 1990s, and in the future will become an envisioner and enabler. While supervision is not new to nursing from an administrative perspective, importantly, traditional nursing supervision has changed to reflect, coincidentally, the participatory nature of the 'new' clinical supervision. This supervision originated from the counselling professions and consists of a supportive relationship for the purpose of teaching and learning psychotherapeutic skills (Ekstein and Wallerstein, 1958). As nursing rejects procedural tasks to embrace a holistic view of the patient (Davies, 1991), developing therapeutic expertise becomes significant for the nurse–patient relationship (Butterworth, 1992).

Further, as nursing moves from a hierarchically dominated apprenticeship vocation to a self-regulating profession, the evolution to safe and competent practitioners who perform without supervision (Australian Nursing Council Inc. [ANCI] 1998) has deemed the term 'supervision' obsolete. The previous Australasian Nurse Registering Authorities Conference [ANRAC] (1990) referred to the registered nurse role as clinical teacher–supervisor synonymously and subsequently, supervision is understood in the contexts of clinical teaching or management. While undoubtedly fuelled by its unfortunate connotations of watching and checking, the difficulty in comprehending what clinical supervision means is further amplified by a generic reference to any number of supervisory practices occurring in the clinical setting. As Kermode (1985: 39) early noted, the term, 'supervision' derives from its 'setting, rather than the practice'. And like the concepts of preceptorship and mentoring introduced into nursing in the early 1980s as clinical teaching strategies, clinical supervision has become a conceptual anomaly. **The most problematic issue** surrounding the contemporary idea of clinical supervision in nursing, both here and overseas, concerns what it actually is – and how it will be articulated, refined and implemented (Yegdich, 1998).

In this chapter I review the Australian perspective on clinical supervision and draw attention to difficulties in clinical teaching generally, and in conceptualizing clinical supervision as an independent entity, in particular.

Emerging trends in clinical education

Essentially, there are three ways of investigating clinical supervision in Australia. First, the curious bystander must search the literature on clinical teaching where supervision is a subsumed activity of preceptorship and mentoring. Second, in its most general sense, clinical supervision or 'clinical facilitation', as is preferred (Dunn and Burnard, 1992), refers to the sequenced course of action on clinical placements (Yarrow, 1993), for undergraduate nursing education, as well as its bedrock activity. The terms 'supervisors', 'facilitators' and 'preceptors' are interchangeable within nursing Academe's reflective curriculum. Fowler's (1996) summary of the UK literature that clinical supervision is both an umbrella and a related term under the rubric of clinical supervision is relevant here. Last, a rudimentary literature within mental health nursing on clinical supervision proper presumes reflectivity and experiential learning.

Cutcliffe and Proctor (1998) observe two separate but confusing perspectives on clinical supervision in the United Kingdom where experienced nurses supervise less experienced nurses, and non-experts supervise experienced nurses. Such discrepancies, it would seem, are responses first to, abate the growing need to bridge the theory–practice gap for inexperienced nurses and second, to address the emerging need for continuous learning for all nurses. Australian clinical teaching models incorporate preceptoring with practice supervision (Brown *et al.*, 1998) for undergraduates and for new graduates beginning practice on formalised Graduate Transition Programs [GNPs] (Commonwealth Department of Human Services and Health [Reid Report], 1994). Clinical supervision models are advocated for and being developed by experienced nurses in mental health settings (Rozelle Hospital, 1996). **Clinical facilitation, preceptorship and mentoring have generally emerged from the academic setting and subsume supervision, while clinical supervision as a distinct practice has primarily been driven by clinicians.**

Table 18.1 outlines the various use of terms and practices of Australian clinical teaching.

At this time, clinical supervision is largely a mental health nursing phenomenon, and marks a significant change in the history and culture of nursing (Jordan, 1999a). There is something alluring about clinical supervision in nursing's history. While capable of arousing distrust and suspicion on name alone (Gill *et al.*, 1999; Teasdale, 1998; Butterworth *et al.*, 1997; Martin *et al.*, 1996; Farrington, 1995; James, 1994), clinical supervision has attracted significant audiences at nursing conferences wholly dedicated to its discussion and

Table 18.1 Models of clinical teaching in Australia: preceptorship, mentorship, clinical supervision, clinical facilitation, reflective practice

	Purpose	Benefits	Elements
Preceptorship	• Transition of new practitioners – work. • Transition of graduates. • Socialisation of nurses. • Promote clinical competence/confidence. • Clinical teaching. • Orientation.	Eases adjustments. Transition from student to RN. Work orientation. Role socialisation. Closer attention – one-to-one. Bridges university-clinical knowledge.	One-to-one teaching. Continuation of education. Apply theory to practice. Provide support. Student assessment. Role modelling. **Supervision***
Mentorship	• Transition into managerial role. • Development of leadership qualities. • Support for promotions. • Nurtures junior colleagues' talent. • Promotes novices. • Transition of values and beliefs. • Retention of active participants.	Professional role modelling. Developing leadership. Development of leaders as future role models. Strengthen professional relationships.	Role modelling. Developing leadership. Confidence building. Supporting and Nurturing. Career counselling. Facilitating acceptance and promotion. Educating. **Supervision***
Supervision*/ clinical supervision*	1. Subsumed generic term under preceptoring and mentorship.* 2. Interchangeable with clinical facilitation.** • Activity of clinical teaching/coaching.	1. As above. Functions of preceptoring, mentoring. 2. Develop higher- order learning – critical thinking. Develop clinical skills. Role socialisation. Interpret clinical experience. Identify learning needs. Alternative frame of reference to institutions.	1. Observation. Explicit demonstration. Explicit instruction. Practice supervision. **Supervision*** • Supportive teaching/learning relationship. • Increase therapeutic skills. • Promote understanding of patients. • Focus on nurse-patient relationship. • Professional growth.

(used in generic terms)	3. Developing in Mental Health Nursing: • Supportive teaching/learning relationship. • Increase therapeutic skills. • Promote understanding of patients. • Focus on nurse–patient relationship.	3. Validates nurse–patient relationship- interactions. Develops therapeutic skills. Promotes accountabilities and autonomy. Protects the patient and nurse. Individualised experiential learning.	3. Supportive supervisee–supervisor relationship: one-to-one, group, peer. Differentiated from managerial supervision and performance appraisal. Clinical supervisor separate from on-line manager/supervisor.
Clinical supervision	• Professional growth.	**Pre-existing education method in therapy training.**	
Clinical facilitation	Preferred term for clinical placement supervision of undergraduate students: • The sequenced course of actions on clinical placements. (In Australia). • Clinical teaching/coaching. Bridge theory-practice gap, knowledge.	As above – 1*, 2**. **Philosophical shift from 'doing' to 'knowing'.**	2. Higher-order thinking. Role-modelling. Student assessment. Liaison – university and hospital. Interpreting clinical experiences. Support. **Supervision***
Reflective practice	• Core Domain (ANCI) Competency. • Make knowledge embedded in expert nursing practice explicit. • Strategy for life-long learning. • Clinical teaching/coaching.	Explicate nursing theories from practice. Identify power relations, oppression, and injustice. Develop nursing knowledge. Empowers practitioner. **Philosophical shift from 'doing' to 'knowing'.**	Links theory to practice. Cyclic – pre and post-conference/ briefing. Reflection-*in*-action. Reflection-*on*-action. Reflection before action

dissemination in North America, the United Kingdom and Australia. The Institute of New York State League of Nurse Education held their annual conference in 1925 on clinical supervision (Schmidt, 1926) with 367 nurses from 61 hospitals in attendance, while in the UK, 519 nurses, midwives and health visitors, UKCC and Department of Health representatives attended a national conference also devoted to clinical supervision (Smith, 1995). In Australia, the Rozelle Hospital, a major mental health service provider in Sydney, in 1996 drew 150 nurses including academics, researchers, clinicians, managers, students and independent practitioners from around Australia and New Zealand at the annual Winter Symposium specifically to debate the need for clinical supervision in mental health nursing (Meehan *et al.*, 1997). That conference featured Tony Butterworth (1996) as key speaker and supporter of clinical supervision implementation in the Australian setting. While Australian academics have railed against the wholesale import of international ideas that neither fit Australian culture nor develop a distinct Australian nursing identity (Lawler, 1991a), Butterworth's ideas have fruitfully interacted with local interpretations. It remains to be seen how idiosyncratically Australians will forge clinical supervision in their own image.

I now view these events within a broader perspective concerning the theory–practice gap (an enduring problem in nursing), and then examine the phenomenon of clinical supervision in mental health nursing.

The changed face of nursing education: the theory–practice gap

According to Ewan and White (1996), every decade brings its own particular focus on the theory–practice gap. The decision in 1984 to transfer funding from state and territory health sectors to the Commonwealth higher education system reflected an impetus to place nursing on a firm theoretical foundation. In the 1970s, higher nursing education had consisted of both universities and colleges of advanced education [CAEs]. As CAEs were considered less scholarly and research-orientated than universities (Roberts, 1995), the transfer from an advanced education discipline to a university discipline as colleges were abolished or upgraded further advanced nursing's professional and educational status. Australian nursing now holds a unique position in education by its demand for a pre-registration bachelor degree. The prevailing expectation of developing a 'different kind of nurse' who would acquire critical thinking abilities and apply them to clinical practice would solve the theory–practice gap. And this would be achieved by better controlling students' clinical experience to match theory, in comparison to hospital-based training (Kermode, 1984).

Prior to the transfer, clinical practice was more valued than theory (Commonwealth of Australia, 1997), and in the early stages of developing the discipline of academic nursing, Reid claimed the danger was to remain too practice-bound: the discipline should 'lead clinical practice rather than being limited by it' (Reid Report, 1994: 314). There is some irony that Australian nursing was moving into Academe at a time when Schön (1983) was criticising the dominant 'technical–rationalist' approach for causing public disenchantment and crisis within the professions. The ensuing need to balance the practical and theoretical ('knowing how' and 'knowing that') and renounce prescriptive rule-driven curricula led to an increasing awareness and beginning acceptance of reflective practice in Australian academic nursing (Davies, 1991). According to Davies, tertiary education's emphasis on critical analysis, problem-solving, decision-making and values clarification would enable students to move beyond rule-governed behaviour and mechanistic approaches to care to develop artistry in professional practice. The reflective practicum promised a central bridge between theory and practice, using reflection on practice as its link (Stockhausen and Creedy, 1992). For nursing, clinical experience completes tertiary education; however, overall quality of nursing education depends on the quality of clinical experience (Reid Report, 1994). Since the transfer, time allocated for clinical placement has diminished (Perry, 1988), with debate extolling the supremacy of *quality* of experience (Battersby and Hemmings, 1991) over *quantity* of time spent in practice – 'learning *from* experience rather than *by* experience' (Sims, 1991: 67).

According to Benner (1984), expertise takes time and cannot be taught, but good theoretical foundations enable graduates to make the best possible use of experience. Nevertheless, later Australian calls for links between academia and industry were highlighted by new graduates experiencing transition difficulties (Sims, 1991). While the role of reflection is critical for identifying expert knowledge embedded in practice – 'untapped knowledge' (Benner, 1984), the recognition that novices do not have enough experience to reflect on (Fowler and Chevannes, 1998; Gray and Forrstrom, 1995) has been harder to accommodate within a system that rewards academic excellence without recognising clinical excellence (Roberts, 1995).

Differing expectations and lack of discussion on workforce needs have resulted in universities and industry becoming separated spheres (Corkhill, 1998) lost in another dimension of the theory–practice gap. Doubtless, reported prejudice and ignorance from hospital nurses toward graduates (Clare *et al.*, 1996) have undermined collaboration, while academic perceptions on cultural differences between the 'professionally socialising university culture' and the 'bureaucratic hospital culture' (Beattie, 1998) along with beliefs that universities emphasise 'learning and self-direction' while hospitals emphasise 'performance and obeying rules' (Crowe, 1994) neither heal rifts, nor revitalise the future growth of the profession (Sellars, 2000).

By the 1990s, the theory–practice gap had come full circle. Where Kermode (1984) believed clinical supervision would integrate theoretical learning with clinical experience, academics now lament the ever-widening separation of clinical knowledge from theory (Gray and Pratt, 1995), and the scant academic attention to skill-mastery (Madjar, 1998). Despite entreaties to return to practice (Lumby, 1995), the implications of acquiring non-reflective embodied knowledge whereby experts rapidly assess situations without reflection has not been fully appreciated. Although Greenwood (1996) implores that teaching by explicit demonstration and supervision must occur in the clinical setting, the teaching and learning of nurse–patient relationship expertise has not been adequately discussed.

Nevertheless, typical solutions to the theory–practice gap have included supervision, preceptorship and mentoring, though little consensus exists on these activities. In fact, there is little clarity on *what* clinical teachers do and even less on *how* they do it (White and Ewan, 1995). It is, after all, a private activity that resents intrusion. Reid (1994) claims that the focus of clinical learning has shifted from 'doing' to 'knowing', and even though clinical teaching is, by nature, active in its demand for students to obtain information directly, the teaching role of clinical supervisors in academia is not clearly defined (Grealish and Carroll, 1998).

Supervision in the academic setting

As nursing is primarily a practice discipline whose core activities are 'acquired, reinforced and consolidated in the actual delivery of care to real people' (Napthine, 1996: 20), it is essential that clinical aspects are taught and supervised by those who are clinically competent (Commonwealth of Australia, 1997). Clinical teachers need to maintain their professional practice competencies (White and Ewan, 1995) and be prepared, up-to-date, objective and available (Ladyshewsky, 1995). The three groups of clinical teachers comprise academics, sessional teachers and clinical staff. However, many academics lack clinical credibility as expert clinicians (Grealish and Carroll, 1998), and tend to adopt a facilitative, rather than teaching role. In the clinical supervision model of facilitation, academic staff are known as either supervisors or facilitators who work on-site with undergraduates for specified periods of time and provide practice supervision and instruction to aid theory-application and psychomotor skill. The advantage in academics offering supervision is their commitment to higher education and research-based practice. In reality, supervision is often delegated to the least experienced, least prepared faculty member or to sessional teachers not familiar with the curriculum (Duke, 1996).

Beattie (1998) claims that ignoring the need to develop clinical teaching skills is to cast clinical teaching as secondary to theoretical teaching and knowledge. A consistent theme in the Australian literature is the poor preparation of clinical teachers and their low status. As tertiary education emphasises research and publication, faculty interest in clinical teaching is minimal. With increasing student numbers, supervisors are spread over several wards and are often unavailable for fundamental learning activities (Duke, 1996), let alone student-centred teaching.

Grealish and Carroll (1998) acknowledge that theory–practice links are more tenuous when the clinical teacher is less experienced and propose a model combining the tasks of supervision and facilitation. They believe that critical thinking is not clearly demonstrated in clinically based preceptors.

Some also lack formal educational training. To overcome weaknesses in either preceptorship or supervision alone, academic supervisors could facilitate learning at higher-order levels while preceptors could enhance clinical skill instruction.

This separation only serves to perpetuate a false dichotomy in viewing universities as responsible for theoretical knowledge and higher-order thinking and clinical settings responsible for skill development and practical knowledge. Ewan and White (1996) consider the belief that clinical teaching is just habit learning and therefore, less demanding than academic teaching, is rooted in an outdated 'learning-by-doing' assumption. The teacher is an important factor (Hart and Rotem, 1993) for the quality of clinical education: within such roles as guide, coach and supporter (Ewan and White, 1996), the ability to steer between helper and challenger is 'one of the most demanding tasks in clinical teaching'(White and Ewan, 1995: 137). To their surprise, Grant *et al.* (1996) discover that hospital-trained experienced nurses feel better prepared to teach than their tertiary-trained contemporaries.

Preceptorship and mentoring

As the formal roles of supervisor, mentor, preceptor and role-model are widely referred to in diverse situations, they are difficult to differentiate. Definitions vary according to the type of relationship established, and it remains contentious whether relationships need to be informal or formal, spontaneous or structured and facilitated (Ross, 1996). Mentoring is often confused with preceptoring. The term 'mentor' is 'enshrouded in a thick veil of conceptual confusion and divergence of opinion' (Wright, 1995: 5), and the term 'preceptor' fares no better (Madison *et al.*, 1994). Barnett (1992) defines preceptoring as a short-term clinically orientated relationship with an expert clinician and role-model linked to particular learning goals, whereas mentoring is career-orientated and therefore, more likely to be longer-term. As mentoring develops leadership skills (Ross, 1996), more nurse managers are mentored than clinical nurse specialists. In a context of its general under-utilisation in Australian nursing, some academic mentoring initiatives exist (James and Proctor, 1992; Madison, 1993), but overall, mentoring is recommended during times of organisational change, personal transition and promotion (Queensland Health, 1999a). Ross (1996) summarises mentoring as a complex concept lacking in thorough detailed research, documentation and debate. It is unclear whether mentors require a facilitated programme of training, support, guidance and feedback.

Preceptorship eases workplace transition (Pelletier and Duffield, 1994) for new graduates on GNPs and new employees to an organisation (Kitchin, 1993), and is used for undergraduates on longer clinical placements. There is no evidence that preceptorship improves nursing care and few Australian studies examine the effects on preceptors after engagement in their role. Where preceptor stress may lead to reduced standards (Beattie, 1998), elsewhere, registered nurses find teaching satisfying (Ives and Rowley, 1991).

Usher *et al.* (1999) identify various pitfalls such as unsuitability, skill deficits, lack of commitment, rewards and incentives, resentment of protégé and lack of time. As preceptors are often selected on availability rather than suitability, it is unrealistic to expect them to establish positive learning environments and student–teacher relationships. Beattie (1998) lists four assumptions under-pinning preceptorship as:

- Clinical experts also make good teachers.
- One-to-one teaching is best.
- Preceptor preparation is sufficient for success of process and relationship.
- All students can use the preceptor model.

These assumptions could equally apply to mentoring and supervision, whereas Ross's queries on whether mentoring requires formal support are relevant for supervision and preceptorship. It is almost a cliché to agree that managerial commitment is required for their success.

Managerial commitment

As well as managerial commitment, educational success in the workplace requires an open climate of collaboration, co-operation and discussion of work with a clear understanding of intended educational purposes (Carruthers, 1993). Strong organisational support alleviates potential problems and increases benefits of formalised clinical teaching. For the 1990s, Caldwell and Carter (1993) define training as no longer work-related, but work-based. The contemporary challenge of workforce preparation is to provide continuous workplace learning that copes with continuous change. In nursing, Pearson (1998) reports disagreement on how nurses' continuous competence should be monitored and whether continuing education enhances practice. McCormick and Marshall (1997) note that in the professions, maintaining competence through mandating continuing education is incompatible with contemporary notions of adult self-directed learning principles. Nevertheless, reflective practice is endorsed as one of eighteen nursing competencies (ANCI, 1993) and becomes one of four domain competencies in the newly reviewed stan-dards (ANCI, 1998). Reflection encompasses elements of critically examining practice, research awareness, professional development of self, ongoing profes-sional development activities that include support networks, role-modelling, coaching and mentoring techniques. The ANCI competencies are central to regulating the profession and frame educational accountability (Reid Report, 1994).

Endorsing clinical supervision in policy

Australian supervisory practice is usually subsumed under clinical teaching but includes supervision of clinical placements and is referred to in relation to meeting pre-registration requirements. Registered nurses work without supervision, but supervise enrolled nurses, where supervision is defined as 'direction and guidance' (Queensland Nursing Council, [QNC] 1998a). It is thus, hierarchical and mandatory for statutory purposes. My recent inquiries to the QNC (1998b), the Nurses Board of Victoria (1998) and New South Wales (1998), the three east-coast state regulating bodies, confirm the lack of a position paper on clinical supervision. All referred to the maintenance of standards, eligibility for registration, supervision of students and mandatory supervision of enrolled nurses. The QNC (1998c), desirous of expanding nursing's scope of practice, was unexpectedly conservative and uninformed, promptly producing glossy brochures on supervising enrolled nurses (QNC, 1997a) and re-entry nurses (QNC, 1997b). The Queensland Nurses' Union (QNU), also committed to advancing nursing as a profession, stated that any formal practice or designated position of clinical supervision would be 'harking back to the dark ages' (personal correspondence). As preceptorship, mentoring and case review had been built into the nursing career structure, adequate provisions exist for clinical supervision. Moreover, any use of the term, 'clinical supervisor' was considered diminishing to the 'professional status nursing has fought to achieve over an extended period' (QNU, 1998). Interestingly, all acknowledged clinical supervision developments in psychiatric nursing.

Clinical supervision in mental health nursing

The Australian Capital Territory (ACT) branch of the Australian and New Zealand College of Mental Health Nurses Inc. (ANZCMHN Inc., 1998) had developed guidelines on clinical supervision to include its definition, the roles and responsibilities of supervisors and supervisees, the college's role in credentialling supervisors and maintaining a database of available supervisors in mental health. These guidelines have yet to be discussed at national level and endorsed Australia-wide, although the college's (ANZCMHN Inc., 1995) standards of practice expressly acknowledge the role of clinical supervision in ongoing education, professional growth and support for therapeutic relationships. It is worth mentioning that prior to becoming the college, the former Australian Congress of Mental Health Nurses (1985) documented national standards that recognised the need for supervision where nurses functioned as primary therapists. Almost a decade transpired before clinical supervision was discussed further at national level (ANZCMHN Inc., 1994). The need to formalise clinical supervision arises from its wider recognition for developing practice and providing support (see Western Australia Mental Health Nursing Education Review Group, 1999). To date, formal arrangements exist in the three main east-coast states in local health districts which have formulated specific clinical supervision policies (Northern Sydney Health, 1999; South Eastern Sydney Mental Health Service, 1999; Royal Brisbane Hospital and District [RBH], 1996; Central Sydney Area Mental Health Service, 1994).

Barriers and resistance from clinicians

Armitage (1997) claims that the emotional impact of working with disturbed patients has necessitated introducing clinical supervision in mental health nursing. Clinical supervision will alleviate distress and provide support for increasing autonomy and the isolation associated with primary nursing. **The promise of support, however, has not been met without resistance from clinicians** (O'Sullivan, 1999), **and among clinical supervisors, it is axiomatic that those who need supervision most are those least likely to attend** (Jordan, 1999b). In considering the enormity of change in nurses' working environments, the perceived need for support in managing organisational change (Queensland Health, 1999b, 1998c), the ever growing demands for professional development, the increased patient acuity and severity seen in shorter hospital stays, professional issues surrounding role definition, erosion, diffusion and confusion, along with the apparently constant threat of burnout, it is remarkable that more nurses do not avail themselves of clinical supervision opportunities when available. Mehrtens' (1996) dismay at nurses' reluctance to obtain 'free' clinical supervision, their subsequent non-attendance and the need to recruit participants during significant organisational change in Victoria underscores the low priority given to clinical supervision, compared with other professional activities (Hughes *et al.*, 1996). Even despite supervision contracts (Moffitt and Abbott, 1996), nurses consistently avoid attendance. I note this theme of resistance throughout my outline of the current state of Australian research and practice development on clinical supervision.

Research and practice of clinical supervision

Not surprisingly, a topical research question on clinical supervision concerns identifying barriers in attending, despite organisational commitment, to explore avenues of increasing attendance (Armitage *et al.*, 1996, 1997). During 1995, Jordan (1996) used multiple methods to conduct clinical supervision workshops and measure nurses' levels of burnout pre- and post-participation in formal clinical supervision at the Rozelle Hospital. The one-day experiential workshops implemented role-play and facilitated discussions on models and definitions of clinical supervision, their application to mental health nursing, associated legal-ethical issues, supervisor characteristics and identifying support for clinical supervision. After the workshops, 81 per cent of participants could acknowledge managerial support for clinical supervision compared with 44.65 per cent before the study, although burnout incidence was more complicated to interpret. Jordan's (1997) statistical analysis of Maslach and Jackson (1981) burnout scales revealed that all nurses scored highly on depersonalisation [DP] and emotional exhaustion [EE] dimensions. These indicate high degrees of burnout, but nurses' higher scores on personal accomplishment [PA] levels indicate low degrees of burnout. According to

Maslach and Jackson (1994), it is the *intensity* of the professional relationship that predisposes to burnout, and this is reflected in the study's findings that clinical nurse specialists/consultants reported the highest levels of burnout, and nursing managers the lowest – matching direct patient contact. Jordan also found those most at risk to burnout were younger and less educated nurses. Although her study demonstrated decrease in burnout levels in two groups receiving clinical supervision, Jordan (1997) is right to point out that burnout is a slow insidious process which does not respond quickly to single interventions. At best, clinical supervision has the potential to act as a buffer, or shock absorber, protecting against burnout.

Cleary's (1997) qualitative aspects of this study sought to identify barriers by clarifying how nurses perceive clinical supervision. She interviewed ten practising clinicians to ascertain their ideas, opinions and attitudes. After first exploring their knowledge of clinical supervision, Cleary introduced a shared definition to enable better understandings between researcher and participant. While all ten participants reported the availability of informal support networks, their need for formal clinical supervision remained ambivalent. Later Cleary *et al.* (1999) relate that many nurses believe teamwork provides a degree of supervision. This perception resonates with ideas that clinical supervision already occurs informally – in supportive networks among colleagues, in friendships outside of work (Cleary, 1996) and in spontaneous debriefing (Jordan, 1994). Clearly, many nurses need to review practice at times of crises, rather than wait for an appointment (Williams, 1996). In Williams' (1996) survey of nurses, seventy-three per cent believed they understood the concept, while fifty-four per cent claimed previous experience of clinical supervision. It is not uncommon to find broad definitions which include clinical reviews, discussions with doctors and even compulsory managerial accountability meetings (Fiorillo and Roche, 1996).

Jordan's (1997: 77) retrospective comment on the Rozelle Hospital study captures the magnitude of introducing formal clinical supervision into a nursing culture that had not established it from inception (Yegdich and Cushing, 1998):

> to attempt to simultaneously educate nurses, to change nursing practice, to challenge the accepted systems of nursing care delivery, and to conduct research was … an overly ambitious undertaking in the same study.

While the study pioneered by placing clinical supervision squarely on the agenda for nurses, it is no exaggeration to claim persistent confusion on differences between clinical, managerial and professional supervision. I have summarised some aspectual features in Table 18.2.

Also pioneering is the work undertaken in Northern Sydney Health by O'Sullivan (1996), who began offering mandatory clinical supervision to in-patient mental health nurses twelve years ago. Although first met with resistance, clinical supervision has been extended to all nurses and its increasing

Table 18.2 Key differences between clinical, managerial and professional supervision

Classification of Supervision			Clinical, Managerial, Professional.
	Outcomes	*Tools*	*Role*
Clinical	• Knowing the *particular* patient. • Develops clinical decision-making, clinical judgment. • Develops psychotherapeutic nurse–patient interactions. • Acknowledges primacy of nurse–patient relationship. • Values individual's work – professional support.	Focus on nurse-supervisee–supervisor–patient triad. Case studies in depth. Exploring nurse–patient interactions. Use a variety of theoretical approaches. **Not** a performance appraisal tool, but can be an objective on performance plan.	Clinical supervisor – No designated position – (e.g. educator, clinician with specialised training). Specialised training includes own supervision of clinical work. Supervisor needs skills in clinical work and clinical teaching. Differentiated from on-line manager / senior professional with managerial authority.
Managerial* Due to mandatory and fundamental nature often a shared responsibility.	• Works within organisational structures. • Promotes accountability. • Maintains policies, procedures and protocols of particular organisation. • Works towards shared vision and philosophy of unit.	Mandatory appraisal Performance appraisal. Organisational policy and procedures. Mission statement. shared vision.	Direct reporting officer – Designated position – (e.g. team leader, on-line manager – CNC, NUM, NPC, ADON, DON). Leadership training. Specialised management skills – enabler and envisioner.
Professional	• Works within structures of particular profession. • Maintains Code of Ethics, Competencies and Standards of profession. • Safeguards practice. • Provides foundation for autonomous practitioner. • Advances profession. • Protects public.	Can be linked to performance appraisal. Statutory bodies. Professional organisations. *Nursing in Australia*: ANCI Inc. Competencies. Public Sector Codes of Conduct. Nurses' Registration Boards, Councils. Nursing Code of Conduct. ANZCMHN Inc. Standards.	Professional senior – usually in conjunction with direct reporting officer, on-line manager (eg. CNC, NUM, NPC, ADON, DON).

*Also referred to as organisational, administrative, operational supervision.

Australian Classifications.
    CNC: Clinical Nurse Consultant.
    NUM: Nursing Unit Manager (Nurse Manager).
    NPC: Nurse Practice Coordinator.
    ADON: Assistant Director of Nursing.
    DON: Director of Nursing.

acceptance has led to voluntary participation. With full support from both nursing and medical management, clinical supervision is formalised on weekly, fortnightly or monthly bases to various specialities including aged psychiatry, community mental health and intensive care, with other specialities soon to commence. Most clinical supervision occurs within group format which suits community settings, whereas shift-workers are more difficult to engage even for individual clinical supervision (O'Sullivan, 1999). Initial staff satisfaction surveys show pleasing results and O'Sullivan intends to pilot a small trial using burnout scales and a locally developed Hope scale (Duffell scale) to measure clinical supervision efficacy. While surely time and resource shortages impact on implementation, passive resistance excuses heavy workloads, low morale and job satisfaction while blaming a lack of clinical supervision culture, benefits, support and supervision for supervisors (Hughes *et al.*, 1996). Needless to say, supervisors as well as managers must give clinical supervision high priority for it to succeed (Neville, 1996).

O'Sullivan conducts training programmes and two-day workshops around New South Wales for nursing and allied health staff. Such information sessions and workshops promote clinical supervision availability and understanding; however, simply saying clinical supervision has value does little to encourage participation (Mehrtens, 1996). Many nurses feel comfortable with their clinical practice (Cleary, 1996), and experienced nurses do not see the need for clinical supervision (Hughes *et al.*, 1996). The opportunity to improve one's ability to be helpful to others (Castles, 1996) may, paradoxically, present helpers with a 'sense of burden' (Jordan, 1996).

Further developments on researching clinical supervision effectiveness are occurring in the South Eastern Sydney Area in collaboration with the Academic Department of Mental Health Nursing, University of Technology, Sydney (Gill *et al.*, 1999). According to Stühlmiller (1999a), widespread demoralisation had occurred among nurses in the past three years. By identifying and elevating good practices, clinical supervision will restore *esprit de corps*. Stühlmiller has trained 33 senior clinical mental health nurses to facilitate group clinical supervision within four major hospitals, thus ensuring clinical supervision access to all mental health nurses (over 200). Her metaphor, 'clinical soup' (Stühlmiller, 1999b) relates to the nourishment a supportive environment provides for nurses to review and advance their repertoire of interactive skills, gain confidence and experience camaraderie. To determine the programme's effectiveness, Stühlmiller has collected demographic information and pre-initiative data using an array of scales that measure work satisfaction, burnout and emotional well-being. She hypothesises that as nurses reflect on practice, they will effectively manage the stress and challenge of interpersonal work and develop work satisfaction.

Whereas most studies focus on clinical supervision efficacy in terms of nurses' stress levels and need for support, my own supervisory work tends to view these factors as secondary to a primary educational role. The reports of resistance would suggest that this purpose is much harder to achieve than providing staff support mechanisms, although clearly, clinical supervision could not flourish without a 'nurturing environment' (Jordan, 1994) – with support at various levels: fundamental professional regulation and accountability, an enabling management that provides access to staff counselling, debriefing, recognition and reward. To help combat resistance, my anecdotal experience informs that clinical supervision needs to be viewed within a whole perspective of education that includes didactic elements. As clinical supervision develops therapeutic skills, it makes sense to situate it and complement it with a formal course of supportive counselling skill development (RBH, 1998), for example, whereby participants are introduced to the notion of discussing their own clinical work. My assessment of clinical supervision effectiveness centres on supervisee progress in 'knowing the patient' (Benner *et al.*, 1996) – this is immediate within an ongoing supervisory process, in contrast to waiting for problematic work events to arise, and can take various forms of both a qualitative and quantitative nature.

Mandating clinical supervision

To meet 'work-related support needs' in Victoria, all mental health services stress the need to enhance professional development through clinical supervision (Garlick, 1996). The mandatory nature of minimum attendance and sharing supervision between on-line managers and discipline seniors to address organisational, professional and personal objectives, suggests that clinical supervision could deteriorate into managerial supervision. Wilson (1996) debates the importance of separating managerial from clinical supervision in terms of progressing supervisees from discussing cases to analysing their own responses within the therapeutic relationship. It is unlikely that such intimate detail would be exposed to supervisors holding administrative authority (Yegdich, 1999a). Indeed, Garlick admits that in the shared-responsibility model, supervisees are uncertain about what issues to take to which supervisor.

Most Australian authors concur that it is imperative to separate clinical supervision from staff appraisal and organisational issues for purposes of learning. Fiorillo and Roche (1996) convey that eighty per cent of nurses surveyed believed clinical supervision should be mandatory and ninety per cent believed there should be a choice about supervisors. As in undergraduate clinical teaching, supervisors' professional credibility is crucial for success (Cross, 1997). The problem with mandating clinical supervision is simply put: one cannot legislate trust, openness or relationships (Madison *et al.*, 1994). Nor does it make sense to offer compulsory support.

Future directions

Clinical supervision has been slow to captivate clinician participation and demand, and even less the attention of academics. So far, professional organisations have neither developed policies or position statements, nor ensued a fundamental understanding of its tenets and role. That academics and clinicians are referring to different meanings of supervision is evident from Hart's (1996) equation of undergraduate clinical facilitation with clinical supervision, in contrast to Wilson's (1996) recommendation to introduce clinical supervision to undergraduates and secure greater acceptance. In its scathing critique of both undergraduate and postgraduate education of future mental health nurses, the recent Scoping Study on Australia's mental health nursing workforce (Commonwealth Department of Health and Aged Care, 1999: 37) completely neglected to mention its struggling existence – while acknowledging that university courses 'lag behind the practice of experienced mental health nurses'. The ACT college branch document (ANZCMHN Inc., 1996) on regulatory practices which notes the loss of psychiatric-mental health endorsement in most states and territories could provide national impetus for more rigorous implementation of clinical supervision for nurses working in mental health areas without specialist education. The college is silent.

Where Wilson (1996) notes lack of agreement on the theoretical and practical aspects of clinical supervision, Jordan (1999a) argues for a range of approaches to meet the demands of the clinical environment. The uniqueness of clinical supervision as an educational strategy is its triadic structure of nurse-supervisee, supervisor and patient (Yegdich, 1999b). Figure 18.1 illustrates this triad and situates managerial and professional supervision as the supporting foundation for clinical supervision.

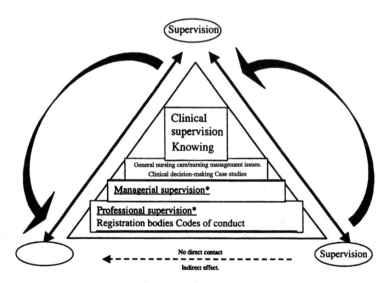

*Clinical supervision is differentiated from managerial and professional supervision although based on their mandatory accountabilities.

Figure 18.1 The triadic structure of clinical supervision

Clearly, supervisory focus is on the nurse (Yegdich, 1994), and not the patient. But nurses are not isolated individuals reflecting on themselves. Clinical supervision emphasises nurses' responses to patients within the nurse-patient relationship, and therefore, the supervisee's privacy is not sacrificed (Kermode, 1985). Understanding the patient emerges from engaging in a process of decentring (Munhall, 1993), that tolerates uncertainty rather than explicating tacitly embedded knowledge. For Chesterson (1996), the nurse's therapeutic use of self in nurse–patient interactions presupposes self-reflection. This is precisely what is impossible (Yegdich, 1996) – and why clinical supervision is needed (Yegdich, 1999c). The first-person nature of our existence means we cannot step outside ourselves to be critical. Supervision provides opportunity to 'oversee' what we cannot see. This is best undertaken within the supportive process of a relationship.

White and Ewan (1995: 139) relate previous experience of students' difficulties in examining what went on interpersonally between patients and themselves; many frankly fudged on 'who said what to whom'. There are many reasons for avoiding discussion of nursing work. Lawler (1991b) refers to nursing's intense privacy 'imbued as it is with body products, death and sexuality'. Therapeutic interaction is no less private or discomforting. The nature of human engagement means the patient's discourse and the nurse's response cannot be known in advance. Human knowing is always in transition (Winnicott, 1967) and thus, the supervisory task lies in developing a disposition of openness to its spontaneity, flexibility and creativity, in contrast to cleverly solving the patient's problems.

Gray and Forrstrom (1995) pose whether reflection on individual practice will have use only for the individual concerned, or will it have meaning for the whole profession. Clinical supervision inquiry brings us closer to the concerns of patients and to explore that place nurses occupy in relation with them. There is constant struggle with narcissism in the effort to 'know the patient'. If the nurse–patient relationship is to become the essence of nursing, nurses need to examine what they say to patients and what they do in the saying.

Conclusion

While little hard data exists to support the importance of clinical supervision for the professional development of those working in caring environments (O'Sullivan, 1999), Stühlmiller (1999a) proposes that clinical supervision establishes conditions under which nurse therapies are effective. This, in turn, increases the viability of a tenuous mental health nursing workforce, counteracts role erosion and demonstrates the central importance of mental health nursing. Indeed, the nurse-patient relationship in all nursing.

Having begun the chapter with reference to a psychoanalytic thinker, I conclude by citing another. Freud (1933: 149) considered teaching one of three impossible professions, noting that, 'education has to find its way between the Scylla of non-interference and the Charybdis of frustration'. For those who would teach, the formidable task of balancing support and challenge creates conditions conducive for the arrival of thought. For those who would learn, the most difficult feat is to learn from one's experience. The supervision encounter invites humility in enjoining both learner and teacher to be instructed by their patients.

Acknowledgements

Acknowledgments are long overdue to Jennifer Carpenter Hall, previous Nursing Director of the Mental Health Centre Royal Brisbane Hospital, whose vision enabled the introduction of clinical supervision, and to Lisa Fawcett, current Nursing Director, who has continued to support the dream and sometimes, nightmare.

My gratitude to Raighne Jordan and Michael Kilshaw.

References

Armitage P (1997) Clinical supervision: Practice gains for the future. Paper presented at the Inaugural Nursing Research Conference: Research for the future, health services and universities in partnership, pp56–59. Health Services and Universities in Partnership, Taree, NSW.

Armitage P Jordan R Cleary M and Cross W (1997) Clinical supervision. Paper presented at the Inaugural Nursing Research Conference: Research for the future, health services and universities in partnership, pp56–83. Health Services and Universities in Partnership, Taree, NSW.

Armitage P Jordan R and Cross W (1996) Clinical supervision in mental health nursing. Paper presented at the Rozelle Annual Winter Symposium: Clinical supervision in mental health nursing, pp123–141. July, Sydney, Australia.

Australian and New Zealand College of Mental Health Nurses Inc. (1994) 20th Annual International Conference: Mental Health – New Directions, October, Brisbane, Qld.

Australian and New Zealand College of Mental Health Nurses Inc. (1995) *Standards of Practice for Mental Health, Nursing in Australia.* Australian and New Zealand College of Mental Health Nurses Inc. ACT Branch, Canberra, ACT.

Australian and New Zealand College of Mental Health Nurses Inc. (ACT branch) (1996) Regulatory practice for mental health nursing (ACT Branch position paper) Australian and New Zealand College of Mental Health Nurses Inc. ACT Branch, Canberra, ACT.

Australian and New Zealand College of Mental Health Nurses Inc. (ACT branch) (1998) Guidelines on clinical supervision (Draft) Australian and New Zealand College of Mental Health Nurses Inc. ACT Branch, Canberra, ACT.

Australian Congress of Mental Health Nurses (1985) *Standards of Mental Health Nursing Practice.* ACMHN, Greenacres, SA.

Australian Nursing Council Inc. (1993) *National Competencies for the Registered and Enrolled Nurse in Recommended Domains.* Australian Nursing Council, Canberra ACT.

Australian Nursing Council Inc. (1998) *ANCI National Competency Standards for the Registered Nurse* (2nd edition draft) August, Australian Nursing Council, Dickson ACT.

Australasian Nurse Registering Authorities Conference (1990) *National Competency Standards for Registered and Enrolled Nurses.* May, ANRAC, Adelaide, SA.

Barnett T (1992) Preceptorship. In *Issues in Australian Nursing* 3, pp245–265 (Gray G and Pratt R eds), Churchill Livingstone: Melbourne.

Battersby D and Hemmings I (1991) A study of university nursing graduates during their first year of nursing. Monograph. Charles Sturt University, Riverina, NSW.

Beattie H (1998) Clinical teaching models: A review of the role of preceptor in the undergraduate nursing programme. *Australian Journal of Advanced Nursing* 15(4), pp14–18.

Benner P (1984) *From Novice to Expert: Excellence and Power in Clinical Nursing Practice*. Menlo Park, California: Addison Wesley.

Benner P Tanner C A and Chesla C A (eds) (1996) *Expertise in Nursing Practice, Caring, Clinical Judgement and Ethics*. New York: Springer.

Brown N Forrest S and Pollock L C (1998) The ideal role of the nurse teacher in the clinical area: A comparison of the perspectives of mental health, learning difficulties and general nurses. *Journal of Psychiatric and Mental Health Nursing* 5, pp11–19.

Butterworth T (1992) Clinical supervision as an emerging idea in nursing. In Butterworth T and Faugier J (eds), *Clinical Supervision and Mentorship in Nursing*, pp3–17, London: Chapman & Hall.

Butterworth T (1996) An introduction to clinical supervision and its evaluation in twenty-three sites in England and Scotland Paper presented at the Rozelle Annual Winter Symposium: Clinical supervision in mental health nursing, July, Sydney, Australia, pp1–18.

Butterworth T Carson J White E Jeacock J Clements A and Bishop V (1997) It *is* good to talk, an evaluation study in England and Scotland. School of Nursing Studies, University of Manchester.

Butterworth T and Faugier J (eds) (1992) *Clinical Supervision and Mentorship in Nursing*. London: Chapman & Hall.

Caldwell B J and Carter E M A (1993) The workplace of the 1990s. In Caldwell B J and Carter E M A (eds), *The Return of the Mentor: Strategies for Workplace Learning*, pp1–8, London: The Falmer Press.

Carruthers J (1993) The principles and practice of mentoring. In Caldwell B J and Carter E M A (eds), *The Return of the Mentor: Strategies for Workplace Learning*, pp9–24, London: The Falmer Press.

Castles M (1996) Peer supervision in community mental health nursing: A personal perspective paper presented at the Rozelle Annual Winter Symposium: Clinical supervision. in mental health nursing, July, Sydney, Australia, pp51–58.

Central Sydney Area Mental Health Service (1997) Policy and Procedures: Clinical supervision. Central Sydney Area Mental Health Service, Sydney, NSW.

Chesterson J (1996) Clinical supervision: The next step paper presented at the Rozelle Annual Winter Symposium: Clinical supervision in mental health nursing, July, Sydney, Australia, pp68–80.

Clare J Longson D Glover P Schubert S and Hofmeyer A (1996) From university student to registered nurse: The perennial enigma. *Contemporary Nurse* 5(4), pp169–176.

Cleary M (1996) Research data from the interviews on clinical supervision. Paper presented at the Rozelle Annual Winter Symposium: Clinical supervision in mental health nursing, July, Sydney, Australia, pp32–39.

Cleary M (1997) Clinical supervision research study. Paper presented at the Inaugural Nursing Research Conference: Research for the Future, Health services and universities in partnership. pp60–65 Health Services and Universities in Partnership, Taree, NSW.

Cleary M Edwards C and Meehan T (1999) Factors influencing nurse-patient interaction in the acute psychiatric setting: An exploratory investigation. *Australian and New Zealand Journal of Mental Health Nursing* 8, pp109–116.

Commonwealth of Australia (1995) *Enterprising Nation: Renewing Australia's Managers to Meet the Challenges of the Asia-Pacific Century – Report of the*

Industry Task Force on Leadership and Management Skills. (Karpin Report). Australian Government Publishing Service, Canberra, ACT.

Commonwealth of Australia (1997) *National Review of Specialist Nurse Education.* Australian Government Publishing Service, Canberra ACT.

Commonwealth Department of Health and Aged Care (1999) *Scoping Study of the Australian Mental Health Nursing Workforce 1999 Report of the Australian and New Zealand College of Mental Health Nurses to the Mental Health Branch of the Commonwealth Department of Health and Aged Care.* Commonwealth Government, Canberra, ACT.

Commonwealth Department of Human Services and Health (1994) *National Review of Nurse Education* (Reid Report) Australian Government Publishing Service, Canberra ACT.

Corkhill M (1998) Undergraduate clinical practicum and the opportunity to practise skills in preparation for the graduate year: A review of the literature. *Contemporary Nurse* 7, pp80–83.

Cross W (1997) The role of the clinical supervisor Paper presented at the Inaugural Nursing Research Conference: Research for the Future pp79–83 Health services and universities in partnership. Health Services and Universities in Partnership, Taree, NSW.

Crowe M (1994) Problem-based learning: A model for graduate transition in nursing. *Contemporary Nurse* 3(3), pp105–109.

Cutcliffe J R and Proctor B (1998) An alternative training approach to clinical supervision: 2. *British Journal of Nursing* 7(6), pp345–340.

Davies E (1991) The relationship between theory and practice in the educative process. In Gray G and Pratt R (eds), *Towards a Discipline of Nursing.* pp149–170 Melbourne: Churchill Livingstone.

Duke M (1996) Clinical evaluation – difficulties experienced by sessional clinical teachers of nursing: A qualitative study. *Journal of Advanced Nursing* 23, pp408–414.

Dunn S and Burnard A (1992) Contextual factors affecting clinical facilitation in undergraduate nursing. In Yarrow A (ed.), *Teaching Role of Supervision in the Practicum: Cross-faculty Perspectives,* pp113–120. Brisbane: QUT Publications and Printery, QUT.

Ekstein R and Wallerstein R S (1958) *The Teaching and Learning of Psychotherapy.* New York: Basic Books.

Ewan C and White R (1996) *Teaching Nursing: A Self-instructional Handbook.* (1st edition 1984) London: Chapman and Hall.

Farrington A (1995) Defining and setting the parameters of clinical supervision. *British Journal of Nursing* 4(15), pp874–875.

Fiorillo P and Roche M (1996) To be or not to be supervised – that is the question Paper presented at the Rozelle Annual Winter Symposium: Clinical supervision in mental health nursing, July, Sydney, Australia, pp114–122.

Fowler J (1996) The organisation of clinical supervision within the nursing profession: A review of the literature. *Journal of Advanced Nursing* 23, pp471–478.

Fowler J and Chevannes M (1998) Evaluating the efficacy of reflective practice within the context of clinical supervision. *Journal of Advanced Nursing* 27, pp379–382.

Freud S (1933) Explanations, applications and orientations. In Strachey J (trans. and ed.), *New Introductory Lectures on Psychoanalysis.* The Pelican Freud Library, Vol.2, pp170–192. London: Penguin Books.

Garlick R (1996) Clinical supervision for psychiatric nursing paper presented at the Rozelle Annual Winter Symposium: Clinical supervision in mental health nursing, July, Sydney, Australia, pp59–67.

Gill K Roser B Roche M and Wilson I (1999) Building the capacity for nursing clinical supervision paper presented at the Rozelle Annual Winter Symposium: The new millennium: Great expectations, July, Sydney, Australia pp58–63.

Grant E Ives G Raybould J and O'Shea M (1996) Clinical nurses as teachers of nursing students. *Australian Journal of Advanced Nursing* 14(2), pp24–30.

Gray G and Forsstrom S (1995) Generating theory from practice: The reflective technique. In *Towards a Discipline of Nursing*, pp355–372. Melbourne: Churchill Livingstone.

Gray G and Pratt R (eds) (1991) *Towards a Discipline of Nursing.* Melbourne: Churchill Livingstone.

Gray G and Pratt R (eds) (1995) *Scholarship in the Discipline of Nursing.* Melbourne: Churchill Livingstone.

Grealish P and Carroll G (1998) Beyond preceptorship and supervision: A third clinical teaching model emerges for Australian nursing education. *Australian Journal of Advanced Nursing* 15(2), pp3–11.

Greenwood J (ed.) (1996) Nursing theories: An introduction to their development and application. In *Nursing Theory in Australia: Development and Application*, pp1–14. Sydney: HarperCollins.

Hart G (1996) Modelling, teaching and evaluating reflective practice. Paper presented at the Rozelle Annual Winter Symposium: Clinical supervision in mental health nursing, July, Sydney, Australia, pp40–46.

Hart G and Rotem A (1993) The best and the worst: Students' experiences of clinical education. *Australian Journal of Advanced Nursing* 11(3), pp26–33.

Hughes M Mostacchi M and Herron B (1996) Clinical supervision for mental health nurses in SWSAHS 'Setting up the process' paper presented at the Rozelle Annual Winter Symposium: Clinical supervision in mental health nursing, July, Sydney, Australia, pp103–109.

Ives G and Rowley G (1991) A clinical learning milieu: Nurse clinicians' attitudes to tertiary education and teaching. *Australian Journal of Advanced Nursing* 7(4), pp29–35.

James J (1994) Case study 5: Stepney neighbourhood nursing team, Steels Lane Health Centre, London. In Kohner N. (ed.), *Clinical Supervision in Practice*, pp31–36. London: King's Fund Centre.

James J and Proctor N (1991) On mentoring. In Gray G and Pratt R (eds), *Issues in Nursing 3*, Melbourne: Churchill Livingstone.

Jordan R (1994) Clinical supervision in psychiatric/mental health nursing paper presented at ANZCMHN Inc. 20th Annual International Conference, October, Brisbane, pp479–493.

Jordan R (1996) Clinical supervision in mental health nursing: Part 2 – Preparation of nurses paper presented at the Rozelle Annual Winter Symposium: Clinical supervision in mental health nursing, July, Sydney, Australia, pp127–133.

Jordan R (1997) Impact evaluation study of a clinical supervision program for nursing staff at The Rozelle Hospital, Central Sydney Area Health Service paper presented at the Inaugural Nursing Research Conference: Research for the future, health services and universities in partnership, pp66–78. Health Services and Universities in Partnership, Taree, NSW.

Jordan R (1999a) Discussion paper: Clinical supervision for mental health nurses in inpatient settings in Central Sydney Area Health Service Rozelle Hospital, Rozelle.

Jordan R (1999b) Letter dated 9th December, 1999.

Kermode S (1984) The role of the clinical supervisor in college programs. *Australian Nursing Journal* 3(6), pp34–35.

Kermode S (1985) Clinical supervision in nurse education: Some parallels with teacher education. *Australian Journal of Advanced Nursing* 2(3), pp29–45.

Kitchin S (1993) Preceptorship in hospitals. In Caldwell B J and Carter E M A (eds), *The Return of the Mentor: Strategies for Workplace Learning*, pp91–111. London: The Falmer Press.

Ladyshewsky R (1995) *Clinical Teaching: HERDSA Gold Guide No. 1.* Higher Education Research and Development Society of Australasia Inc., ACT, Australia.

Lawler J (1991a) In search of an Australian identity. In Gray G and Pratt R (eds), *Towards a Discipline of Nursing*, pp211–228. Melbourne: Churchill Livingstone.

Lawler J (1991b) *Behind the Screens: Nursing, Somology, and the Problem of the Body.* Melbourne: Churchill Livingstone.

Lumby J (1995) The power of one: The changer and the changed. In Gray G and Pratt R (eds), *Scholarship in the Discipline of Nursing*, pp191–209. Melbourne: Churchill Livingstone.

Madison J (1993) Collaboration through a mentoring experience. Paper presented at Charles Sturt National Nursing Conference, Effective collaboration: Effective practice in nursing April/May 1993.

Madison J Watson K and Knight B A (1994) Mentors and preceptors in the nursing profession. *Contemporary Nurse* 3(3), pp121–126.

Madjar I (1998) Project to review and examine expectations of beginning registered nurses in the workforce 1997: Executive summary. Newcastle: University of Newcastle.

Martin J Simpson F Marchant C Hampson J Baden S and Munday E (1996) Clinical supervision. *Practice Nurse* 11(3), pp159–162.

Maslach C and Jackson S E (1994) *Maslach Burnout Inventory: Human Services Survey* (2nd edition). Palo Alto, California: Consulting Psychologists Press.

Maslach C and Jackson S E (1981) *Human Services Survey* (2nd edition). Consulting Psychologists Press, Palo Alto, California.

McCormick G and Marshall E (1997) Mandatory continuing professional education: A review. *Australian Journal of Physiotherapy* 40(1), pp17–22.

Meehan T Delaney J and Jordan R (1997) Conference Report: The Rozelle Hospital Winter Symposium: Clinical supervision in mental health nursing. *Australian and New Zealand Journal of Mental Health Nursing* 6, pp44–45.

Mehrtens J (1996) Introducing clinical supervision for psychiatric nurses: Experiences of two projects. Paper presented at the Rozelle Annual Winter Symposium: Clinical supervision in mental health nursing, July, Sydney, Australia, pp142–147.

Moffitt C and Abbott E (1996) Developing a clinical supervision system in an acute mental health unit paper presented at the Rozelle Annual Winter Symposium: Clinical supervision in mental health nursing, July, Sydney, Australia, pp29–31.

Munhall P (1993) 'Unknowing': Toward another pattern of knowing in nursing. *Nursing Outlook* 41(3), pp125–128.

Napthine R (1996) Clinical education: A system under pressure. *Australian Nursing Journal* 3(9), pp20–24.

Neville C (1996) Clinical supervision for community mental health nurses: The experiences of a supervisor. Paper presented at the Rozelle Annual Winter Symposium: Clinical supervision in mental health nursing, July, Sydney, Australia, pp47–50.

New South Wales Nurses Registration Board (1998) Letter dated 7 May 1998.

Northern Sydney Health (1999) Area mental health nursing policy on clinical supervision, 4th Draft. Northern Sydney Health, NSW Govt., Sydney.

Nurses Board of Victoria (1998) Letter dated 11 May 1998.

O'Sullivan S (1996) Clinical supervision paper presented at the Rozelle Annual Winter Symposium: Clinical supervision in mental health nursing, July, Sydney, Australia, pp81–86.

O'Sullivan S (1999) Letter dated 16 December, 1999.

Pearson A (1998) Editorial: The competent nurse and continuing education: Is there a relationship between the two? *International Journal of Nursing Practice* 4, p143.

Pelletier D and Duffield C (1994) Is there enough mentoring in nursing? *Australian Journal of Advanced Nursing* 11(4), pp6–11.

Perry M (1988) Preceptorship in clinical nursing education: A social learning theory approach. *Australian Journal of Advanced Nursing* 5(3), pp19–25.

Queensland Health (1999a) *Ministerial Taskforce: Nursing Recruitment, Retention.* QHealth, Qld Govt. Brisbane, Qld.

Queensland Health (1999b) *Supporting Employees Through Organizational Change: 'How To' Guide.* QHealth, Qld Govt. Brisbane, Qld.

Queensland Health (1998) *Managing Organizational Change: 'How To' Guide.* QHealth, Qld Govt. Brisbane, Qld.

Queensland Nursing Council (1997a) *The Role and Functions of the Enrolled Nurse in Queensland.* September, QNC, Brisbane, Qld.

Queensland Nursing Council (1997b) *Policy Statement: Recency of Practice and Fitness and Competence to Practise Nursing.* April, QNC, Brisbane, Qld.

Queensland Nursing Council (1998a) *Registration and Enrolment of Nurses and the ANCI Competencies* October, QNC, Brisbane, Qld.

Queensland Nursing Council (1998b) Letter dated 3 April 1998.

Queensland Nursing Council (1998c) *Scope of Nursing Practice: Decision Making Framework.* August, QNC, Brisbane, Qld.

Queensland Nursing Union (1998) Letter dated 17 April 1998.

Roberts K (1995) Theoretical, clinical and research scholarship: Connections and distinctions. In Gray G and Pratt R (eds), *Scholarship in the Discipline of Nursing,* pp211–226. Melbourne: Churchill Livingstone.

Ross K (1996) Follow the leader. *Australian Nursing Journal* 3(11), pp35–37.

Royal Brisbane Hospital (1996) Clinical supervision: Policy and procedures Mental Health Centre, Royal Brisbane Hospital, Brisbane (Revised 1999).

Royal Brisbane Hospital (1998) Supportive counselling for nurses and mental health nurses Mental Health Centre, Royal Brisbane Hospital, Brisbane.

Rozelle Hospital Winter Symposium (1996) *Clinical Supervision in Mental Health Nursing.* July, The Rozelle Hospital, Sydney.

Saville J and Higgins M (1990) *Supervision in Australia.* (2nd edition). South Melbourne, Victoria: Macmillan.

Schmidt E (1926) Principles and practice of supervision. *American Journal of Nursing* 27(2), pp119–120.

Schön D A (1983) *The Reflective Practitioner, How Professionals Think in Action.* New York: Basic Books.

Sellars E T (2000) Revitalise to survive. *Collegian* 7(1), pp16–22.

Sims S E R (1991) The nature and relevance of theory for practice In Gray G and Pratt R (eds), *Towards a Discipline of Nursing,* pp54–72. Melbourne: Churchill Livingstone.

Smith J P (1995) Conference report: clinical supervision: conference organized by the National Health Service Executives on 29 November 1994 at the National Motorcycle Museum, Solihull, West Midlands, England. *Journal of Advanced Nursing* 21, pp1029–1031.

South Eastern Sydney Area Health Service and Academic Department of Mental Health Nursing University of Technology, Sydney (1999) Area Mental Health Nursing Clinical Supervision Policy SESAHS and ADMHN, UTS, Sydney.

Stockhausen L and Creedy D (1992) Promoting reflection in clinical practice. In Yarrow A (ed.), *Teaching Role of Supervision in the Practicum: Cross-faculty Perspectives,* pp9–21. QUT Publications and Printery, QUT, Brisbane.

Stühlmiller C (1999a) Embracing foundations of nursing in mental health nursing. 25th Annual International Conference: Looking forward – looking back, September, Launceston, Tasmania.

Stühlmiller C (1999b) Clinical soup: Nourishment for mental health nurses paper presented at the ANZCMHN Inc. August, Winter Symposium, Queensland Branch, Gold Coast, Qld.

Sutton F and Smith C (1995) Advanced nursing practice: Different ways of knowing and seeing. In Gray G and Pratt R (eds), *Scholarship in the Discipline of Nursing,* pp133–150. Melbourne: Churchill Livingstone.

Taylor B (1997) Big battles for small gains: A cautionary note for teaching reflective processes in nursing and midwifery practice. *Nursing Inquiry* 4(1), pp19–26.

Teasdale K (1998) Clinical supervision for all. *Professional Nurse* 13(5), p278.

Usher K Nolan C Reser P Owens J and Tollefson J (1999) An exploration of the preceptor role: Preceptors' perceptions of benefits, rewards, supports and commitment to the preceptor role. *Journal of Advanced Nursing* 29(2), pp506–514.

Western Australia Mental Health Nursing Education Review Group (1999) Report of the Review of Mental Health Nursing Education in Western Australia April, Graylands Hospital, WA.

White R and Ewan C (1995) *Clinical Teaching in Nursing.* London: Chapman and Hall.

Williams J (1996) The flight of clinical supervision … pointing or propelling the way forward paper presented at the Rozelle Annual Winter Symposium: Clinical supervision in mental health nursing, July, Sydney, Australia, pp110–113.

Wilson I (1996) Clinical supervision: An essential requirement for mental health nurses or an unnecessary luxury? Paper presented at the Rozelle Annual Winter Symposium: Clinical supervision in mental health nursing, July, Sydney, Australia, pp19–28.

Winnicott D W (1967) The location of cultural experience. In *Playing and Reality.* pp112–121. London: Penguin.

Wright C (1995) Critical issues in nursing: The need for a change in the work environment. *Collegian* 2, pp5–13.

Yarrow A (ed.) (1993) *Teaching Role of Supervision in the Practicum: Cross-faculty Perspectives.* QUT Publications and Printery, QUT, Brisbane.

Yegdich T (1994) Parallels, paradigms, boundaries and barriers: On learning-from the patient and thinking-about the nurse–patient relationship in clinical supervision. Paper presented at ANZCMHN Inc. October, 20th Annual International Conference, Brisbane, Qld. pp459–478.

Yegdich T (1996) Borne to be free: enduring the unthought known in supervision and therapy paper presented at the Rozelle Annual Winter Symposium: Clinical supervision in mental health nursing, July, Sydney, NSW, Australia pp95–102.

Yegdich T (1998) How not to do clinical supervision in nursing. *Journal of Advanced Nursing* 28(1), pp193–202.

Yegdich T (1999a) Clinical supervision and managerial supervision: Some historical and conceptual considerations. *Journal of Advanced Nursing* 30(5), pp1195–1204.

Yegdich T (1999b) Lost in the crucible of supportive clinical supervision: supervision is not therapy. *Journal of Advanced Nursing* 29(5), pp1265–1275.

Yegdich T (1999c) Clinical supervision: Work and play. Paper presented at the ANZCMHN Inc. August, Winter Symposium, Queensland Branch, Gold Coast, Qld.

Yegdich T and Cushing A (1998) A historical perspective on clinical supervision in nursing. *Australian and New Zealand Journal of Mental Health Nursing* 7(1), pp3–24.

19 Clinical supervision in Finland – history, education, research and theory

Marita Paunonen and Kristiina Hyrkäs

Editorial

This chapter focuses on the Finnish perspectives of clinical supervision. It highlights the development of clinical supervision training and provides a summary of the research on clinical supervision that has been undertaken in Finland. The chapter then describes the SUED model of quality assurance: a model that integrates clinical supervision, in service training and further education. The material contained in this chapter appears to indicate that the theory and practice of clinical supervision is well developed in Finland and that like Britain, Finland appears to be providing a lead that other countries may choose to follow.

Introduction

For two decades clinical supervision has been a subject for discussion in Scandinavian countries and as a result a multitude of studies have been published in Finland. Research endeavours have covered, for instance, the effects of clinical supervision on work satisfaction, professional identity and quality of care (see Hyrkäs *et al.*, 1999). Since the majority of these research reports have not been translated into English, their examination is of interest to readers. In Finland, clinical supervision is accepted as a natural part of nursing practice, and official recommendations regarding its organisation have been given. Clinical supervision refers to systematic action after vocational education aiming at developing the supervisees' professional knowledge and skills as well as supporting, clarifying and strengthening professional identity.

In Finland the history of clinical supervision in nursing spans three decades (Niskanen *et al.*, 1988; Paunonen, 1989c). An examination of the studies available shows a close connection to clinical supervisor training. Given this history, more extensive empirical research on the subject dates back to the 1990s (Paunonen, 1989c). So far many of the studies are various academic theses (e.g. master's theses and dissertations), which employ a specific perspective on the topic. Most of the articles published in Finnish discuss clinical supervision at a general level, as opinions and experiences, which seems to be common also in the English speaking countries (Hyrkäs *et al.*, 1999). The current research and literature serve as the foundation for the prevailing practice of clinical supervision and contribute to further research.

In this chapter, the history of clinical supervision is first briefly reviewed as it forms the basis for the practice. The development of clinical supervisor education in nursing is then examined as the training provided by the field itself has also been a significant step forward, from the viewpoint of research. The academic research reports are examined more closely and the difficulties as well as challenges to further research are discussed. As a result of this development span the SUED model is introduced. The model is now in an official proposal state in the Ministry of Social Affairs and Health in Finland to be used as a national obligation to develop health care practitioners' cognitive preparedness in working life (Terveydenhuollon ammatillisten ..., 1999).

The development of clinical supervision in nursing and the beginning of clinical supervisor training for nurses

Clinical supervision started at a slow pace in the Finnish health care system at the end of the 1950s. At that time psychoanalysts, trained abroad, began to organise the practice. Experiments on clinical supervision were launched in the 1960s in psychiatric hospitals, and in the 1970s minor trials were carried out by Balint groups for health centre physicians, in clinical supervisor training for psychiatrists and in allied fields of health care. Clinical supervision expanded to cover the whole field of health care in the 1980s (Niskanen *et al.*, 1988; Paunonen, 1989c)

The beginning of the 1980s was a turning point in Finnish clinical supervision. An extensive survey conducted by a working group appointed by the Ministry of Social Affairs and Health revealed that the need for clinical supervision for example in psychiatric nursing was twice as great as its supply. The lack of suitable clinical supervisors inhibited the efforts to correct the situation (Sosiaali-ja terveysministeriö, 1983). Based on the survey, the Ministry of Social Affairs and Health issued the first recommendation concerning the organisation of clinical supervision. The qualifications required for clinical supervisors were defined as well as the different models of clinical supervision and the healthcare sectors that seemed to be in need of clinical supervision. According to the recommendation, the organisational models of clinical supervision included one-to-one, group, case-load, peer supervision for managers and multidisciplinary team supervision. A distinction was made between real-time and delayed clinical supervision, that is, whether the supervisor was present at the situation or whether the supervisee described the situation to the supervisor. Internal arrangements within the organisation were suggested as preferable and economical ways to organise supervision. Having clinical managers acting as clinical supervisors was considered complex and difficult due to the possible role conflicts. The recommendation stated that clinical supervision should be available by the year 1990 for all who wished to participate (Sosiaali-ja terveysministeriö, 1983).

Originally, clinical supervision for nursing staff was provided mainly by other healthcare professionals, such as doctors, psychologists, hospital chaplains and social workers. It became evident that the nursing profession's own expertise would empower clinical supervisor training. This resulted in a model and training being developed specifically for nurses, which was evaluated in 1989 (Paunonen, 1989c, 1991d).

The original clinical supervisor training programme for nurses consisted of lectures and training (360 hours), extending over a period of two years. The purpose of the training was defined as providing specially trained nurses with the basic skills and knowledge required in the supervisor's role. The effort was guided by a theoretical framework emphasising, for instance, different theories of supervision, promotion of personal growth and professional qualifications as well as alleviation and prevention of job fatigue. Apart from studying clinical supervision, participants themselves also provide clinical supervision and are obliged to undergo supervision provided by an experienced supervisor (Paunonen, 1989c, 1991d).

So far, different programmes for supervisor training have been developed and applied for nurses. These have been organised as internal training within hospital organisations in the 1980s and 1990s among others at the Tampere University Hospital. National courses in clinical supervision have also been organised for different occupational groups in healthcare in the 1980s and 1990s at the Open University and in the university institutes for extension studies (see e.g. Leijala, 1988; Oksa, 1997).

In spite of the educational efforts the access to and organisation of clinical supervision has progressed quite slowly. The results from a limited survey (n=110) at the beginning of the 1980s indicate that four per cent of the nurses working in physical health care received clinical supervision (Paunonen, 1982a). The more recent study of Koivula *et al.* (1998) of one of the largest hospital districts in Finland shows that fourteen per cent (n=723) of the nurses with varying educational backgrounds received clinical supervision at the end of the 1990s.

Review of the published research

For the purposes of this chapter, a systematic search of studies and articles on clinical supervision was carried out using Finnish databases. The time period covered was from 1970 to the present. The search yielded 190 references, mainly various academic theses in nursing science, educational studies and medicine as well as in psychology and social work, reports, articles in journals and books, textbooks and books. The academic studies of clinical supervision in nursing were chosen for a closer examination (Table 19.1).

Follow-up studies have been employed to investigate the efficacy of clinical supervision. Paunonen (1989c) using experimental and control groups to investigate the effects of clinical supervision provided weekly sessions for one year in three different health care organisations. The study focused on the nursing

Table 19.1 Summary of the Finnish research on clinical supervision in nursing

Researcher	Data collection, methods of analysis, data	Main results
Paunonen (1989a)	Questionnaire: baseline and at the end Statistical methods and content analysis. Supervisees, experimental group n=113, control group n=88	**CS** clarified nursing towards a more theoretical emphasis, served to expand self-knowledge, make self-image more realistic, enhance professionalism, decrease burnout and develop working climate in a more positive direction.
Korhonen (1990)	Questionnaire Content analysis Supervisees, n=28 Future supervisors, n=28	**CS** was considered useful: its main function is to alleviate workers' psychological pressures and facilitate coping with work. CS is important with regard to the development of nursing. CS provoked both positive and negative feelings. Nurses with supervisor training had a stronger professional identity and self-image than the supervisees.
Paunonen (1991b)	Questionnaire: baseline, at the end and one year later. Statistical methods nurses undergoing supervisor training, n=26	**Changes that took place in nurses' action** during a two-year supervisor training: CS enhanced willingness and freedom to act in nursing and improved nursing action as such.
Aavarinne et al. (1992)	Questionnaire Statistical methods Supervisees, n=171	**CS** is an interactive process, support for mental health, nursing experts' action, promotion of knowledge and skills. One third reported the goal to be personal growth, one fourth the development of collaboration. Haste at work, distressing relations with patients and relatives as well as with other staff, and the exacting nature of nursing gave rise to the need for CS.
Swanljung (1995)	Open interviews Qualitative content analysis Supervisors, n=7	**The dimensions of CS**: examining the characteristics of nursing, analysing care relationships, supporting professional growth and learning, supporting growth as a nursing manager, supporting collegiality and caring.
Kilpiä and Virta (1997)	Questionnaire Statistical descriptive methods Supervisees from five working communities, n=80	Career development is supported by self-appreciation, challenging work, appreciating success in work, commitment, awareness of the goals of the care community, willingness to develop work and support from colleagues. Support for personal development and promotion of collaborative skills were expected of **working community based CS**, but of these were not seen very important with regard to professional development. About half of the respondents were dissatisfied with consistency and sufficiency of training, and with the possibility to attend training during working hours.
Pajala (1997)	Theme interviews Qualitative content analysis Supervisors, n=4	Professional ethics denoted the ability to identify and meet the difficult situations emerging during CS. The supervisor strives for high-quality action, understands the importance of education and of his or her own supervision. Professional ethic denotes identifying the bases for one's action and the goals for CS.

practice and the nurse practitioners' personality and professional identity. Specialist nurses undergoing a two-year supervisor training, designed by the researcher (see in more detail: Paunonen, 1991d), acted as clinical supervisors. The subjects had on average over ten years' experience of nursing. Data were collected simultaneously from experimental and control groups using a questionnaire. The experimental group received clinical supervision and the control group did not. The results showed that clinical supervision had influenced the development of personal characteristics, but had less impact on professional identity. Clinical supervision had promoted the quality of care and especially documentation. As for the reliability of the research, it is noteworthy that rivalry between the groups complicated the research.

The effects of clinical supervision (Paunonen, 1991a) have been studied in conjunction with the clinical supervision associated with a two-year supervisor training. The effects were studied with regard to the nursing practice of the qualified nurses who had completed clinical supervisor training. The focus of interest was on changes in self-reported freedom of actions and willingness to act in attending to the patient's needs. Changes in nursing were examined based on the theory of Yura and Walsh (1983). Data collection was by means of a questionnaire. The results indicate that clinical supervision had promoted the nurses' willingness to act, but also their freedom of action in clinical practice and as a result the nursing care had improved (see also Paunonen, 1991c).

The content and goals of clinical supervision have been described over a period of one year from the perspective of nurses in supervisor training and from that of their supervisees (Korhonen, 1990). Data were collected using a questionnaire from three different types of hospital organisations. **The results indicate that supervisors and their supervisees considered clinical supervision necessary. The most important gain was the decrease in work-related pressures and enhanced coping with work.** Clinical supervision provoked both positive and negative feelings. The supervisors and the supervisees had different goals. Supervisors' goals concerned the supervisory group and its dynamics. Correspondingly, supervisees' goals mainly related to human relations within the teams. Both the supervisors and their supervisees saw the development of nursing practice as important. The supervisors had a stronger professional identity and self-concept than the supervisees.

The content of clinical supervision has been studied also from the supervisors' perspective. Characteristics of clinical supervision in nursing have been described by investigating the conceptions of experienced nurse-supervisors of their work (Swanljung, 1995). The study yielded six main themes. The first theme was nursing and the care relationship, including problematic situations, ethical dilemmas, issues related to the quality of care as well as the supervisee's own expertise and strategies in relation to these. The second was professional growth and learning, incorporating personal knowledge, self-assessment skills and their development as they emerged during clinical supervision. Lastly, clinical supervision as a support for nursing management concerned coping with a variety of tasks and clinical problems in everyday management relationships, and the clarification of the goals of nursing. An important field in clinical supervision in nursing was in developing a collegiate support and caring culture, which requires learning to give and receive support, listening to others and being heard.

The ethical bases of supervisors' professional practice have been studied by interviewing experienced nurse-supervisors (Pajala, 1997). According to the results, the supervisor's self-reflection skills can be considered an important component of professional practice of an ethically high standard. Professional ethic refers to scrutinising and analysing one's actions, outlining and encountering problematic situations (e.g. accountability) as well as the pursuit of high-quality practice (e.g. self-development through education and own personal clinical supervision). The foundation for ethical practice is profound scrutiny of the bases of one's action and of the goals of clinical supervision.

Aavarinne *et al.* (1992) have made an extensive inquiry into the nursing staff's need for clinical supervision. The study was implemented on neurology and medical wards of a Finnish university hospital. Data were collected using a questionnaire. The results showed that the need for clinical supervision was induced by haste, distressing relations with patients and relatives, relations among staff and factors causing uncertainty in work as well as by various administrative factors. **Clinical supervision was described as solving clinical problems, as an interactive process between supervisor and supervisee, as support to mental health and expert practice, as growth in knowledge and skills required by work.** Personal growth, solving of administrative issues and especially the development of collaboration between different occupational groups were seen as the aims of clinical supervision. Ward sisters, assistant ward sisters and specialist nurses, representing different levels of nurse education, considered clinical supervision more necessary than did registered nurses and practical nurses.

Clinical supervision in multiprofessional teams and the effects of clinical supervision on career development were explored on five wards of a university hospital (Kilpiä and Virta, 1997). Data collection was by a questionnaire. The results showed that multidisciplinary supervision teams regarded self-respect, appreciation of colleagues and their work, support provided by colleagues, a challenging job, and a continuous possibility to learn as important with regard to career development. As for personal characteristics, commitment to work was seen as pivotal. First-line managers clearly failed to provide support for the staff, and various problems related to human relations seemed to complicate work, which was considered an impediment to career development, as well. As for career development, participants expressed dissatisfaction with their in-service training. Multidisciplinary teams expected to acquire support for personal development and for improving collaboration skills through clinical supervision. The importance of clinical supervision with regard to professional development was not considered important.

To sum up, the clinical supervision research has focused on two perspectives: supervisees and supervisors. From these points of view the empirical research has covered the different models of supervision, that is, one-to-one, group and team supervisions. Research interests have focused on the effectiveness, content and ethical issues of and need for clinical supervision and support. Both qualitative and quantitative approaches have been applied. **Support provided by clinical supervision for developing personal characteristics seems clearly to emerge as a result from the studies, as does clinical supervision with regard to relationships and team dynamics as well as collaboration between different occupational groups.** However, the results of the studies are partly contradictory with regard to the effects of clinical supervision on e.g. professional identity, professional development, the quality of care and quality management.

Difficulties and challenges to research

Research on clinical supervision is a complex endeavour. So far Finnish researchers have themselves strongly criticised the fact that there is no precise definition of the concept of clinical supervision. (e.g. Hyyppä, 1983; Paunonen, 1989b). If we look at the existing definitions of clinical supervision in the literature (Ojanen, 1983; Niskanen *et al.*, 1988; Paunonen, 1989c; see also Hyrkäs *et al.*, 1999), three major perspectives seem to emerge: the emphasis on the goals, activities and participants of clinical supervision. The critique implies that the core of the concept is missing. It has been explained that in pursuing a definite description definitions have remained rather superficial, and the characteristics and substance of clinical supervision have not been covered. The examination of the literature enables also the conclusion that there are four differing perspectives on the practice of clinical supervision: pedagogical, learning and training, clinical practice and personal growth. What all this means is that the conceptual and theoretical ambiguity is reflected as *confusion in the practice* of clinical supervision, but most of all *in research* (Hyrkäs *et al.*, 1999). The critique is (e.g. Karvinen, 1991) that if the scientific framing of research questions remains inadequate because of the difficulty in defining the concept, then study designs have probably remained insubstantial and the results are an uncritical apology for clinical supervision with no scientific validity. Looking back to the research reports reviewed here, it is easy to expose the problems in defining the concept, but these have also been pointed out and criticised by the researchers themselves. It seems that conceptual clarification presents one of the main challenges for clinical supervision research in Finland.

Data collection for clinical supervision research presents problems of its own. Although hospitals and hospital districts usually have a person or group responsible for the planning, co-ordination and organisation of clinical supervision (Sosiaali-ja terveysministeriö, 1983), there is no extensive or national register of trained supervisors. What this means for research is that hospital districts offer varying information on supervisors and current supervisory relationships, which is found in varying sources and documents (e.g. written agreements on clinical supervision between supervisor and supervisee). Tracking down supervisory relationships is a laborious and slow process. Furthermore, nursing supervisors often work in a different organisation from their supervisees. The use of the so-called external supervisors aims at guaranteeing confidentiality, objectivity and impartiality in supervision (Sosiaali-ja terveysministeriö, 1983; Niskanen *et al.*, 1988). However, with regard to data collection, networking supervisory relationships in different organisations may be confusing when applying for ethical clearance. The number of applications may increase greatly in proportion to the number of supervisees in different organisations.

Both quantitative and qualitative research methods (see Table 19.1) have been employed in the studies of clinical supervision. Qualitative methods are well founded and suitable, if the aim is to explicate supervisees' experiences, conceptions, subjective interpretations or reactions to clinical supervision. As it is known that the generalisation of qualitative research results is not possible, their contribution to the development of clinical supervision is of little importance. Quantitative research has problems of its own. The approach is based on researchers' theoretical assumptions about clinical supervision and its essence. Also generalisation of results, one of the strengths of quantitative research, is not simple. Collection of the large samples needed and the organisation of experimental and control designs is laborious, almost impossible, as was shown earlier. This means for example, that it is hard to scientifically show the efficacy of clinical supervision. Another difficulty with quantitative research has been the absence of suitable instruments. So far the researchers have designed a questionnaire for each study, which makes it impossible to make, e.g. broader comparisons. In addition to this, national surveys of the current situation into clinical supervision have not been made since the survey by the Ministry of Social Affairs and Health in 1983.

The process-like nature of clinical supervision seems to complicate the study of the phenomenon. In the literature (e.g. Niskanen *et al.*, 1988) clinical supervision is most often described as occurring in three different stages: the introductory, the implementation and the consolidation stages. In this process the supervisee is assumed to review together with another person/persons (supervisor and optionally with other supervisees) his or her clinical work and relevant aspects of reactions to that work. However, it is not possible to determine the pace and duration of the process, since the process might be interrupted or even fail to start properly. An additional difficulty is that clinical supervision is a multi-layered process of thought and practice concerning both the supervisor and supervisee, the explication of which is hard by means of research. In the Finnish literature, clinical supervision has also been considered a research method in itself, which has further served to confuse the matter while exploring phenomena and questions during the process. The point here is that as clinical supervision is a reflective process related to professional practice, the boundaries with regard to action research are easily blurred (see e.g. Karvinen, 1991). Empirical research is a challenge from this point of view, that is, the research method employed needs to be critically selected, but the chosen method also needs to be evaluated across the study process to maintain scientific rigour.

A number of clinical supervision models can be found in the literature (e.g. Niskanen *et al.*, 1988), but also included are several assumptions which have not been studied empirically. For example, one-to-one supervision is assumed to offer more opportunities for participants, team supervision (cross-discipline) is described as inexpensive and attractive in terms of time, but demanding for the supervisor in terms of knowledge from different fields and experience of group dynamics. Group supervision (within one's own discipline) is described as an opportunity to present collectively, for instance, patient cases and discuss nursing care. This approach has come under criticism as too demanding in terms of supervisors' experience of clinical practice as well as having group leader skills and knowledge of group dynamics. Peer supervision for nursing managers and ward sisters, the various models described above, their effects and the comparison of these, the strengths and weaknesses or cost-effectiveness have not been addressed using empirical research. These themes are a challenge to future research with regard to the development and intensification of clinical supervision, but first of all with regard to resource acquisition.

Future prospects: the SUED model as quality assurance in healthcare services

The SUED model as quality assurance in healthcare services presented here suggests that integration of clinical supervision, in-service training and further education would be most beneficial in order to support and promote the nursing practitioners' professional development as a continuous process. Paunonen's model, hereafter the 'SUED' model, takes its name from concepts *succeed, supervision and education*. The first concept refers to quality assurance, the second to the principles of clinical supervision, and the third to the principles of education: experiential learning and critical thinking. Apart from establishing the efficacy of clinical supervision and education, the model strives to gain synergy in multidisciplinary teams. The development, planning and testing of the model dates back to the late 1980s (Paunonen, 1989c). It was first tested and published in an academic dissertation (Paunonen, 1989c), and its suitability has been further tested in the 1990s at Tampere University Hospital alongside a cost–benefit analysis.

In Finland, administrative studies (e.g. Paunonen *et al.*, 1996) have found that collaboration in multidisciplinary teams is defective and problematic. The fact that healthcare practitioners are trained in separate educational programmes may be the reason for this. However, it is expected that all parties are familiar and ready to collaborate. The different disciplines may have no experience of working together and in addition, individual team members' competence profiles may not have been outlined. Multidisciplinary clinical supervision brings out the competence of a team, thus yielding the possibility to gain synergy.

Nursing practitioners' further education and in-service training after initial nurse training are taken as necessary and in part for granted. Here the in-service training refers to that which is organised at workplaces or outside organisations and financed by healthcare organisations or units on the basis of the practitioner's perceived needs. Further education is more formal, relating to the development of work tasks in particular, the prerequisite for which is constant updating and maintenance of knowledge and skills. However, the examination of further education and in-service training in Finland shows their fragmentary nature. There is no co-ordination at the national, that is, macro level, and no exact regulations have been given, which often results in inconsistencies. There are no exact statistics available regarding the target groups, the amount, duration or content areas of education and clinical supervision. Similar lack of co-ordination manifests itself in individual healthcare organisations and their units. Organisations and their different units are forced to purchase courses in further education based on supply instead of real needs. The practitioners try to find training they perceive as necessary among the supply, but due to the lack of co-ordination at both macro and micro levels this has proven to be difficult, as research has stated (e.g. Työvoimaministeriö, 1981; Sosiaali-ja terveysministeriö, 1983; Suomen Kaupunkiliitto, 1988a).

Further education as well as in-service training can be external but they do not necessarily meet the staff's real needs (e.g. Työpaikkakoulutustoimikunta, 1990) within their own unit, focusing on the substance of the practice. External training may increase theoretical knowledge and be appropriate in this sense, but this is not necessarily always the case. The cost–benefit ratio fails to reach the level of well-planned training and clinical supervision. As the system is rather random in nature it fails to systematically support the professional development of healthcare practitioners.

One central shortcoming is that further education and in-service training are commonly organised separately. However, the ideal would be to integrate all education and clinical supervision so that clinical supervision would be part of the health care practitioners' work and focused towards identifying those areas which need to be addressed through reflection upon work and oneself. This would make quality management, education and clinical supervision more systematic and focus on the content of practice as well as allow continuous professional development and growth.

Introducing the SUED model

The idea and the bases of the model are crystallised in the problems mentioned above. The SUED model has been planned and implemented in health-care organisations (Paunonen, 1989c, 1993b; Terveydenhuollon ammatillisten ... 1999), and it is currently being tested for the second time on five wards at the Tampere University Hospital. The nursing staff and physicians from these five units have participated in the latest research. Final report of the test is now being written and the model's cost–benefit testing is also in progress. Preliminary results clearly show that the model contributes to the quality of practice and practitioners' satisfaction with work, which supports the findings of earlier Finnish research (e.g. Kaltiala and Sorri, 1989; Paunonen, 1989a; Aavarinne *et al.*, 1992; Jakonen-Kaasalainen, 1983; Moilanen, 1994).

The starting point of this model is the idea that the aims, implementation and definition of the quality of practice are specified together with the manager in each unit (Figure 19.1). This also involves the specification of individual practitioners' expertise and its development. Thus, it is possible to draw an individual plan for the implementation in accordance with the person's motivation and commitment to develop the unit's clinical expertise.

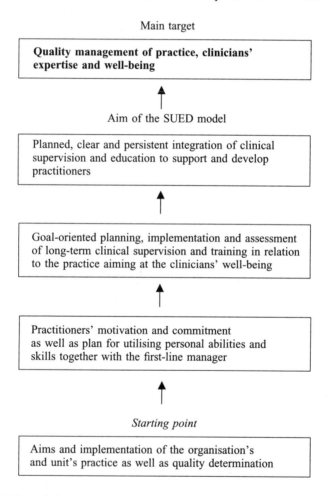

Main target

**Quality management of practice, clinicians'
expertise and well-being**

↑

Aim of the SUED model

Planned, clear and persistent integration of clinical
supervision and education to support and develop
practitioners

↑

Goal-oriented planning, implementation and assessment
of long-term clinical supervision and training in relation
to the practice aiming at the clinicians' well-being

↑

Practitioners' motivation and commitment
as well as plan for utilising personal abilities and
skills together with the first-line manager

↑

Starting point

Aims and implementation of the organisation's
and unit's practice as well as quality determination

Figure 19.1 Description of the general structure of the SUED model

In the long run this process will have a beneficial effect on practice as a whole, as well as on quality and the healthcare practitioners' well-being.

The implementation of the aims of the SUED model emphasises the integration of clinical supervision and in-service training so that clinical supervision is included as a process in each practitioner's work on regular intervals. Clinical supervision identifies areas for development in the practitioner's practice and workload management. In-service training is therefore designed to provide the opportunity to develop the skills and expertise required thus making training and education integrated and purposeful in relation to the practitioner's own work as perceived self-perception (Figure 19.2). Therefore, in-service training and the substance of practice do not remain random. In-service training becomes integral with educational programmes and supports the individual's professional growth as well as meeting the organisational goals.

At present, the implementation of the model may present problems due to the lack of suitably trained supervisors. This can be amended by training supervisors based on needs analysis. Networks can be applied to recruit or train supervisors, by employing educators or educational institutions and by setting up and implementing tailor-made training. It would be advisable to use the network model at least in small organisations to create adequate distance according to the principles of clinical supervision (Figure 19.3). This network system would also include purchased tailor-made services.

In the network model, organisations A, B, C, D etc. jointly implement clinical supervisor training in an appropriate way and implement clinical supervision on the network principle. This indicates that, for example, in the organisation A, clinical supervisors from units A1, A2 and A3 supervise units B1, B2 and B3 from the organisation B etc., or, in a big organisation A, its unit A1 supervises the unit A3, but not other units.

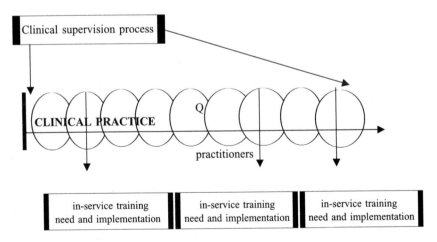

Figure 19.2 Integration of clinical supervision and in-service training to assure the quality of the practice and the healthcare practitioners' well-being

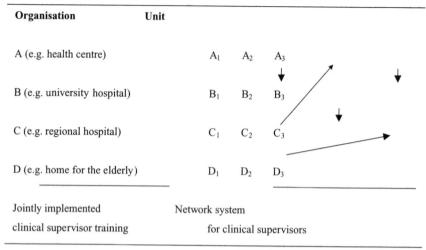

Figure 19.3 Network model for training and clinical supervision of clinical supervisors

It is the task of nursing managers to plan the implementation of clinical supervision and in-service training in collaboration with the practitioners. This involves:

- yearly plan for long-term clinical supervision and appropriate training;
- nominating persons and groups responsible for co-ordination, follow-up, assessment and development of practice;
- definition of the aims of and need for clinical supervision and training in the organisation and its units;
- organising clinical supervision and associated training according to the network model presented above;
- follow-up and assessment of and research into the effects of clinical supervision and education, as well as further development of this practice.

Summary

Clinical supervision, its research and theoretical development in nursing in Finland seems to be entering a new era. Although clinical supervision has been accepted as part of nursing, its popularity and utilisation for professional growth have expanded at a relatively slow pace among healthcare practitioners. Except for individual experiments, utilisation of clinical supervision, for example, in the development of multi-professional collaboration and quality improvement in nursing, has remained scarce. Finnish healthcare staff have not necessarily made the best use of the possibilities offered by clinical supervision. Conceptual ambiguity might be one of the reasons for this. This has led to the fact that while talking about clinical supervision in the press and in the literature, the tone and emphasis used have varied greatly. This has brought about ambiguous conceptions of clinical supervision, partly on account of its roots being embedded in psychiatry and partly because of insufficient knowledge of the phenomenon itself. Future nursing practitioners will probably have a clearer idea of the meaning and value of clinical supervision, because at the moment clinical supervision is incorporated in healthcare education and its curricula. The practice is, however, still heterogeneous, since it is up to the educational institutions to decide the way they wish to include clinical supervision in the training they provide.

So far, the extent of research into clinical supervision in nursing in Finland is not great, which is probably caused by the slow expansion of the popularity of clinical supervision. Research interests have included, for example, the effects and content of and the need for clinical supervision, as well as ethical issues. More research into these areas is needed to generate deeper knowledge. Furthermore, experiments on various new methods (e.g. empathy-based stories) present a challenge for future research. Additionally, clinical supervision has several topical areas, which have yet not been addressed by means of empirical research. The most interesting and challenging areas are, for example, various modes of clinical supervision and their efficacy as well as analysis of the cost–benefit ratio of clinical supervision.

Development work on theories and models of clinical supervision in Finland in nursing science seems to be in progress. So far, models generated in other disciplines have been utilised (e.g. Vienola, 1995), for example, the systems theoretical model of clinical supervision developed in educational studies by Hyyppä (1983). The development of the SUED model, applicable to health care, was launched at the end of the 1980s and it has been tested more extensively at the end of the 1990s. The central idea of the model is to incorporate clinical supervision, in-service and further training in each practitioner's work as a continuous process, whose aim is to support the staff, professional development and quality improvement in nursing. Encouraged by the good experiences of the model and by the research results obtained, the Ministry of Social Affairs and Health has showed increasing interest in the model so that by the time this chapter was written, it had appointed a committee to consider proposals for the national introduction of the SUED model as part of the system of in-service training in hospitals and health centres. The model will be further developed on the basis of experiments in health care and of pilot studies directed at allied fields (e.g. social work).

References

Aavarinne H Halvari H and Piri R (1992) Työnohjauksen lähtötilanteen selvittäminen: Hoitohenki-lökunnan käsityksiä työnohjauksesta ja sen tarpeesta (Analysis of the initial situation of clinical supervision: nursing staff's views of supervision and its necessity). Hoitotiede 4 (1), pp9–16.
Hyrkäs K Koivula M and Paunonen M (1999) Clinical supervision in nursing in the

1990s – current state of concepts, theory and research. *Journal of Nursing Management* (7), pp177–187.

Hyyppä H (1983) Avointen järjestelmien teoria työohjauksen viitekehyksenä (The theory of open systems as a framework for work counselling). Oulun yliopiston kasvatustieteiden tiedekunnan tutkimuksia 17, Oulu.

Jakonen-Kaasalainen E (1983) Ryhmän työnohjauksen vaikutukset sosiaali-ja terveydenhuoltoalan työntekijöihin (The effects of group clinical supervision on welfare and health workers). Turun yliopisto, Psykologian laitos, Turku.

Kaltiala R and Sorri P (1989) Lääkärien työnohjaus yleissairaalassa (Clinical supervision for physicians in a general hospital) *Suomen Lääkärilehti* 25, pp2454–2459.

Karvinen S (1991) Työnohjaus sosiaalityön ammatillisuuden vaalijana (Clinical supervision as preservation of professionalism in social work). In: Sosiaalityö ja työnohjaus. Sosiaalityön vuosikirja Helsinki: VAPK-kustannus, pp7–53.

Kilpiä P and Virta M (1997) Urakehitys moniammatillisessa hoitoyhteisössä työnohjauksen tukemana. Alkumittaus urakehitysmallin testaamisessa (Career development in a multiprofessional healthcare team supported by clinical supervision. The preliminary study of the career development model). Pro gradu-tutkielma Tampereen yliopiston hoitotieteen laitos Tampere.

Korhonen T (1990) Työnohjaus hoitohenkilökunnan näkökulmasta (Clinical supervision from the nursing staff's perspective). Pro gradu-tutkielma. Kuopion yliopiston hoitotieteen ja terveydenhuollon laitos. Kuopio.

Leijala H (toim) (1988) Etelä-Pohjanmaan Keskussairaalan työnohjaajakoulutuksessa olevien työntekijöiden seminaarityöt työnohjauksesta (Written assignments of the workers participating in clinical supervisor training at Southern Ostrobothnia Central Hospital). Seinäjoki.

Niskanen P Sorri P and Ojanen M (1988) Auta auttamaan – käsikirja työnohjauksesta (Helping to help – Clinical supervision manual). Werner Söderström Oy, Porvoo.

Ojanen S (1983) Työnohjauksen teoriat (Theories of clinical supervision). In: Siltala P 1983 (ed.) 1983 Työnohjaus terveydenhuollossa ja opetustyössä. Weilinand and Göös, Espoo pp19–35.

Oksa L (1997) Hoitotyön työnohjaus. Hoitotyön työnohjauksen kehittäminen 1991–1997 (Clinical supervision in nursing. The development of clinical supervision in nursing in 1991–1997). Pirkanmaan sairaanhoitopiirin julkaisuja. Tampereen yliopistollinen sairaala. Nokia.

Pajala H (1997) Hoitotyön työnohjaajan ammattietiikka (The professional ethic of a supervisor in nursing). Pro gradu -tutkielma. Tampereen yliopiston hoitotieteen laitos. Tampere.

Paunonen M (1982a) Sairaalan toimipaikkakoulutuksen ja työnohjauksen nykytilasta ja kehittämis-tarpeesta (Current state and need for developing on-the-job training and clinical supervision in a hospital setting). Pro gradu -tutkielma. Turun yliopisto kasvatustieteiden laitos. Turku.

Paunonen M (1991a) Changes initiated by a nursing supervision programme: An analysis based on loglinear models. *Journal of Advanced Nursing* 16, pp982–986.

Paunonen M (1991c) Promoting nursing quality through supervision. *Journal of Nursing Staff Development* 87 (5), pp229–233.

Paunonen M (1991d) Testing a model for counsellor supervision in three public health care organizations *Nurse Education Today* 11, pp270–277.

Paunonen M (1993b) Terveydenhuollon koulutuksen ja potilaan hoidon kehittäminen terveyden ja hyvinvoinnin edistämiseksi (Developing health care education and patient care to promote health and well-being). In: Salminen H (ed.) Haasteita sosiaali-ja terveudenhuollon koulutukselle. Opetushallitus, Helsinki pp84–90.

Paunonen M Hyrkäs K and Laakso H (1996) URA-projekti – hoidon laadun hallinta työnohjausinterventiona. Hoitamisen näyttämö – mitä siellä tapahtuu. (The CAREER project – quality management of care as a supervisory intervention. The scene of caring – what is happening). IV kansallinen hoitotieteellinen konferenssi 27–28.9.1996. Hoitotiede. Pro Nursing ry:n vuosikirja. Julkaisusarja A 10 pp184–191.

Sosiaali-ja terveysministeriö (1983) Työnohjautyöryhmän muistio. (Ministry of Social Affairs and Health. Report of the working group on clinical supervision). Helsinki.

Swanljung S (1995) Hoitotyön työnohjaus työnohjaajina toimivien sairaanhoitajien kokemana (Supervision in nursing – the experiences of supervising nurses). Pro gradu-tutkielma. Tampereen yliopiston hoitotieteen laitos. Tampere.

Työvoimaministeriö (1981) Työohjaus työvoimahallinnossa (Clinical supervision in labour administration). Helsinki.

Vienola V (1995) Systeemiteoriaan pohjautuva kaksivuotinen työnohjaajakoulutus – toiminta-tutkimuksellinen tapaustutkimus (System theoretical two year supervisor training course – case study and action research). Joensuun yliopiston kasvatustieteellisiä julkaisuja No 23, Oulu.

Literature and reports in Finnish

Aalto K (1985) Työnohjaus, ammatillisen kasvun avain (Clinical supervision, the key to professional growth). Kirjapaja, Hämeenlinna.

Aalto M (1986) Työnohjauksen tarve ja merkitys terveydenhuollossa (The need for and meaning of clinical supervision in health care). *Sairaala* (49), 2, pp52–54.

Aalto M (1988) Työnohjaus tänään (Clinical supervision today) In: Sairaalaliitto, Työnohjaus, Vammalan Kirjapaino Oy, Vammala.

Antikainen P (1995) Tarvitseeko anstesiahoitaja työnohjausta? (Does an anaesthetic nurse need clinical supervision). *Spirium* (29), 4, pp5–6.

Brettschneider G (1983) Työnohjaus ja sen tavoitteet (Clinical supervision and its goals). In: Siltala P *Työnohjaus terveydenhuollossa ja opetustyössä*. Weilin and Göös, Espoo.

Ehrnrooth A (1985) Hoitohenkilökunnan työnohjaus (Clinical supervision of nursing staff). *Ylihoitajalehti* (13), 4, pp8–10.

Himanen M-R and Närväinen K (1985) Työnohjauksen tarpeeseen johtavien ongelmien kartoittamista anestesia-ja leikkausosastoilla (An exploration of the problems leading to the need for clinical supervision in anaesthetic and operating units). Turun sairaanhoito-oppilaitoksen julkaisuja A Turkuoitotyön työnohjaus. (Clinical supervision in nursing) *Ylihoitajalehti* (17), 2, pp74–78.

Karila I (1987) Ehdotus työnohjauksen periaate-ja toteuttamissuunnitelmaksi Helsingin kaupungin terveysvirastossa (Proposal for the implementation of clinical supervision in the health care administration of the city of Helsinki). Helsingin kaupungin terveysviraston raportteja B Helsinki.

Karpoff H-R (1997) Terveydenhoitajien kokemuksia psyykkisestä työkyvystään sekä työnohjauksen merkityksestä siihen (Public health nurses' experiences of their mental work ability and the impact of clinical supervision). Espoon-Vantaan ammattikorkeakoulun julkaisusarja A Vantaa.

Koivula M, Paunonen M and Laippala P (1998) Prerequisites for quality improvement in nursing. *Journal of Nursing Management* 6, pp333–342.

Kukkola H (1990) Työnohjaus työyhteisön kehittämistyössä: vanhainkodin kehittämisprojektin eräs toimintamuoto (Clinical supervision in the development of working communities: a strategy of a development project in a home for the elderly). Vanhus-ja lähimmäispalvelun liitto Helsinki.

Kukkola H (1993) Consultation in developing the working community: one way of developing the old people's homes. Association of services for the old-aged and neighbours. Helsinki (Työnohjaus vanhustenhoidossa).

300   *Marita Paunonen and Kristiina Hyrkäs*

Lahti P (1981a) Työnohjaus tarpeen terveydenhuoltoalalla (The healthcare sector needs supervision). *Tehy* 1, pp30–33.

Lahti P (1981b) Työnohjaus työterveyshoitajan työssä (Clinical supervision in occupational nurse's work). *Työterveyshoitaja* 1, pp6–8.

Moilanen L (1994) Työnohjausryhmät toimintakyvyn tukena (Clinical supervisory groups as support for functional capacity). In: Lindström K (ed.) (1994) *Terve työyhteisö – kehittämisen malleja ja menetelmiä*. Työterveyslaitos, Helsinki pp138–153.

Outinen M, Haverinen R and Maaniitty M *et al.* (1995) Laadunhallinta sosiaali-ja terveydenhuollossa. Valtakunnallinen suositus sosiaali-ja terveydenhuollon laadunhallinnan järjestämisestä ja sisällöstä (Quality management in social welfare and health care. National recommendation for the organisation and content of quality management in social welfare and health care). STAKES, Helsinki.

Palmgren H (1980) Osaston hallinnon työnohjaus ja osastonhoitaja (Managerial supervision and the ward nurse). *Sairaanhoitaja* (56), 16, pp30–31.

Paunonen M (1982b) Työnohjaus terveydenhoitajan ammatti-identiteetin selkeyttäjänä ja vahvistajana (Clinical supervision and the public health nurse's professional identity) *Terveydenhoitaja – Hälsovårdaren* 4, pp11–13.

Paunonen M (1983a) Ammatti-identiteetti ja työnohjaus. (Professional identity and clinical supervision). *Ylihoitaja* 8, pp4–10.

Paunonen M (1983b) Sairaalan toimipaikkakoulutuksen teoreettisten lähtökohtien tarkastelua ja empiirinen tutkimus sen nykytilasta ja kehittämistarpeista (Examination of the theoretical bases of on-the-job training in a hospital and an empirical study of its current state and development needs). *Sairaanhoidon vuosikirja* XIX, pp327–361.

Paunonen M (1985) Hoitotyöntekijöiden toimipaikkakoulutus ja työnohjaus (On-the-job training for nursing practitioners and clinical supervision). Kaupunkiliiton julkaisu C 71. Kaupunkientalon painatuskeskus, Helsinki.

Paunonen M (1987a) Työnohjaus hoitotyön laadun varmistajana (Clinical supervision as quality assurance in nursing). Pro Nursing ry:n vuosikirja. *Julkaisusarja* A:1, pp58–67.

Paunonen M (1987b) Johtajuus ja inhimillinen kasvu ja luovaan kasvuun kannustava työyhteisö (Leadership, growth and a working community supportive of creativity). In: Nores T (ed.) and working group: Grön K, Koskinen S, Lindqvist M, Rauhala L, Siltala P and Wilenius R *Inhimillinen kasvu*. Otava, Helsinki pp226–247.

Paunonen M (1988a Hoitoyhteisö (The care community). Sairaanhoitajien koulutussäätiö. Helsinki.

Paunonen M (1988b) Työnohjauksen vaikuttavuus terveydenhuollon työnohjaustutkimukseen osallistuneiden kokemana (Efficacy of clinical supervision as experienced by participants in clinical supervision research). In: Sairaalaliitto (ed.) *Työnohjaus*, Vammalan kirjapaino Oy, Vammala pp77–94.

Paunonen M (1989a) Hoitotyön työnohjauksen ulottuvuuksia (Dimensions of clinical supervision in nursing). Lapin korkeakoulun täydennyskoulutuskeskuksen julkaisuja 30. Lapin korkeakoulu. Rovaniemi.

Paunonen M (1989b) Hoitotyön työnohjaus hallinto-ja koulutuskeinona hoitotyön kehittämisessä (Clinical supervision in nursing as an administrative and educational method in developing nursing care). *Hoitotiede* (2), 1, pp74–78.

Paunonen M (1989c) Hoitotyön työnohjaus. Empiirinen tutkimus työnohjauksen kehittämisohjelman käynnistämistä muutoksista (Supervision in nursing. An empirical study of the changes initiated by a supervision development programme). Kuopion yliopisto. Yhteiskuntatieteellinen tiedekunta. Sairaanhoitajien koulutussäätiö. Turun yliopiston offsetpaino. Turku (Doctoral thesis).

Paunonen M (1989d) Hoitotyön työnohjaus (Supervision in nursing). *Perushoitaja* 1, pp17–20.

Paunonen M (1990) Handledning i vårdarbetet: Definition av handledningen och des innebörd och arbetshandledningens utveckling i framtiden. Psyche – psykiatrisk vördstidskrift 4, 24.

Paunonen M (1991b) Koulutus ja työnohjaus hoitotyön kehittämisessä (Education and clinical supervision in developing nursing care) Hoitotiede 3 (3), pp90–95.

Paunonen M (1993a) Hoitoyhteisöjen toimivuus hyvän hoidon edellytyksenä (Functioning care communities as prerequisites for good care). Hoitotiede 5, pp78–84.

Paunonen M (1994a) Työnohjaus hoidon laadun varmistajana ja jatkuvan koulutuksen perustana (Clinical supervision as quality assurance of care and as the basis for continuous education). In: Salo, Sirpa (ed.) Muutoksen johtaminen terveydenhuollossa. Opetushallitus. Yliopistopaino, Helsinki pp53–58.

Paunonen M (1996) Työnohjaus henkilöstön huolenpidon välineenä (Clinical supervision as a tool for caring for the staff). Ylihoitaja Marja Seppäsen juhlakirja "Huolenpito hoitotyössä". Pohjois-Savon sairaanhoitopiirin julkaisusarja pp27–34.

Paunonen M and Braathen R (1994) Veiledning som stötte i sykepleiearbeid og i utvikling av faglig-personligt identitet. Sykepleien fag 6, pp41–43.

Paunonen M, Laakso H, Lehti K, Harisalo R, Uusitalo A and Nieminen H (1996) Vuorovaikutuksen toimivuus suuressa sairaalaorganisaatiossa. (Functionality of interaction in a large hospital organisation). Suomen lääkärilehti 11: pp1211–1215.

Rasimus R (1978) Yksilöterapia ja työnohjaus yhteisössä (Individual therapy and clinical supervision in a community). Terveydenhuoltotyö (41), 9, pp20–25.

Rekola J (1994) Hoitosuhteen kehittäminen. Balint-ryhmätoiminnan kokemuksia perusterveydenhuollossa (The development of care relationships. Experiences of the Balint group action in primary health care). Sosiaali-ja terveysalan tutkimus-ja kehittämiskeskuksen raportteja. STAKES Helsinki.

Ruotsalainen S (1980) Työnohjaus psykiatrisessa hoitotyössä (Clinical supervision in psychiatric nursing). Työterveydenhuoltotyö (43), 11, pp8–12.

Sailo K (1993) Työnohjauksesta hyvinvointia? (Well-being through clinical supervision?). Sairaanhoitaja (66), 5, pp13–14.

Sairaalaliitto (toim.) (1988) Työnohjaus. (Clinical supervision). Vammalan kirjapaino Oy, Vammala.

Sihvonen M (1992) Työnohjauksen edellytyksenä työn tuntemus (Knowledge of work as the prerequisite for clinical supervision). Terveydenhoitaja 2/42.

Siltala P (toim) (1983) Työnohjaus terveydenhuollossa ja opetustyössä (Clinical supervision in health care and education). Weilin and Göös, Espoo.

Siltala P (1990) Ruumiillisten sairauksien hoitoyhteisöjen ja niiden työnohjauksen ongelmia (Problems in care communities caring for somatic diseases and in their clinical supervision). Psykoterapia-lehti. 2.

Siltala P (1991) Ruumiillisten sairauksien hoitoyhteisöjen ja niiden työnohjauksen ongelmia (Problems in care communities caring for somatic diseases and in their clinical supervision). In: Lindfors O, Paakkola E and Pylkkänen K Yhteisödynamiikka. Atena kustannus Oy, Jyväskylä.

Siltala P Hilpelä J Karkama A Kyhäräinen J Kyhäräinen T Riikonen K and Ruponen R (1993) Kasvu ja kehittyminen työnohjaajaksi. Raportti työnohjaajakoulutuksesta (Growth and development as a clinical supervisor. A report on clinical supervisor training). Sosiaali-ja terveysalan tutkimus-ja kehittämiskeskus. Raportteja 82.

Sinkkonen S and Paunonen M (1983) Työnohjaus hoitotyön ja hoitotyöntekijöiden kehittämisessä (Clinical supervision in the development of nursing and nursing staff). In: Sairaanhoidon vuosikirja pp404–427.

Suomen kaupunkiliitto (1988a) Työpaikkakoulutuksen suunnittelu terveyskeskuksessa. (Planning of on-the-job training in a health centre). Helsinki.

Suomen Kuntaliitto (1998a) Laadunhallinta kuntien ylläpitämissä ja hankkimissa terveyspalveluissa (Quality management in health care services provided or purchased by municipalities). Helsinki.

Suomen Kaupunkiliitto, Suomen Kunnallisliitto, Finlands Svenska Kommunförbund and

Sairaalaliitto (1988b) Yleiset periaatteet työnohjauksen järjestämiseksi kunnissa ja kuntainliitoissa (General principles for organising clinical supervision in communes and federations of municipalities). 12.10.1988 Helsinki.

Suominen T (1991) Työnohjaus – teho-osasto (Clinical supervision in an intensive care unit). Tehohoito (9), 1, pp51–60.

Tavia I Saari P and Lindberg V (1981) Kokemuksia työnohjauksesta mielenterveystoimistossa (Experiences of clinical supervision in a mental health clinic). Työterveyshoitaja 1, pp9–10.

Terveydenhuollon ammatillisten valmiuksien kehittäminen työelämässä (1999) (The development of cognitive preparedness in working life). Monisteita Sosiaali-ja terveysministeriö, Helsinki.

Tikkanen E and Munnukka T (1998) Ajatellaanpa ääneen!: hoitotyön työnohjauksen käsite kirjallisuuden valossa (Think out loud: the concept of clinical supervision in nursing in the light of the literature). Sairaanhoitaja (71), 7, pp9–11.

Työpaikkakoulutustoimikunta (1990) Työpaikkakoulutustoimikunnan mietintö (Committee report on on-the-job training). Opetusministeriö, Helsinki.

Valkeinen M-L (1996) Työnohjaus terveydenhoitajan työn kehittämisessä (Clinical supervision in the development of a public health nurse's work). Terveydenhoitaja (28), 5, pp13–15.

20 A North American perspective on clinical supervision

Linda R. Rounds

Editorial

This chapter provides a North American perspective of clinical supervision. It notes that within the United States of America (USA), the term clinical supervisor is synonymous with the relationship between an administrator or supervisor and another. However, professional relationships that share the underpinning philosophies and many of the dynamics of (British) clinical supervision are to be found in the USA, in both education and practice. The author points out that if clinical supervision is interpreted in its broadest sense, the experiences of a preceptor and nurse practitioner student are comparable to the experiences of a clinical supervisor and a nurse supervisee. The expected outcomes for both include growth in the professional role, increased knowledge of possible solutions to clinical problems, increased confidence, and increased self-awareness. The author also points out that clinical supervision and the process of preceptoring nurse practitioners also share common difficulties, such as a lack of formal standardised training. The chapter also includes a summary of the North American research in this area.

We believe that given that such similarities appear to exist, then perhaps there is much to learn from examining the experiences of North American practitioners and inversely, perhaps North American practitioners could learn much by studying clinical supervision in Britain. The lessons learned from examining the processes, dynamics, systems and research findings evident in another country can then be seen to be adding to the worldwide knowledge base on clinical supervision, and hopefully contributing to improved client care in each of these countries.

Introduction

The issues and challenges of nursing are not bound by the geopolitical lines of countries, differences in language, or even the culture of the people. As one travels the world, it becomes obvious that nurses face the same questions and problems – only the setting has changed.

One such challenge is the definition and usefulness of clinical supervision in the education and development of new and experienced nurses. The term clinical supervision has been discussed and debated in the literature of the United Kingdom throughout the 1990s (Butterworth and Faugier, 1992; Butterworth *et al.*, 1996; Cutcliffe and Burns, 1998; Cutcliffe and Proctor, 1998a; Playle and Mullarkey, 1998; White *et al.*, 1998). From the perspective of an outside observer, it seems one persistent question is indeed the definition of clinical supervision. Is it a unique term or an umbrella term encompassing several other relationships? Butterworth (1992) proposes 'that it is possible to differentiate between clinical supervision, mentorship and role of assessor and preceptor' (p 11). Cutcliffe and Proctor (1998a) clearly describe the central purpose and primary benefit of clinical supervision as the improvement of patient care.

The use of clinical supervision in the United States

The term clinical supervision is used in the United States primarily to define relationships between an administrator or superior and another. It is used with a connotation of supervisory responsibility for the performance of the supervisee rather than a relationship of peers or colleagues. For example, the nurses caring for patients on a given hospital unit report problems or concerns to their supervisor, seek guidance in administrative matters, and receive performance evaluations from the supervisor. In advanced practice, physicians have often sought to be clinical supervisors for nurse anaesthetists, midwives, or nurse practitioners, which would give physicians the authority to control the practice of these advanced practice nurses. One might add that this attempt at supervisory control of advanced practice has not been successful.

The professional relationships that have developed in the USA that are akin to clinical supervision are found in both education and practice. Undergraduate nursing students are often assigned to a preceptor in one of the last clinical experiences of a programme (Hagopian *et al.*, 1992; Meng and Morris, 1995). The intent is to aid the student in synthesising the multiple elements in the role of the professional nurse into a reality-based practice. It is a one-on-one experience giving the student the opportunity to function more fully in the nursing role, often in the clinical area of the student's choice. More recently, preceptors and mentors have been used in assisting the new graduate to adjust to the realities of practice. This involves a one-on-one relationship with an experienced nurse who provides guidance, support, and instruction as needed. Unfortunately, the fiscal constraints in the US healthcare system and resulting decreases in available staff have made some of these programmes less widespread. Finally, preceptors are commonly used in the education of advanced practice nurses, including nurse practitioners. The role of the preceptor in this situation is to guide the nurse practitioner student through a clinical experience in primary care. The preceptor 'facilitates and evaluates student learning in the real world of the clinical area.' (Hayes and Harrell, 1994, p 220). In some situations, the preceptor may actually become a mentor.

Mentoring, a technique used by many professions, is an ancient term arising in Homer's *Odyssey*. Athena, Greek Goddess of Wisdom, disguised herself as the man, Mentor. In this role she cared for Telemachus, son of Odysseus, and prepared him for his future role as king while his father was absent fighting the Trojan war (Hayes, 1999). In the US literature, several authors have explored the meaning and value of mentoring for nursing (Pardue, 1983; Darling, 1985; Valadez and Lund, 1993). Pardue looked at the relationship of students and mentors in a graduate teaching practicum. She developed a tool identifying expected behaviours of mentors and asked students to evaluate the mentors using this framework. Students found the tool useful in defining the goals of the practicum and validating the role of the expert teacher. Darling, when asked, 'What do nurses want in a mentor?' responded with three characteristics: attraction, action, and affect. Attraction was associated with admiration for the mentor. Action indicated a need for an investment of time and energy. Finally, affect referred to a need for respect, encouragement, and support. Darling also developed a list of characteristics nurses found useful in mentors. **In developing a preceptor training programme, Valadez and Lund discovered a higher level of accomplishment evolved when a mentoring relationship developed rather than a purely preceptor-trainee format. The authors noted, in particular, the achievement of a mentoring relationship when the mentor attempted to match human needs with work needs.**

Comparison of clinical supervision and the preceptor experience for nurse practitioner students

If clinical supervision is interpreted in its broadest sense, as an umbrella term with a goal of developing professional skills, the preceptor experience for nurse practitioners in the USA might be considered a form of clinical supervision. Nurse practitioners in the USA, with few exceptions, are educated to master's level. The students are experienced professional nurses before entering a nurse practitioner programme, bringing with them varied knowledge and diverse skills. In the USA, the vast majority of nurse practitioner programmes are in primary care with the recent addition of a small number of acute care programmes. The educational approach tends to prepare a generalist rather than a practitioner with speciality skills such as asthma or cardiovascular care. Clinical experiences are generally with a nurse practitioner or physician preceptor. Faculty members are responsible for overseeing the experience.

Because these students are skilled and knowledgeable nurses, they do not need the same kind of clinical instruction that a novice nurse or nursing student requires. Additionally, the intent of the education is different. The clinical teacher is faced with the task of helping the student make a transition that requires the student to retain strong nursing skills while incorporating selected medical knowledge and skills. Because of this, a major difference in the clinical education of nurse practitioners is that one is trying to teach a new role, not fundamental nursing. Many of the same skills required in clinical supervision can be applied to the clinical experience of the preceptor and nurse practitioner student. Faugier (1992) offers guidelines for the supervisory relationship and highlights those areas for which the supervisor is responsible. **Essential qualities in the approach of the supervisor include generosity, rewarding, openness, willingness to learn, thoughtful and thought provoking, humanity, sensitivity, uncompromising, personal, practical, orientation, relationship, and trust. Many of these parallel the characteristics that create a successful relationship between a preceptor and nurse practitioner student.**

The qualities outlined by Faugier (1992) can be applied to the approach needed by the preceptor for a nurse practitioner student. It is essential that the preceptor be *generous*, especially of time. Teaching nurse practitioner students requires time, time that is taken away from seeing patients or other related tasks. This is particularly difficult in the current US healthcare scheme, where generation of income is paramount. When preceptors do not have time, clinical education suffers and the student feels unwelcome. As with all teacher–student relationships, the approach must be *rewarding*. In attempting such a new role, many students feel very uncertain and full of doubt. Rewarding them with praise and positive feedback helps the student to gain confidence. *Openness* is a skill the nurse practitioner must have for safe practice. The ability to say 'I don't know' or 'I don't understand' is essential when entering unfamiliar territory such as medical diagnosis. The preceptor can effectively model such behaviour. The relationship between preceptor and student requires from both, a *willingness to learn*. The preceptor must be willing to learn the skill of teaching and may also learn new clinical information from a student. Students may share their own expertise or new clinical developments from the didactic portion of the programme with the preceptor. Students, of course, must be willing to learn from a preceptor. Otherwise, a rich opportunity and the whole purpose of the experience are lost. The preceptor who is *thought provoking* often gets high marks from students. Students are quick to spot the preceptor who lacks current knowledge and soon ask to be removed from that clinical placement. *Humanity* is fundamental to any nursing relationship. Preceptors can model the caring, confidentiality, and dignity for patients and extend the same qualities to students. *Sensitivity* from a preceptor permits a student to make mistakes and learn from them. Recognition that personal feelings and self-confidence are integrated with the student's performance allows the preceptor to see the whole student, not just a single performance. *Uncompromising* standards in patient care and role implementation are requirements for any nurse practitioner, but especially for the preceptor who is a role model for the student. The practice of nurse practitioners is often subjected to scrutiny because it remains a controversial role in some parts of the medical community. Adherence to standards of both practice and role is essential in rebutting the challenges of medicine and other disciplines.

Understanding that *personal* qualities are part of any relationship is important for the preceptor. This quality is modelled in encounters with both patients and students. Occasionally, it is necessary to acknowledge that one cannot work with a particular patient or a given student. The same is true for the student. One of the greatest lessons a student can learn from a preceptor is the *practical* knowledge and skill of primary care practice. Clinical experiences are intended to allow the student to apply the didactic and theoretical lessons of the classroom. The preceptor who can translate his/her own ability into practical lessons is highly valued. Establishing an *orientation* to the setting and the values of a practice at the beginning of an experience avoids later problems. This permits the student to understand the priorities for patient care in a given setting. This is especially helpful as students in the USA often work with several preceptors during the educational programme. Of course, all these qualities contribute to a relationship, but acknowledging the necessity of an *open relationship* at the beginning sets the stage for the learning experience. It is important that a preceptor can both give and receive feedback. Often an uncomfortable role for the preceptor, the ability to give feedback and evaluate a student is highly valued by the teaching instructor. Finally, as in the nurse–patient relationship, *trust* is fundamental to the preceptor–student relationship. Students need to trust preceptors to give them reasonable assignments, correct information, and honest evaluations.

Using a broad definition of clinical supervision and the above comparison, it seems reasonable that one could also compare the experience of a preceptor and nurse practitioner student to the experience of a clinical supervisor and a nurse supervisee. The expected outcomes for both include growth in the professional role, increased knowledge of possible solutions to clinical problems, increased confidence, and increased self-awareness (Cutcliffe and Proctor, 1998a; Hayes, 1999).

The role of the preceptor for nurse practitioner students

In the USA, the most common method of providing clinical education for nurse practitioner students is for a faculty member to assign students to a preceptor who is experienced in the role and practice of a nurse practitioner. Occasionally, students select their own preceptor with approval from a faculty member. The faculty teacher has overall responsibility for the learning experience and guides the preceptor in the goals of the experience.

Preceptors who work with nurse practitioner students are preferably master's level nurse practitioners themselves who have had experience in primary care practice and the role of the nurse practitioner. However, due to a lack of available nurse practitioners, physicians are commonly used in the role of preceptor. This paper addresses the expectations of preceptors who are nurse practitioners although skilled physician preceptors may also conduct themselves in a similar fashion. The primary concern with physician preceptors is their inability to teach the role of the nurse practitioner.

Preceptors are charged with the responsibility of creating a productive and positive learning environment that results in professional growth, self-confidence, and clinical competence for the student (Hayes and Harrell, 1994). The knowledge and skills required of the preceptor include clinical competence, a thorough understanding of the nurse practitioner role, skill in clinical teaching, and a recognition of the strengths and limitations of the clinical setting in which he or she practises (Sloand *et al.*, 1998). One of the primary functions of the preceptor at master's level is to facilitate new learning and role socialisation (Hayes and Harrell, 1994). The student, an adult, should be more experienced, self-directed, and autonomous in his/her learning (O'Shea, 1994; Meng and Morris, 1995). Thus the teaching should be facilitative rather than directive.

Lack of training for preceptors

One of the major difficulties faced by preceptors is the lack of formal or standardised training for the role of preceptor. The underlying assumption is that because an individual is competent in the role, this knowledge can easily be transferred or shared with another. This is an incorrect assumption. 'Expert clinicians will not intuitively grow into expert preceptors' (Meng and Morris, 1995, p 184). Although students have been exposed to the qualities of good and poor preceptors, this does not necessarily influence their own skills as preceptors upon graduation. Similar to the proposal of Cutcliffe and Proctor (1998b), student exposure to the expectations, skills, and criteria for selection of preceptors might result in improved teaching and enhanced preceptor–student relationships.

Many preceptors express discomfort in the role of teaching and evaluating nurse practitioner students, many of whom are experienced and highly educated prior to entering the nurse practitioner programme (Hagopian *et al.*, 1992; Hayes and Harrell, 1994). In addition, adequate support from the employing agency, faculty support, and personal identity in the role all affect the preceptor's ability to teach (Hayes and Harrell, 1994). Much as in the discussion by White *et al.* (1998) of clinical supervision, preceptors are not aware of theoretical models of teaching and set about the process blindly. In addition to formal training, success of preceptors as clinical teachers is dependent upon faculty involvement. It is vital that faculty teachers make regular visits to the clinical agency and discuss the student's progress with the preceptor. In the case where this is not possible, communication via telephone or other electronic means may be adequate.

In an attempt to correct the lack of training for preceptors, faculty members have developed educational programmes and other innovative support techniques. Several master's level programmes have developed continuing education offerings that focus on the needs of the preceptor as teacher (Hagopian *et al.*, 1992; Meng and Morris, 1995). Others have developed manuals to guide the preceptor in the teaching process and the expectations in the role of preceptor (Hagopian *et al.*, 1992). Currently, there are proposals for web-based courses that would guide the preceptor in the teaching role and provide tutorials in teaching skills.

The role of the faculty member

The increasing number of students entering nurse practitioner programmes and the standards set by national organisations for low faculty-student ratios in nurse practitioner programmes have limited the ability of faculty to directly provide clinical instruction to students. The current National Organization of Nurse Practitioner Faculties Programme Standards (1995) permit no more than six students per faculty member when the students are with a preceptor. If in clinical instruction with the faculty member, the required ratio is two students to one faculty member. Such a high cost for clinical education necessitates the use of preceptors rather than teaching faculty for clinical instruction. This is supported by similar experiences in undergraduate education. In addition, the scholarly demands of teaching, practice, and research also take away from faculty member's ability to precept students (Nehls *et al.*, 1997).

Since it is impractical for faculty members to supervise a student directly in a clinical experience, then what is the role of the faculty member? Certainly, faculty members are responsible for teaching didactic and theoretical content and for assuring students a quality clinical experience. However, for nurse practitioner students, one of the most difficult aspects of their education is the role transition (Anderson *et al.*, 1974; Sloand *et al.*, 1998; Hayes, 1999). This is typically a very difficult transition highlighted by a role crisis. Experienced, confident nurses return to school to take on a new role and with that role, novice status in the role. This is a particularly difficult and challenging experience. The role crisis is further complicated by the uncertainty of integrating medical aspects of patient care into an already established nursing framework. Assisting students in this role transition is one of the major tasks of faculty in nurse practitioner programmes

One method used by faculty to help students gain insight into the role transition is the critical incident. The faculty teacher asks students to describe a particularly difficult situation from clinical practice. It may involve a patient care or a role issue. Often it is presented in a group situation where other students may also benefit from the discussion. The discussion of critical incidents is similar to that described by White *et al.* (1998) as a practice theme in clinical supervision. Unquestionably, this role transition is a recurring theme for nurse practitioner students, and a successful role transition for the nurse practitioner student necessitates the guidance of the faculty and the preceptor.

Research related to preceptors and students

As the nurse practitioner movement in the USA has matured, the need for research has become evident – in both education and practice. Several faculty members have undertaken the task of analysing the preceptor role, role transition for new nurse practitioner graduates, and the skills of expert preceptors.

Mentoring

Recent results include the work of Hayes (1998a, 1998b) who describes nurse practitioner students' perceptions of mentoring by their preceptors and associated self-efficacy of the students. Hayes proposes that a mentoring model rather than a preceptor model may be more appropriate to the learning needs of the nurse practitioner student. She defines mentoring as 'a longer term, voluntary relationship between a student and an expert, willing, committed preceptor' (1998a, p 522).

In her study, Hayes (1998a) used several instruments to measure both mentoring and self-efficacy (a sense of confidence in one's ability to reach a given outcome). Her results included a positive correlation between mentoring and the student's self-efficacy, and significant differences in the mentoring scores of students who personally selected their preceptor compared to those for whom faculty assigned a preceptor. Regression analysis also revealed length of the clinical experience and the experience of the preceptor in that role as predictive of positive mentoring. This research showed potential benefit for students when a mentoring model, rather than a preceptor model, of clinical education is used. **Further, students might also benefit from choosing a preceptor whom they already know and admire. Permitting or encouraging students to select their own preceptors has not been the usual process in many programmes.** Programmes may also need to rethink the practice of rotating students through a variety of experiences rather than allowing them to stay with one preceptor for an extended period.

The above outcomes may also have implications for clinical supervision. Self-efficacy and self-confidence in practice are certainly goals of clinical supervision. Is there value in permitting the supervisee to select a supervisor who is familiar and admired? The literature from the UK (Faugier, 1992; White *et al.*, 1998; Andrews and Wallace, 1999) would also indicate a need for a long-term relationship as well as experience and knowledge for the individual in the supervisory role.

Hayes's (1999) report of additional research in this area focused on the experiences of mentored and non-mentored nurse practitioner students. This qualitative study explored the relationship of preceptors and students, the meaning of the relationship to the student, and the experience of mentoring or non-mentoring by the students in these relationships. The students who considered themselves mentored described several themes of the experience or characteristics of the preceptor in this relationship. These themes included nine characteristics and many share common ground with those described by Faugier (1992) as the elements of a good supervisory relationship. First, students described a *vested interest* by the preceptor as a commitment, similar to Faugier's description of generosity. In this situation, preceptors wanted to see the student succeed and were willing to give time, energy, and resources to meet this goal. Students described mentoring preceptors as *loving to teach*, a characteristic that included both expert knowledge and concern for the student. One might consider this similar to the combination of willingness to learn, practical, and thought provoking behaviours in the supervisory relationship. Hayes described giving students an *opportunity* through trust and feedback as a third characteristic of mentoring. Preceptors who gave students an opportunity demonstrated confidence in the students' abilities even when students had little confidence in themselves. This relates closely to the trust and rewarding behaviours described by Faugier. *Openness*, described by Hayes, is identical to the term used by Faugier. Students valued preceptors who permitted open communication, allowing preceptors and students to learn about one another. Students also reported that openness led to *friendship*, the fifth characteristic of mentoring, which is similar to relationship in the supervisory model. Friendship engendered energy, enthusiasm, and excitement about their future role. Students described a *life jacket* as a preceptor who helped them get through the most difficult parts of the nurse practitioner programme. There is no similar characteristic in the supervisory relationship, possibly because clinical supervision typically takes place with graduate nurses rather than students. Nurse practitioner students described *patience, kindness, and valuing the beginner* as the seventh characteristic of a mentoring relationship. This became especially important in view of the difficult role transition experienced by many students. Faugier's description of humanity and sensitivity are closely related to this characteristic. Students also described *job advice* as a valued characteristic of a preceptor. In a new role with many uncertainties, advice included the importance of selecting a position where other nurse practitioners worked and could provide support. Nothing in the supervisory relationship compares to this characteristic. Finally, nurse practitioner students found modelling of *confident, competent, empathic patient care* a characteristic of mentoring. Students valued the preceptor's ability to listen and understand the patient's experience. This has similar qualities to the characteristics of humanity and relationship in the supervisory role. Provision of such competent, quality nursing care is one of the purposes of both mentoring and clinical supervision.

The work of Hayes (1998a, 1999) has implications for the methods used for clinical education of nurse practitioners. The characteristics of mentoring described by the students may be those that faculty members should seek in preceptors. However, this may be difficult to evaluate in a new preceptor. A more useful tactic would be to include these skills in the orientation and education of preceptors. This research also has relevance for clinical supervision as so many of the characteristics of a positive mentoring experience for nurse practitioner students relate closely to the growth and support model of clinical supervision described by Faugier (1992). The results of Hayes's studies lend additional credibility to beliefs about the need for such mentoring to achieve quality care and independent and accountable practice, one of the goals of clinical supervision (Butterworth, 1992).

Role transition

The transition from student nurse practitioner to primary care provider is both exciting and intimidating. How best to make this transition has often been discussed by educators, employers, and graduates. Brown and Olshansky (1998) developed a research-based model, entitled 'Limbo to Legitimacy', to describe the stages of this transition. The non-linear stages of the model include laying the foundation, launching, meeting the challenge, and broadening the perspective. The first stage, *laying the foundation*, focuses on recovery from school and obtaining credentials and a job. In the *launching* stage, the new nurse practitioner dealt primarily with adjusting to the realities of a new position and developing a feeling of legitimacy in the role. In this stage, the availability of a colleague to share timesaving tips and verbal support helped the new nurse practitioner to succeed and flourish. Dealing with anxiety related to personal confidence in his/her knowledge and skill was an important element of this stage. In the third stage, *meeting the challenge*, these practitioners were more realistic in their expectations for their professional development. Competence and confidence increased and they were also able to acknowledge problems originating in the healthcare system that interfered or affected their new role. Finally, the last stage, *broadening the perspective*, occurred near the end of the first year of practice for many study participants. At this point, they could reflect on their accomplishments and acknowledge progress. They were better able to deal with system problems and accept positive comments regarding their work. It set the stage for life-long learning.

In addition to the identified stages of progress in practice, one major implication from the study was the need for mentoring (Brown and Olshansky, 1998). Based on the data from the study, the authors identified mentoring as an essential component of practice for a new nurse practitioner. Mentors in this situation are analogous to supervisors in clinical supervision. According to the authors, mentors need to be skilful guides, assisting new nurse practitioners through difficult experiences. The mentors also serve as a source of information and support. They can provide reality checks, helping the beginning practitioner to refocus expectations. The authors believe that mentoring became particularly important during the launching stage, a time when new practitioners are especially vulnerable to the stress of practice. Additionally, the authors recommended regular, planned meeting times between the mentor and new practitioner. This reduced unscheduled interruptions by the beginning practitioner and offered regular, anticipatory guidance.

Preceptor skills

Other recent research related to nurse practitioner development centres on techniques used by successful preceptors. Davis *et al.* (1993) reported on effective teaching strategies of expert preceptors. In a qualitative study, they identified four major strategies used by the expert preceptors participating in the study. These included orientation strategies, overall strategies used for all levels of learners, ongoing strategies specific to the level of the learner, and finally strategies for letting go. These expert preceptors incorporated many of the same characteristics outlined by Hayes (1999) and Faugier (1992) into their teaching strategies. Among these were orientation, patience and kindness, thought-provoking behaviour, trust, and modelling of good patient care. A critical difference in this study compared to Hayes is that these results are from the perspective of the preceptor rather than the student. Important to note, many of the characteristics are the same.

Other relevant research

Hill *et al.* (1999) conducted another relevant study focusing on the rewarding and discouraging experiences of being a preceptor. This study sampled preceptors of allied health students (health information management, physiotherapy, radiologic technology, dietetics, and respiratory therapy). The results were not surprising. The most rewarding experience was observing the student grow and work toward independence. The most discouraging experience was low motivation of students. The growth and increasing autonomy of nurses and nurse practitioners are also rewarding and are cited by Brown and Olshansky (1998) and Davis *et al.* (1993) as important characteristics to beginning practitioners and mentors alike. Low motivation may be present among nurses and nurse practitioners, but this offers an additional reason for mentoring or clinical supervision to determine the source of poor motivation and to modify it if possible.

Other current research in the USA relevant to preceptors, mentoring, or clinical supervision looks at undergraduate nursing programmes. Nehls *et al.* (1997) report a qualitative study on the lived experience of students, preceptors, and faculty using the preceptor model of clinical instruction. One of the essential themes identified by all participants was the importance of 'learning nursing thinking' (p. 222). Students sought to learn how nurses think. Faculty and preceptors attempted to discover how this thinking is taught and learned. This is not unlike what preceptors are attempting to teach nurse practitioner students. The primary difference is that nurse practitioners need to learn advanced nursing thinking and use it in a different role. Clinical supervision may necessitate a similar goal – helping nurses to experience and refine the thinking of nursing. The authors also suggested that preceptor roles be clearly defined and that preceptors be invited to participate in curriculum development.

Nordgren *et al.* (1998) described the use of preceptors for beginning level undergraduate students. Students were in a one-on-one teaching relationship with an experienced nurse. The authors reported characteristics of positive experiences for the students as well as positive approaches by the preceptors. Part of the study required that students learn about the student–preceptor relationship. The exposure of students to this model of teaching will begin to prepare them for future experiences serving as a preceptor or mentor or as the recipient of such experiences. Cutcliffe and Proctor (1998b) propose that students exposed to the role of the supervisee will derive future benefit when participating in clinical supervision.

Summary

Although clinical supervision, by strict definition, is not commonly used in the US, other experiences are clearly related, particularly in the education of nurse practitioners. The value of this type of relationship is identified in both practical application and current research. The lessons learned in the education of nurse practitioners may be useful in further development of clinical supervision. As discussed in this chapter, there are already many similarities between the preceptor/mentor for nurse practitioner students and the supervisory experience in clinical supervision. Researchers have also identified this type of relationship as a valued part of the transition to primary care provider.

The ongoing research and lessons learned in both the USA and UK regarding clinical supervision, mentoring, or the education of nurse practitioners have obvious value to nursing in these and other countries. The goal of achieving clinical excellence and role autonomy is one many nurses hope to attain and one the global community of nurses should strive to realise. The use of mentoring and clinical supervision offers one step in reaching that goal.

References

Anderson E, Leonard B and Yates J (1974) Epigenesis of the nurse practitioner role. *American Journal of Nursing* 74(10), pp1812–6.

Andrews M and Wallis M (1999) Mentorship in nursing: a literature review. *Journal of Advanced Nursing* 29(1), pp201–207.

Brown M A and Olshansky E (1998) Becoming a primary care nurse practitioner: challenges of the initial year of practice. *The Nurse Practitioner* 23(7), pp46, 52, 54–56, 58, 61–62, 64, 66.

Butterworth T (1992) Clinical supervision as an emerging idea in nursing. In: Butterworth T and Faugier J (eds) *Clinical Supervision and Mentorship in Nursing* London: Chapman and Hall.

Butterworth T and Faugier J (eds) (1992) *Clinical Supervision and Mentorship in Nursing.* London: Chapman and Hall.

Butterworth T, Bishop V and Carson J (1996) First steps toward evaluating clinical supervision in nursing and health visiting. I. Theory, policy and practice development. *Journal of Clinical Nursing* 5(2), pp127–132.

Cutcliffe J and Burns J (1998) Personal, professional and practice development: clinical supervision. *British Journal of Nursing* 7(21), pp1318–1322.

Cutcliffe J and Proctor B (1998a) An alternative training approach to clinical supervision: 1. *British Journal of Nursing* 7(5), pp280–285.

Cutcliffe J and Proctor B (1998b) An alternative training approach to clinical supervision: 2. *British Journal of Nursing* 7(6), pp344–350.

Darling L (1985) What do nurses want in a mentor? *Journal of Nursing Administration* 14(10), pp42–44.

Davis M Sawin K and Dunn M (1993) Teaching strategies used by expert nurse practitioner preceptors: a qualitative study. *Journal of the American Academy of Nurse Practitioners* 5(1), pp27–33.

Faugier J (1992) The supervisory relationship. In: *Clinical Supervision and Mentorship in Nursing* (Butterworth T and Faugier J eds) London: Chapman and Hall.

Hagopian G Ferszt G Jacobs L and McCorkle R (1992) Preparing clinical preceptors to teach master's-level students in oncology nursing. *Journal of Professional Nursing* 8(5), pp295–300.

Hayes E (1998a) Mentoring and nurse practitioner student self-efficacy. *Western Journal of Nursing Research* 20(5), pp521–535.

Hayes E (1998b) Mentoring and self-efficacy for advanced nursing practice: a philosophical approach for nurse practitioner preceptors. *Journal of the American Academy of Nurse Practitioners* 10(2), pp53–57.

Hayes E (1999) Athena found or lost: the precepting experience of mentored and non-mentored nurse practitioner students. *Journal of the American Academy of Nurse Practitioners* 11(8), pp335–342.

Hayes E and Harrell C (1994) On being a mentor to nurse practitioner students: the preceptor-student relationship. *Nurse Practitioner Forum* 5(4), pp220–226.

Hill N Wolf K Bossetti B and Saddam A (1999) Preceptor appraisals of rewards and student preparedness in the clinical setting. *Journal of Allied Health* 28(2), pp86–90.

Meng A and Morris D (1995) Continuing education for advanced nurse practitioners: preparing nurse-midwives as clinical preceptors. *Journal of Continuing Education in Nursing* 26(4), pp180–184.

National Organization of Nurse Practitioner Faculties (1995) *Advanced Nursing Practice: Curriculum Guidelines and Program Standards for Nurse Practitioner Education.* Washington, DC: NONPF.

Nehls N Rather M and Guyette M (1997) The preceptor model of clinical instruction: the lived experiences of students, preceptors, and faculty-of-record. *Journal of Nursing Education* 36(5), pp220–227.

Nordgren J Richardson S and Laurella V (1998) A collaborative preceptor model for clinical teaching of beginning nursing students. *Nurse Educator* 23(3), pp27–32.

O'Shea H (1994) Clinical preceptorships: strategies to enhance teaching and learning *Journal of Wound, Ostomy, and Continence Nursing* 21(3), pp98–105.

Pardue S (1983) The who-what-why of mentor teach/graduate student relationships. *Journal of Nursing Education* 22(1), pp32–37.

Playle J and Mullarkey K (1998) Parallel process in clinical supervision: enhancing learning and providing support. *Nurse Education Today* 18(7), pp558–566.

Sloand E Feroli K Bearss N and Beecher J (1998) Preparing the next generation: precepting nurse practitioner students. *Journal of the American Academy of Nurse Practitioners* 10(2), pp65–69.

Valadez A and Lund C (1993) Mentorship: Maslow and me. *Journal of Continuing Education in Nursing* 24(6), pp259–263.

White E Butterworth T Bishop V Carson J Jeacock J and Clements (1998) A clinical supervision: insider reports of a private world. *Journal of Advanced Nursing* 28(1), pp185–192.

21 Clinical supervision and clinical governance for the twenty-first century

An end or just the beginning?

Tony Butterworth

Editorial

This chapter identifies and then draws together some of the threads which run throughout this book, and then uses these as the basis for speculating on the immediate future for clinical supervision. It draws attention to the obvious relationship between clinical supervision and clinical governance and points out that as a result, we have, for perhaps the first time, a formal link between the individual and the organisation in a framework for ensuring the quality of clinical services. It offers a brief strategy for implementing, maintaining and evaluating clinical supervision and suggests good practice for employers.

In considering the future of clinical supervision, we believe that this chapter highlights a significant issue that needs consideration. Given the changing nature of some health care, and the resulting 'brief' nature of contact with some health care professionals (e.g. day case surgery, NHS Direct), models of clinical supervision, designed specifically to address the restorative, formative and normative needs of these practitioners need to be developed. This is just one example of the issues that will need to be addressed in the future of clinical supervision. Whilst much has been learned about clinical supervision and whilst many developments have occurred over the past ten years, the next ten years promise to be equally challenging and, hopefully, enlightening.

Introduction

The volume of material available which describes and analyses clinical supervision is self evident from this book and its collected references. New patterns of work are beginning to emerge and the once contentious issues of cost benefit and 'proof of value' are no longer the problems to implementing clinical supervision that they once were. Clinical supervision has new champions and a spirit of enthusiasm surrounds it, generated by the demands of clinical governance and continuous professional development. This chapter draws together some of these threads and speculates on the immediate future for clinical supervision.

Professional self-regulations and clinical governance are hallmarks of a new spirit of individual accountability and corporate responsibility in the helping professions. The well-publicised cases of negligence in the UK National Health Service and the lessons of the Harold Shipman case carry echoes from the Beverly Allitt case of a decade ago but the outcomes for patients and families are the same. They raise questions such as – 'How could this happen without anyone knowing?' – 'Why are fellow professionals still fearful of whistleblowing bad practice?' – 'How can healthcare professionals be so out of date in their practices that they actively harm patients?'

The answers are of course, that continuous professional development is unevenly funded, individual 'professional' arrogance sometimes overrides patient needs and some individual performance simply does not deliver safe, let alone 'best' practice.

The government response to organisational and individual deficiencies has been to put in place a range of checks in the system, which it is hoped will prevent the serious shortcomings that have led to such well-publicised cases.

Clinical governance and its attendant requirements are now purposefully located in NHS trusts and accountability for development is being carried by the National Health Service Executive. National standards for service are being established through the National Institute for Clinical Excellence and the National Service Frameworks. Standards will be monitored through the Commission for Health Improvement.

Researchers and clinicians are being pressed constantly to use an evidence-based approach to care, and databases established through Cochran Centres allow practitioners to interrogate the most reliable research available and make use of it in their practice. These measures are to be applauded and will make a significant impact on the provision of health care. There is also every reason to believe that they will mitigate the problems of poor practice reported in the media. However, there still remains a bridge to be built between the measures which the government imposes and the personal response to accountability.

Clinical governance and clinical supervision

There is an obvious relationship between the good practice of clinical supervision and the responsibilities necessary for effective clinical governance. Clinical supervision has been properly secured in many health care trusts and can therefore inform and be part of the systems of clinical governance which must be established and in place in all NHS trusts. It is possible to summarise the relationship between the two and the natural alliance which can grow from them.

Clinical governance can be defined as:

> '*a framework through which NHS organisations are accountable for continuously improving the quality of their services and safe-guarding high standards of care by creating an environment in which excellence in clinical care will flourish.*' (DOH, 1998)

More simply put, clinical governance is:

'the means by which organisations ensure the provision of quality clinical care by making individuals accountable for setting, maintaining and monitoring performance standards.'

(NHSE North Thames Regional office, 1998)

Clinical governance places the responsibility for the quality of care jointly on organisations and on individuals within organisations. Clinical care is increasingly complex and requires professionals to develop an intricate network of relationships so that they may appropriately exercise their clinical responsibilities in a collective and joint way. The exercise of individual accountability in a multi-professional clinical environment has never been more relevant.

A clinician is responsible for providing individual care of high quality and being able to demonstrate this by setting and monitoring acceptable standards. This will require joint standard setting where there is more than one clinician involved in the care. An institution is responsible for providing services of high quality and being able to demonstrate this by setting and monitoring standards for the system set up to provide the services and by ensuring that individual clinicians fulfil their individual responsibilities. **We have thus for perhaps the first time a formal link between the individual and the organisation in a framework for ensuring the quality of clinical services.** This relationship is further strengthened by the individual accountability that chief executives of NHS trusts have for the quality of clinical care in their organisations.

Clinical supervision is '**a formal process of professional support and learning which enables individual practitioners to develop knowledge and competence, assume responsibility for their own practice and enhance consumer protection and safety of care in complex clinical situations.**' (DOH, 1993)

Clinical supervision for nurses has been purposefully developed and implemented in many healthcare trusts across the United Kingdom. Helpful direction from NHS policy development and recent research evidence demonstrating its acceptability by the profession, focus on clinical work and skill development shows that there is a well developed mechanism already in place which supports some of the central requirements of clinical governance. Other emerging evidence suggests that tools can be developed which competently assess the impact and focus of clinical supervision so that it can be properly evaluated, benchmarked and compared across a number of service providers. The value of clinical supervision to clinical governance is summarised in Table 21.1.

A summary of good practice for implementing, maintaining and evaluating clinical supervision

Whilst there is no one universally correct way or method to implement, maintain and evaluate clinical supervision, the following strategy indicates key aspects of this process:

Table 21.1 A summary of the value of clinical supervision to clinical governance

---

Clinical supervision **focuses** on matters of central importance in the provision of safe and accountable practice.
The **content** of clinical supervision is focused on:
- organisational and management issues
- clinical casework
- professional development
- educational support
- confidence building
- interpersonal problems

Implementing

- thorough preparation of clinical supervisors
- making sufficient time available for clinical supervision to happen
- enabling trusting relationships between supervisors and supervisees

Maintaining

- making clinical supervision part of the Trust 'culture' and a requirement for practising professionals

Evaluating

- evaluating the provision and the product of clinical supervision on a regular basis.

Suggested good practice for employers

In conjunction with the steps outlined above, further good practice for employers who wish to be seen to fully embrace clinical supervision includes:

- gathering data for the trusts who demonstrate continuing investment in the preparation and development of clinical supervisors;
- reviewing the process and product of clinical supervision activity in the trust;
- establishing the means by which clinical supervision can be drawn into the required responsibilities of clinical governance.

Work continues at the University of Manchester in developing a standardised evaluation tool (the Manchester Clinical Supervision Scale). Researchers are using a number of experimental sites and results continue to show that clinical supervision is addressing improvements in skills, encouraging reflective practice and attending to personal development.

Participating in clinical supervision in an active way is a clear demonstration of an individual exercising his or her responsibility under clinical governance. Organisations have a clear responsibility to ensure that individual clinicians have access to appropriate supervision and support in the exercise of their joint and individual responsibility. Clinical supervision should properly seen as an activity that takes place in a wider framework of activities that are designed to manage, enhance and monitor the delivery of high quality clinical services.

Examples of these wider activities are:

- clinical audit;
- clinically effective practice;
- clinical risk management;
- quality assurance monitoring frameworks;
- continual professional development;
- organisational development.

Hence, clinical supervision should take place in the context of an overall framework rather than being seen as an individual activity carried out in isolation.

Delivering clinical supervision

Early attempts at defining the 'right amount' of clinical supervision have been produced and 'ideal types' are described elsewhere in this book. The patterns of care emerging in the UK Health Service mean that the opportunity to express care through, for example, a nurse–patient relationship requires some further thought. A large section of the workforce still engages with patients and families who will receive care over a prolonged period of time. Psychiatric care and care of older people are striking examples of this. Equally, however, there are others who will have only a brief contact with health professionals. The most striking example here is that where people receive day patient or 24-hour 'short stay' surgical care. Even more interesting are the new telephone contact and consultation services available through NHS Direct and phone line services set up by NHS trusts. **These new ways of working will demand new models of clinical supervision, which can embrace new and more traditional forms of care and helping relationships.**

An example serves to make that point. One of the characteristics of 'good nursing' has been seen as the ability to form a therapeutic relationship with patients and families. A whole section of the education curriculum is devoted to establishing relationships, developing interpersonal skills and 'the key helping relationship'. This anticipates that relationships are meaningful and can be used as an integral part of the delivery of health care and changing health behaviour. Clinical supervision attempts to recognise this and develop it to the mutual satisfaction of nurse and patient alike. Short-term, brief interactions are different and will need educational preparation and clinical supervision, which accommodates it. There remains much work to be done in this area of brief intervention and contact between professionals and people who use services. The consequences of these new ways of working are as yet unclear.

Patients and families as beneficiaries of clinical supervision

Discussion on the effects of clinical supervision on patients and their families continues. At its most simple the effects are clear, a well educated, acceptable and 'open' healthcare professional should lead to a safe and well informed patient. To attempt to disentangle the 'effect' of clinical supervision on patient and families may well result in years of tortured attempts to seek a cause and effect which is impossible to locate. **Of course patients and their families *must* be the beneficiaries of clinical supervision, it is after all a system to support and develop the professionals offering care to them and does not exist to merely advance the cause of the professions themselves.**

What next for clinical supervision?

To speculate on the future of clinical supervision is always difficult. It has arrived and it is probably here to stay. Most practising nurses accept its value, at least in theory. Only a decade ago it would not have been possible to find much reference to it in the professional literature for nurses. This book, although in its own way unique, is now one of several produced which can offer insights into professional development and clinical supervision and the influence it is having on research, clinical practice and international collaboration.

It has been absorbed into the nomenclature of the profession and for nurses it offers a real opportunity to debate practice and its consequences on both the professional and the patient and family. Clinical governance has provided an organisational 'location' for the activity which surrounds clinical supervision and it can make a demonstrable contribution to professional practice and patients' safety. The true test of its acceptance will be when it is no longer necessary to see it as a separate activity and it has become part of the normal business of professional practice for all nurses.

References

Department of Health (1993) *A Vision for the Future*. Report of the Chief Nursing Officer.
Department of Health (1994) CNO letter 94(5) *Clinical Supervision for the Nursing and Health Visiting Professions*.
Department of Health (1998) *A First Class Service Quality in the New NHS*. Health Services circular (1998)/113.
NHSE North Thames Region Office, London. Clinical Governance in North Thames, A paper for discussion and consultation (1998) The Department of Public Health.

Index